The 3-Day Headache "Cure"

By

Jeremy Orozco

Copyright © 2015 Jeremy Orozco

All rights reserved.

ISBN: 151950134X
ISBN-13: 9781519501349

For my wife and closest migraine sufferer, Sondra,
who told me to quit a secure government job and head for the unknown.

And for our family, who agreed.

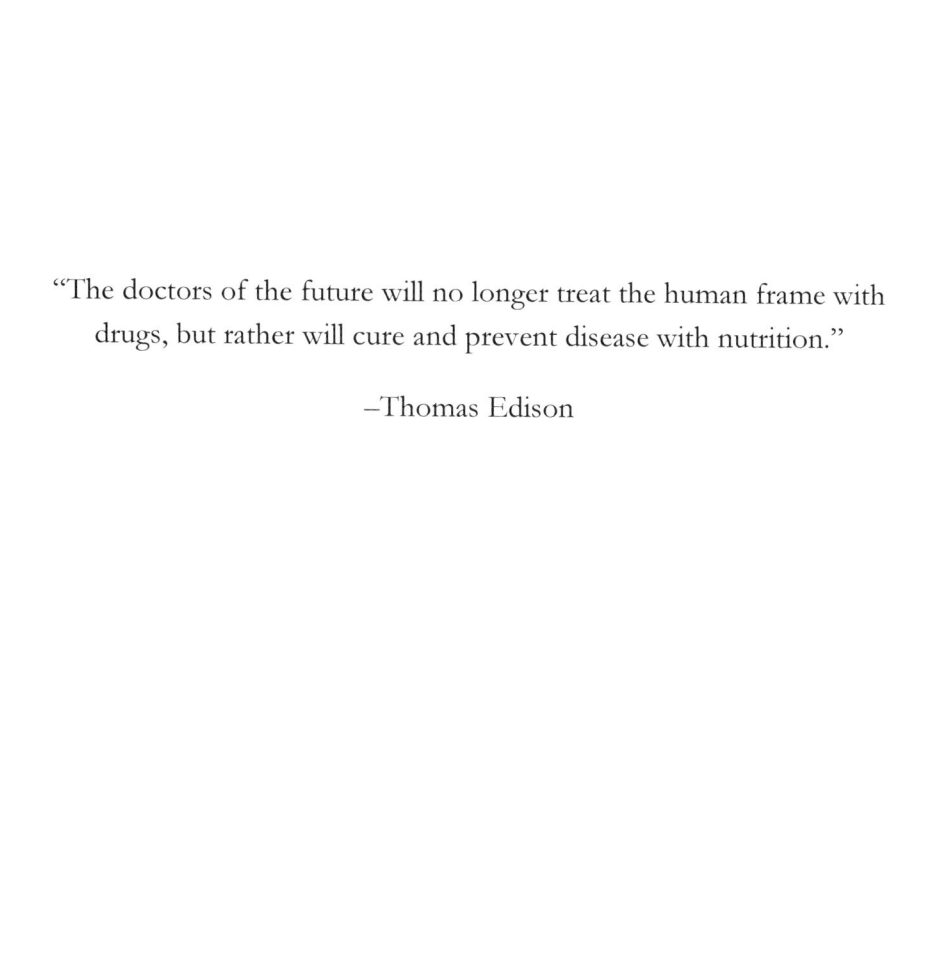

"The doctors of the future will no longer treat the human frame with drugs, but rather will cure and prevent disease with nutrition."

–Thomas Edison

Contents

THE 3-DAY HEADACHE "CURE" I
   WHY I WROTE THIS BOOK 1
      Treat the Cause First 3
      It's All About Headache Triggers 6
      Yes, Virginia, There Is a Migraine Gene 7
      What's in the Book 9

LET'S GET REAL ABOUT HEADACHES 3
   MIGRAINES BY DEFINITION 14
      The Four Phases of a Migraine 16
      The Headache Threshold 19
   MIGRAINE TREATMENTS IN HISTORY 20
   FAMOUS MIGRAINE SUFFERERS 24
   TWO MIGRAINE STUDIES THAT WILL BLOW YOUR MIND 26
      The 1983 Migraine Study 26
      The 1979 Migraine Study 30
   THE STRATEGY AND TACTICS OF FOOD ELIMINATIONS 33
      The 2010 IHS Study 34
      The 2007 Food Allergen Study 35
      Cross-Reactions 38
   IS GLUTEN-FREE HEADACHE-FREE? 47
      Getting High on Gluten 49
      More Damning Evidence 53
      Down with the Food Pyramid! 56
      The Benefits of Being Gluten-Free 57
   MEN, WOMEN, AND CHILDREN 59
      Migraines and Female Hormones 60
      Children 61
      The First Migraine Gene 63
      The Glutamate/Estrogen Factor 66
   MIGRAINES PER POUND 71
      The Bariatric Surgery Study 71
      Hara Hachi Bu 72
      The Johns Hopkins Study 73

One Pound, One Trigger at a Time *74*
Let's Talk About Poop *75*

HEADACHE TRIGGERS **81**
THE HEAVY-HITTING HEADACHE TRIGGERS 82
Heavy Hitting Trigger #1: Foods that Inflame *84*
Heavy-Hitting Trigger #2: MSG *96*
Heavy-Hitting Trigger #3: Gluten, Glutamate, Glutamine, and MSG *105*
Heavy Hitting Trigger #4: GMOs *116*
Heavy Hitting Trigger #5: OJ, the Killer *121*
THE CHRONIC HEADACHE TRIGGERS 128
Chronic Trigger #1: Cooking Oils *131*
Chronic Trigger #2: Trans Fats *134*
Chronic Trigger #3: Sugar *136*
Chronic Trigger #4: Refined Grains *139*
Chronic Trigger #5: Milk *145*
Chronic Trigger #6: Artificial Sweeteners *149*
Chronic Trigger #7: Inflammatory Meats *155*
Chronic Trigger #8: Alcohol *159*
Chronic Trigger #9: Corn *173*
Chronic Trigger #10: Soy *179*
OTHER HEADACHE TRIGGERS TO AVOID 181
Headache Trigger #1: Biogenic Amines *182*
Headache Trigger #2: Rice *209*
Headache Trigger #3: Eggs *215*
Headache Trigger #4: Chocolate *220*
Headache Trigger #5: Sulfites *225*
Headache Trigger #6: Nitrites *231*
Headache Trigger #7: Weather, Mold, Allergies, and Other Airborne Triggers *237*
Headache Trigger #8: Smells *243*
Headache Trigger #9: Smoking *247*
Headache Trigger #10: Artificial Sweeteners *249*
Headache Trigger #11: Ice Cream *258*
Headache Trigger #12: Caffeine *261*
Headache Trigger #13: Blue Light *267*
Headache Trigger #14: Poor Sleep Patterns *270*

WTF CAN I EAT? 279
THE ELIMINATION DIET PROCESS 280
Dear Diary 282
Step 1: Choose Your Elimination Diet Option 285
Step 2: Figure Out WTF You Can Eat During Your Elimination Diet 294
Step 3: Reintroduce Possible Headache Triggers 298
THE HEADACHE HELP CHECKLIST 302
Before You Begin 302
My Headaches in a Nutshell 303

PREVENTIVE MEDICINE 317
HYDRATE 318
Water and Weight Loss 320
Next Stop: Hydration Station 321
Sodium, the Other Part of Hydration 326
JUICING 333
Juicing Drawbacks 334
Juicer or Blender? 336
What to Buy 337
Juicing Recipe Sources 338
KETOGENIC DIETS 340
The Easiest Way to Burn Ketones 341
Risks 342
MIGRAINE VITAMINS AND HERBS 344
Magnesium 345
Butterbur 350
Coenzyme Q10 350
B Vitamins 353
Vitamin D 364
Feverfew 370
Omega-3 371
5-Hydroxytryptophan (5-HTP) 374
STRESS LESS 378
Stress and Migraines 385
GET BLISSED ON YOUR OWN CHEMICALS 387
Dopamine 388
Serotonin 390
Oxytocin, the True Love Drug 391

Endorphins *392*
   Make a Stop at Motivation Station *392*
EXERCISE 397
   Exercise or Drugs? *397*
   Don't Go Overboard *398*
   The Dark Side: When Exercise Causes a Migraine *400*
MEDITATION 402
   Meditation Techniques *403*
BINAURAL BEATS 406
   What's a Frequency Got to Do with My Brain? *406*
   Placebo Effect or Relaxation Effect? *407*
   Could Binaural Beats Cause a Headache? *407*
   Volume *408*
   Apps *408*

ACUTE PAIN RELIEF **411**
MASSAGE IT AWAY 412
   Want to Learn More? *413*
SEX—CURE OR CURSE? 414
   Sex During a Migraine *415*
   Headaches and Your Relationship *415*
CANNABIS 417
   Cannabis Drawbacks *419*
   Cannabis Strains and Types *421*
TOP-RATED MIGRAINE PRODUCTS 424

PAIN RELIEF + PREVENTION **429**
ACUPUNCTURE 430
   Acupuncture for Migraines *431*
   Does It Hurt? Does It Really Work? *433*
CHIROPRACTIC CARE 435
   What the Big Studies Say *436*
   My Experience with Chiropractic Care *436*
   Is It Safe? *437*
NERVE BLOCKS AND SURGERIES 441
   Nerve Blocks *441*
   Surgeries *446*

VISITING YOUR DOCTOR **449**
YOUR DOCTOR, YOUR PARTNER IN RESEARCH 450

>   *The Medical Evaluation* *453*
>   DRUGS 459
>   *Beware of Money Drugs* *459*
>   *Drugs for Acute Pain Relief* *461*
>   *Rescue Medications* *474*
>   *Preventative Medications* *480*
>   *The Future of Migraine Drugs* *491*
> **CONCLUSION** **495**
> **CITATIONS** **499**

Why I Wrote This Book

Even the little headaches can hold you back. My fellow firefighters and I were helping a woman who was unconscious on the floor. I pricked her finger and the blood glucose monitor read 78 mg/dl. My head ached. I couldn't think straight. I reached for the dextrose to hand it to the medic and I stalled. I started to feel hot, and my head throbbed as if it were drumming to the sound of my panic—I couldn't remember our very basic medication protocol.

Somehow, amidst my haze, I realized that this unconscious patient could have a brain bleed from a fall, which would require a completely different course of action. It wasn't a horrible headache—just a headache—but it put me in a state of confusion while working as a firefighter and EMT, while answering a 911 call, while a person's life was at stake. Had this been one of my severe headaches, I wouldn't have been thinking at all, and I wouldn't have been able to drive to this emergency in the first place.

I snapped out of my fog when the patient woke up with a drooping left cheek and incoherent speech—signs of stroke. Any 20-second mental fumble could be deadly for a patient who needs to get to the hospital to stop an intracerebral hemorrhage, the most destructive form of stroke. I checked over the radio to get an ETA for the helicopter ambulance, ensured that the police closed the road for a landing zone, and had about a minute left to document a long list of vital signs and medications before the transporting ground ambulance arrived to take the patient to the landing zone. The patient, suddenly able to speak more clearly, said, "I'm not going, and I'm not paying any more medical bills."

"Is this normal?" my paramedic partner asked the patient.

"Yes," she replied. "I'm just having a migraine. It happens a lot. I go to the hospital and they can't do anything about it."

After she adamantly refused medical treatment but still promised to have a friend take her to the emergency room to get checked out, I canceled the helicopter and room full of surgeons waiting for her arrival (an event with a $100,000 on-average price tag).

As a firefighter, I responded to these medical emergencies on a regular basis. We took migraines very seriously, because they often cause debilitating symptoms that are associated with many other life-threatening neurological conditions. Aside from that, migraines can destroy someone's life. Some migraineurs fear leaving the house alone because there's a chance they will get a migraine, become paralyzed in the street, and be unable to communicate.

Having migraines—even having chronic, debilitating headaches that don't qualify as migraines—is no way to live your life. There was one thing I could see clearly from all of these 911 calls for migraines: People needed help. And from what I could tell, they weren't finding it.

So I started researching. I reviewed thousands of headache articles and edited hundreds. I worked with two MIT grads, Dr. Dani and my wife, Sondra Orozco, to develop a website called understandmigraines.org. Our aim was to find the answers to headaches and bring them all to one place. There was just one problem: The answers didn't add up.

After researching for a year and a half, what I found was a shocking mixture of conflicting information. I would find one headache cure on a respected medical site only to discover that it was listed as a headache trigger on another—two very different answers from top medical authorities. It wasn't just an internet problem; it was *the problem*. Sixty percent of migraine sufferers walk out of the hospital dissatisfied, and very few ever stop having migraines despite treatment.[1] So I started thinking about how we could look at migraine treatment from a different angle.

Treat the Cause First

Through the course of writing this book, I came to understand just how broken our medical system is. And I learned how the same headache triggers that are most likely responsible for catastrophic migraines were also responsible for my headaches. I wrote this book because I don't believe in a system that allows someone with unimaginable pain to walk into a hospital and walk out with pills that can cause more headaches and absolutely no knowledge of the long list of headache triggers that are most likely causing the pain. And as a firefighter and EMT, I was part of this system I don't believe in. I've treated numerous migraine patients and sent them off to the hospital knowing they would probably not find help. I want to change that. I'm not against hospitals. I'm simply dumbfounded that the majority of people with debilitating headaches don't leave hospitals with any kind of game plan for actually stopping—rather than masking—their pain.

I have realized that part of the problem is in how we approach treating our headaches: Instead of trying to heal the *cause* of the headache, our focus goes directly to stopping the pain. But what if you figured out what causes your headaches so you could stop them before they start?

Migraineurs often rate the pain of their migraines as 10 out of 10, with 10 being the worst pain they have ever endured. I experienced my 10 on the pain scale after I accidentally chopped off the tip of my thumb one day while trying to cut a plastic mount for a car stereo. I made several failed attempts with an old, rusty razor blade before throwing it away and getting a new one. The shiny new blade sliced all the way through the plastic mount like butter, stopping only after an abrupt collision with the bone of my thumb, leaving the tip dangling by the nail. The clean incision through my most sensitive touch receptors was the easy part; the real pain started when I got to the ER. I remember uncontrollably shaking as the doctor pried open the interior of my thumb to give seven slow, painful injections of anesthetic. It was pure torture.

I've had excruciating headaches, but none rated that high on my pain scale. That could explain why I was never diagnosed with migraines. Get this: A migraine sufferer may feel a pain level of 10 multiple times a month, and migraines can last for days. I've never been able to say that, and I was still fed up with my headache pain. And to make it worse, I'd watched my wife Sondra suffer from migraines for years.

While we have receptors for pain all over our bodies, pain is subjective to our brain's interpretation. Think of your level-10 pain. Astonishing, right? But what's even more astonishing is the number of migraine sufferers who sit beside us. Migraines have been ranked among the top 20 most disabling conditions in the world, and there is a migraine sufferer in one out of four American households. In 2013, *The Journal of Headache and Pain* ranked migraines as the leading cause of disability among neurological disorders, accounting for over half of all the time lost to neurological disabilities globally.[2] This is shocking because most nonmigraineurs think of migraines as "just headaches."

You may have migraines depending on how your doctor diagnoses (or misdiagnoses) them. It's agreed that doctors have a wide interpretation of what a migraine is, making it one of the most largely misdiagnosed conditions. Some migraines cannot be distinguished from regular headaches. Partly due to this, I use "headache" as an inclusive (or umbrella) term that includes migraines as one type of headache, though I do not think that migraines are "just headaches." But also, it's not only migraineurs who can benefit from the information and research in this book. Anyone who suffers from chronic or debilitating headaches will find help here, no matter how those headaches are described. Besides, the term doesn't really matter, does it? A debilitating headache is, well, debilitating. No one wants that. With or without a diagnosis, the information I found will help you heal your headaches and become healthier in the long run.

And if you have headaches regularly, you've probably already done some Googling. You have probably tried more than a few prescription medications, and you have probably given a few home remedies a try. And, in doing so, you may have realized some things: You don't want just the drug company's answer or the article from a journalist who has no clue. You don't want the natural remedy unless there are hard facts that it actually works. You don't want to sift through hundreds of costly studies that practically use a different language. What you want is to be headache-free. Today. And you might have done this research yourself if your head didn't hurt so badly, and so often, that instead, you regularly imagined actually taking it off and rolling it down the street like a bowling ball.

What we all need is real headache help.

It's All About Headache Triggers

Headaches and migraines are extremely common, and they're becoming more common as typical Americans continue to increase their consumption of headache triggers. Here's the lowdown: Some 90% of the population gets headaches,[3] many migraine sufferers would choose death over a life with migraines, and there is no list of the best headache help.[4]

Not only that, but headaches are expensive. Chronic headaches cost even more. How much does a headache cost you? Do you miss days of work? Does it interfere with your social or family life? How often do they keep you from feeling 100%? What does less productivity cost you? If you were to actually track the hours and days you lost to headaches and sum them, I bet you would be surprised. Multiply the hours by what your time is worth, and the dollar figure might make you swoon. Finding out why you have headaches is well worth your time.

It was definitely well worth mine. I couldn't get over how debilitating migraines are and how many of us suffer from them, so I quit my job to research and work on this book full time. Here's what I did: I took a summary of the last 50 years of headache research and put it with the last few years of exciting breakthroughs in neurological understanding. And what I learned is a little sad: that following a simple checklist could prevent all of our headache pain.

The one thing headache sufferers all have in common is that we are unaware of our worst headache triggers. This is where things get interesting. Very interesting.

The most successful studies on migraines and headaches have involved the elimination of headache triggers. Aside from being extremely difficult to read, these studies practically use a different language. And to make matters worse, no migraine study has ever researched the commonalities between the top headache triggers. It's a medical fact that there is a headache threshold that is affected by multiple headache triggers, yet no one has asked, "What do these headache triggers have in common?"

I had to know the answer to that question because it defines the headache problem. It took me over three years, including the two years writing this book, to find my answer. It wasn't a difficult question to answer: It was tedious. I evaluated every headache trigger for its likelihood to cause migraines, the success of its elimination, and most importantly, the correlation between the triggers and other deadly conditions—because it is true that migraines can be signs of other health problems.

The information you'll find here has changed my life and my wife's. While migraines can be boundlessly more painful than regular headaches, or can cause no pain at all, both are caused by the same triggers. When we eliminated our top headache triggers, my severe headaches were gone and so were my wife's migraines.

Yes, Virginia, There Is a Migraine Gene

Some people say, "There's nothing you can do about migraines—they're genetic." But there is a way to completely bypass the migraine gene. This is important because a large percentage of the population has this mutated gene, including people who do not get migraines.

Even so, there is no such thing as a "medical cure" to headaches, nor will there ever be. So why the quotation marks in *The*

3-Day Headache "Cure"? The word "cure" is a term that has perpetuated the overuse of medication in a broken medical system. The medical definition of "cure" is "to recover from a disease."[5] I don't believe that migraine sufferers are diseased. And because migraines are often precursors to other, sometimes severe, medical conditions, "curing" these warning signs isn't actually what anyone needs. What we really need is to find out what's triggering the headaches so we can heed the warning signs our bodies are giving us.

There is, however, a common definition of "cure" that does apply to this book: "something that ends a problem or improves a bad situation" (*Merriam-Webster Online Dictionary*).[6] When doctors tell patients that there is no "cure" for migraines, patients think there is nothing they can do about them. The American Diabetes Association, with its mission "to cure diabetes," has recently evaluated the same lexical dilemma.[7] High blood sugar, diabetes, and migraines are unlike bacterial infections that can be medically *cured* with antibiotics, because both are affected by a continuum of everyday events (e.g., diet, exercise, medications, stress, and illness). So we aren't looking for a medical cure, we're looking for what triggers and prevents migraines to end the headache problem. Forever.

Fortunately, it doesn't matter what your headache problems are, because learning about your headache triggers and moderating your consumption of them has a great side effect: It will make you feel incredible. This book is a combination of the best headache "cures" on Earth based on the most reliable research out there, and it's easy to read and comes with a very simple Headache Help Checklist and a free guide. I believe that sharing this vast amount of information in the form of a book will help more people than any other headache help has.

What's in the Book

This book looks deeply into the large failure rate of headache help. Why have so many headache elimination diets failed? Why do so many people ridden with headaches become sick and fat from foods that we deem healthy? What are the "unhealthy foods" that *promote* weight loss and headache health? What are the biggest headache triggers and how did they become "safe" in the first place? Why aren't most migraineurs and healthcare professionals familiar with the most successful medications and treatments? While writing this book, I confronted all of these questions and many, many more. And I didn't take a noncommittal shrug for an answer.

Here you will find quick summaries of hundreds of headache studies and the testimonials of many migraine sufferers. The studies I referenced do more than simply explain how to eliminate the headaches that warn us of life-threatening conditions. The studies show that participants who learned how to eliminate the things that trigger their headaches enjoyed improved clarity, energy, health, strength, stamina, and sleep. And it's about more than just diet. You'll soon find out how the simple steps to improve your health are also the best ways to become headache-free.

I can't provide you with an immediate, quick-fix answer to stopping your headaches, though you've probably suffered enough already to deserve a quick fix. What's causing your headaches is personal and very specific to you, so instead, this book will take you on a journey to discover what you might be putting in your body that's causing them.

This book is filled with scary terms like "elimination diet" and "gluten-free." If you have gluten-free friends, or if you've tried elimination diets yourself, or if you've just heard enough about elimination diets to have a healthy skepticism, you may already think this book isn't for you—but it is. Elimination diets aren't as bad as you might think, and what they can teach you is remarkable. More than that, they are a key to helping you unlock what's causing your headaches. Your elimination diet is the most successful path to your own three-day "cure." Use the Headache Help Checklist to help you find out what's causing your headaches so you can make more informed choices about what you eat so you can control your migraines—so you can get your life back.

I'll tell you now that gluten is a villain to your body—and to your headache threshold. But I'm not going to tell you that you should give up gluten forever if it turns out to be one of your triggers. That choice is up to you. I will, instead, show you what gluten does in your body and in your brain so you can make the most informed choices possible about what you eat and when you eat it. At its best, reading this book will help you eliminate your headaches forever. At its worst, this book will make you more self-aware and able to make more informed choices that will help you reduce your headaches.

Disclaimer: I am obviously not a doctor, and this is not medical advice. I'm a headache sufferer who did thousands of hours of research to find the best information available on how to stop suffering. Each person who reads this book will come to it with individualized health conditions, so read this book, do some of your own research, and talk to your healthcare professionals about the path that's right for you. This is your life. You only get one.

You'll find the free guide to this book at www.3dayheadachecure.com.

Let's Get Real about Headaches

Migraines by Definition

What actually *is* a migraine? A migraine is a severe headache with specific symptoms, but the definition is still subjective, which may be why only 50% of physicians accurately diagnose them.[8] How do doctors accumulatively earn such an outstanding failure rate? For one, most doctors treating migraine patients are not specialists. And only 4% of migraine sufferers consult a headache specialist.

Is it really that hard to find good help? Yes. According to the United Council for Neurologic Subspecialties, there are only 416 certified headache subspecialists in the United States who have demonstrated competence in neurological headache healthcare.[9] There are 320 million Americans, so that's one specialist for every 769,000 people—and many migraine sufferers live in states with no headache subspecialists. And that's why good help is hard to find.

Even most neurosurgeons are not specialists, because it's almost impossible to fully understand a complex condition with so many triggers and variables hidden deep within unpopular research. It's no wonder the International Headache Society's criteria for migraines is so general:[10]

- Headache attacks last 4–72 hours
- Headaches include at least two of the following characteristics:
    - Unilateral location
    - Pulsating quality
    - Moderate or severe pain intensity

- - Aggravation or avoidance of routine physical activity
- During a headache, at least one of the following:
  - Nausea and/or vomiting
  - Photophobia and phonophobia

The IHS criteria for migraines also explains that, because it's often difficult to differentiate between migraines without auras and occasional tension headaches, in order for your headaches to be considered migraines, you must have had at least five attacks that cannot be attributed to another disorder.

This diagnosis is 100% subjective to the individual and the interpretation of his or her doctor, who is probably not—a *big* probably not—a specialist. Most people get headaches, and some would say they are moderately painful and last for hours and that bright light and noise make them worse. Some people would also say they've had to stop doing some activities because of them. Meanwhile, a migraine sufferer is grounded with low blood pressure, hallucinations, and what feels like an ice pick jammed in the temporal lobe—possibly, this migraineur is ready to jump off a bridge.

The IHS definition of a migraine says that migraines aren't attributed to other disorders, but they often are—and those migraines are still migraines, right? Not according to the IHS. If MSG triggers a migraine, it's not called a migraine. It is classified as an 8.1.5.1 monosodium glutamate-induced headache.[11] This conflicts with the concept of the headache threshold and the fact that there are multiple triggers that could cause a migraine—the more triggers you induce or experience, the more likely you are to break that headache threshold and get a migraine. So here's my definition of a migraine: a severely painful and misunderstood neurological condition that is triggered by the sum of various types of inflammation and that could be a warning sign of far more deadly conditions that result from prolonged exposure to those sources of inflammation.

We definitely need a new formal definition of what migraines are because so much of the general public thinks migraines are just headaches, and so do many healthcare professionals. Maybe the government thinks the same thing since government research funding for migraines is a pathetic $15 million per year. To give you an idea of just how underfunded migraine research is, asthma receives $244 million, and diabetes receives over a billion dollars per year in research funds.[12]

But migraines are ranked the seventh-highest disability among specific causes,[13] costing the United States over $20 billion in healthcare costs and lost workdays, and migraines affect roughly 13% of the population. Of course, those statistics are just rough estimates due to a lack of research, an abundance of misdiagnoses, and a mess of a healthcare system. The latest research, which is from 2015, marks 14.2% of the adult population with migraines. That's somewhere around 45 million Americans.[14] Migraines are a big deal, and people are really suffering.

The Four Phases of a Migraine

You may not experience all four migraine phases and may only present a few symptoms, but that doesn't mean you don't get migraines. And yes, this only adds to the confusion and misdiagnosis rates. Understanding the four distinct phases of a migraine, however, and knowing which phases you experience can help you get to know your own headache pattern better. For example, the wisdom you can gain by experimenting with preventative measures during the prodrome, or warning, phase could help you stop a migraine before it hits you really hard.

Prodrome Phase

The prodrome phase is first—this is the "Oh crap, oh no, oh here it comes" phase. Some people know that a migraine is coming based on any number of specific sensations. And some migraine sufferers can only say, "I just know it's coming" about this phase. Prodrome sensations may include: fatigue, excessive energy, difficulty finding words, euphoria, restlessness, an irritable mood, a food craving, a loss of concentration, neck pain, and a sensitivity of the senses. If you subtract the excessive energy from that list, it sounds like a typical Monday morning, right? But the list goes to show that the warning can be just about anything, and it typically happens anywhere from a few hours to 24 hours ahead of time. Relaxation and meditation teach you how to hone in on these senses in an effort to prevent the migraine before it really gets its grips on you.

Aura Phase

The aura phase is generally thought of as a visual disturbance that anticipates the migraine. It can happen before or during the headache and usually lasts minutes, but in some cases it can last hours. An aura is associated with the destruction caused from an influx of glutamate, calcium, and inflammation.[15] It's an electrical thunderstorm in the brain. The possible symptoms of the aura phase include: distorted vision; allodynia (painful sensations from heightened sensitivity); sound hallucinations; confusion; dizziness; mixing odors, sounds, sensations, and visions; vertigo; and one-sided paralysis or stroke-like symptoms.

Attack Phase

After the aura phase comes the attack phase, which is the actual headache. The typical symptoms of a migraine may come with the secondary effects of inflammation. Because migraines are neurological problems set in place by stress, they can create painful stress in the face, head, neck, and stomach—really, they can create pain in the entire human body. Your attack phase symptoms may include: confusion, dehydration, depression, diarrhea, high blood pressure, sinus pain, nausea, allodynia, vertigo, eye pain, disinterest in social interaction, tingling extremities, hallucinations, broken speech, weakness, extreme thirst, insomnia, cold feet, hot flashes, mood swings, jaw pain, neck pain, blindness, paranoia, fainting, stroke symptoms, poor balance, stabbing pain, or you may feel as if there's a vise squeezing your head.

Postdrome Phase

The postdrome phase, which is also referred to as the "headache hangover," is the last phase. In a study of over 800 migraineurs, 68% of patients reported feeling a "headache hangover." As with any booze-induced hangover, symptoms can last a few hours to days. In the case of migraines, many people don't notice the hangover after experiencing the relief of a headache passing. How good we feel is often subjective to how bad we felt. Postdrome symptoms may include the following: tiredness, sluggishness, confusion, a poor mood, euphoria, and poor concentration.[16,17]

The Headache Threshold

We can stop all of these phases from starting by paying attention to the headache threshold. This book is based on the headache threshold theory, which is the idea that single events do not cause migraines; rather, an accumulation of foods and events are responsible for provoking migraines. We all have a headache threshold that we don't want to break. Some have a lower threshold than others, so while one person may be able to handle consuming a large number of headache triggers, you may only be able to handle one or two before you break your threshold.

This book was designed to help you discover what breaks your headache threshold. Through this process, you'll also learn which foods you can eat to help you raise your threshold, so you can handle more headache triggers. Doing this requires eliminating known headache triggers to see which are doing you the most harm and causing you the most pain. If the threshold image isn't working for you, think of the headache threshold as a cup. There are multiple ingredients that increase the contents of that cup (and break the headache threshold) or decrease the contents. Reading this book will show you how to turn that cup into a giant jug so your headache triggers never reach the top and spill over.

JEREMY OROZCO

Migraine Treatments in History

As far back as 7000 BC, there were signs of a popular procedure called trepanation, which involved removing a piece of a person's skull. Ancient man believed this procedure could help relieve headaches. While it makes perfect sense that cracking open the skull would relieve pressure, the procedure was actually intended to release the evil spirits causing the trouble.

Jump forward to the seventeenth century. Physicians replaced stones with less barbaric hand-powered drills to perform the well-known procedure on migraine patients, hopefully with a more scientific reasoning. But don't think history won't continue to repeat itself; experimental surgeries are being performed today on headache sufferers who would rather have their skulls opened up than live with the pressure within. Doctors are getting even more creative now by using electric stimulation within the skull to stop headaches. But don't get too excited yet unless you want to become a guinea pig—this high-risk procedure is a last resort and doesn't have a lot of evidence behind it.

Let's take our modern perception to Egypt in 1500 BC. Although the pyramids remain a mystery of unmatched architectural design, we know exactly how ancient Egyptians dealt with the worst headaches. Egyptians remedied their migraines by firmly binding a clay crocodile to their heads using linen inscribed with the names of the gods they believed would help cure the ailment. Three thousand years later, migraineurs are still using cloth (scarves, bandanas) to put pressure around their heads as they lie in darkness. Some swap the clay crocodile for cold or hot packs.

Hippocrates described the aura of a migraine in 400 BC. He said that it was followed by immense pain that could be brought on by a number of activities, including sex.

Switching the clock over to AD, the Roman physician Galen attributed migraines to digestive disturbances. He noticed that stomach fluid (bile) was yellow during a migraine and pain decreased after this fluid was vomited.

Galen influenced the sciences that would later be known as anatomy, physiology, pathology, pharmacology, and neurology. The guy was kind of a big deal. He believed that a healthy gut could lead to a healthy brain. Finally, neurology is catching up with Galen as we're learning how important the gut is for not only our neurotransmitters, but also for our health in general. That "gut feeling" is almost making sense.

In medieval times, they used a headache treatment of opium and vinegar. Others in the Middle Ages tied a dead mole to the head of a headache sufferer to suppress pressure. Perhaps that sparked the next brilliant idea of using a hot iron to subdue the pain surrounding the head. This wouldn't be too far off from today's experimental treatment of removing muscles around the head. These methods stem from a very scientific theory that goes a little something like this: "Hey, this hurts! Let's get rid of it."

Hildegard von Bingen may have been history's most famous migraineur, as her migraine auras have named her the first migraine-inspired artist. This also led her to write several books on medicine and natural remedies. Of course, some historians just say she was crazy—because only crazy people have visions.

Even the Greek gods weren't exempt from migraines. Zeus, god of gods, had the mother of all headaches and howled so loudly that it could be heard throughout the earth. Hephaestus helped Zeus out by taking a wedge and splitting his head open. Then Athena, goddess of war and wisdom, was born, fully clothed in armor and intellect. Today, doctors are still interested in opening the skull to fix the problem, as if the answer were just waiting to jump out with all of its wisdom.

In the late 1800s, William Gowers mentioned migraines in a book that would one day earn him the title "the father of modern day neurology." He invented the headache treatment of a nitroglycerin and alcohol mixture—but it was a very temporary solution, if not a problem in itself for migraineurs. One of his treatments is still used every day in the United States for migraine sufferers—medical marijuana.

Gowers was also an advocate of following a healthy diet to prevent migraines. While a handful of medications have been used to successfully stop migraines, like Sigmund Freud's prescription of cocaine, not a single medication has been overwhelmingly successful in the prevention of them. Long-term medication use will almost always lead to more problems and more medication—with side effects that include more headaches. Gowers's prescription to eliminate the problem and aid headache prevention with nutrition will be the most successful headache cure of the twenty-first century.[18]

There was also Hua Tuo. This surgeon's second-century treatment may help you today. I don't know what he thought he was doing practicing surgery in 100 AD, but his successful alternative treatment—using the Yongquan acupuncture point to relieve headaches—may still be able to change your life. You just need to turn a few pages.

Famous Migraine Sufferers

Sometimes, at least, it's comforting to know you're not alone in your suffering. Even better, we can compare ourselves to these people who've accomplished impressive things and say to ourselves, "I'm not weak because I have migraines—look at all of these people." So, yes, look at all of these people. Dwyane Wade of the Miami Heat has missed games from his debilitating migraines. He had an especially hard time during the 2011 playoffs. Former Denver Broncos running back Terrell Davis lost his vision because of a migraine during Super Bowl XXXII. His vision returned, he scored the game-winning touchdown in the second half, and he was named MVP of the Super Bowl.[19] Migraines can happen to *anyone* at any time.

Other famous migraine sufferers in sports include:[20]

Freddie Ljungberg	J. R. Redmond
Ryan Giggs	David Bell
Michael Dawson	Dwight Gooden
Ian Wright	Eric Milton
Percy Harvin	Jose Canseco
Kareem Abdul-Jabbar	Jason Williams
Serena Williams	Se Ri Pak
Troy Aikman	Kathryn Marshall
Marquez Pope	Fred Couples
Scottie Pippen	Jordan Ada
Rohan Davey	

Other famous migraine sufferers:

Famous Migraine Sufferers

Elvis Presley
Kanye West
Carly Simon
Loretta Lynn
Susanne Shaw
Victoria Beckham
Gareth Gates
Janet Jackson
Jeff Tweedy
Michael John Coleman
Janet McKenzie
Trevor Southey
Dennis Frings
B. J. Anderson
Ben Affleck
Elle Macpherson
Susan Olsen
Star Jones
Whoopi Goldberg
Elizabeth Taylor
James Cromwell
Lisa Kudrow
Lee Grant
Kristin Chenoweth
Virginia Madsen
Hugh Jackman
Marcia Cross

Dani Harmer
Jessica Fox
Sammy Winward
Cindy McCain
Michele Bachmann
Princess Margaret
Fred Norris
Jennifer Ringley
Annie Glenn
Lewis Carroll
Thomas Jefferson
Vincent Van Gogh
Charles Seurat
Sigmund Freud
Claude Monet
Virginia Woolf
Miguel de Cervantes
Julius Caesar
Napoleon Bonaparte
Ulysses S. Grant
Robert E. Lee
Mary Todd Lincoln
Friedrich Nietzsche
Charles Darwin
John F. Kennedy
Albert Einstein
Emily Dickinson

Two Migraine Studies That Will Blow Your Mind

Maybe migraines aren't the cause of migraines. Maybe there is nothing wrong with you. Maybe a debilitating headache is the only way that your body can tell you something is wrong with the food you eat. The 1983 study I reference here reinvented the "cause" of headaches, and the 1979 study was 100% effective at reducing migraines. If you're reluctant to try an elimination diet, beware—reading about these two studies might change your mind! Today, the 1983 study is referenced by hundreds of headache resources as one of the most successful migraine studies ever conducted.

The 1983 Migraine Study

Is a migraine a food allergy? That's a great question; it's also the title of this 30-year-old study, which is still relevant today.[21] It wasn't until 10 years later that the first migraine-specific drug came on the market. Triptans, nicknamed a "miracle medication," show an effectiveness of 50–60% and are prescribed every day in hospitals across the globe.[22]

An acute migraine medication with a 50% success rate is a top-of-the-line drug. The 1983 elimination diet makes a success rate of 50% look like the grade it deserves: an F. You wouldn't put an exam with a big, fat, red F on your fridge. Why would you settle for an F from a headache treatment?

Two Migraine Studies That Will Blow Your Mind

The 1983 study eliminated top food triggers from the diets of 88 children who had suffered from migraines for an average of about four years. Of the 88 children, 78 stopped having migraines completely! For a drug to be successful, it must be able to simply *reduce* migraines. The 1983 study did way more than that. Four of the remaining patients who still suffered from migraines had far fewer attacks than they did before. This study is the first cobblestone in a path that leads to one headache answer.

The headache diet the children followed consisted of:

- One meat (lamb or chicken)
- One carb (rice or potato)
- One fruit (banana or apple)
- Water
- Vitamin supplements

After the patients stopped having headaches, certain foods were reintroduced to see what foods were problems and what foods could be added to a nutritionally and socially acceptable diet. Some patients recovered in one day, while others took up to three weeks. Reactions to the reintroduction of a trigger food occurred in two days, on average. This is incredible, considering that most people (including many doctors) think that food triggers cause immediate headaches. This suggests that eliminating food triggers may leave you headache-free in three days.

The study also suggests that processed foods may provoke migraines. Some patients reacted to bacon but not pork, or white wheat flour but not brown. Other triggers, like stress and noise, had no effect on patients after they started the diet. This supports the threshold theory that single events do not cause migraines; rather an accumulation of foods and events are responsible for provoking migraines. Researchers also witnessed that reintroducing foods that were once triggers no longer provoked migraines after significant migraine triggers had been removed.

As successful as the study was, it failed six patients and left doubt for millions of headache sufferers. Why did it fail those patients? The study mentioned that three of the six failed patients tested positive for extraneous allergies (pollen, cats, outside allergens, etc.). While allergies are a factor in headaches, the diet introduced problems from the start. Inflammatory meats may provoke headaches, depending on the known headache triggers the animal is fed or injected with. Additionally, massive amounts of white rice can lower your headache threshold (not good) but can make you feel so good during a headache.

The 1983 study showed an elimination diet to be highly effective on its own. Imagine if you combined the elimination diet with foods that are proven to support a healthy brain—foods that do exactly what our best drugs attempt to mimic—or imagine if you cheated and used supplements that are proven more effective than the strongest medications. Now add in exercise, which you will soon learn is extremely powerful for headache prevention. Then eliminate the top headache triggers documented in the last 30 years of research (and in the Headache Help Checklist). How do you think you would feel if you tried all of that? It could help you live a life without headaches and feel better than you ever have.

This study only managed one type of headache trigger. Impressively, by eliminating major food triggers, the other triggers, such as light, sound, and stress, became irrelevant. Yet, the study had one major flaw in its elimination of headache triggers. It only focused on acute (fast-acting) triggers, rather than chronic triggers. Ideally, this study would have looked for triggers that chronically lower the headache threshold—those that stay in your system and continue to give you headaches. Luckily the researchers happened to stumble upon a trigger that is both acute and chronic: wheat.

You may be thinking, "Oh great, I was looking for headache help, and this book looks like it's going to give some hippy bull hooey about how food is the voodoo that's killing us—the same food our grandparents ate and lived to be 100 years old." But really, this book is largely about the top headache triggers that have been proven by multiple studies. You'll learn how much wine it takes before it goes from being an anti-inflammatory to becoming a headache trigger. And sure, if you want to give up all the headache triggers causing you grief and do it forever, you can. But I've found that approaching the information in this book more moderately works best for me.

And if you don't believe diet is related to migraines, take a look rural Tanzania in Africa, where the population has very few headache triggers and hardly any processed food consumption. Researchers went door to door to survey 7,412 individuals about migraines under the criteria set forth by the International Headache Society. They found the area to have a migraine prevalence of only 2.5%. Could it be a fluke? Tanzania's extremely low migraine prevalence is not unusual for rural Africa where people eat local and natural food. According to the study, it's smack dab in the middle.[23] And then we have Parma, Italy, where 24.7% of its citizens experienced migraines within the last year.[24] Yes, Parma, like Parmesan cheese or Parma ham—perhaps the only true prosciutto. Aged cheeses and cured meats are migraine triggers—and we can't discount Italy's love for that villain, wheat.

Taking stock of the most common headache triggers and eliminating them from your diet are simple choices that will change the way you feel today—especially if you start with wheat. Your mind will begin to clear. Your energy will skyrocket. You'll sleep better. Your immune system will improve. You'll feel great, simply from eliminating that one top headache trigger from the 1983 study.

The 1979 Migraine Study

Do you want to use the most successful migraine diet in history? I don't think I can put into words how extraordinary this study was. This elimination diet is more likely to help people than any other single headache "cure" on earth. Let's take it back to 1979, a time when some studies aimed to find the "cause" of migraines instead of treating the "effect" of headaches with expensive drugs. The study was published in the May 1979 issue of *The Lancet*. Researchers advised 186 migraine patients while they embarked on a two-year elimination diet. The first 60 migraineurs who completed the diet were the focus of this report.[25] The 1983 diet was profoundly successful, but it is second best—this elimination diet is the most successful headache "cure."

Patients in this study had suffered for an average of 20 years. The patients started out with a five-day diet of only two low-risk foods (usually lamb and pears). What a challenge to eat only two foods for five straight days! One patient had to substitute fish for lamb because of her migraine reaction. It's these individual food reactions that make finding that perfect diet difficult. Reactions for the majority of patients went like this:

Day 1 = Migraines

Day 2 = Migraines

Day 3 = Some migraines

Day 4 = No migraines

Day 5 = No migraines

In *only three days*, most of these migraine veterans were migraine-free. This gives people real hope. Most food triggers take two or three days to cause a migraine. Eliminate those triggers and migraines are gone in three days.

After the first five days, the researchers reintroduced foods and observed the patients for reactions. Those 60 patients had a total of 624 reactions to different foods, with an average of about 10 food reactions per patient. These reactions were observed by a change in pulse, and the top triggers caused additional symptoms and/or pulse changes.

The 1979 study's top migraine triggers:
- Wheat
- Oranges
- Eggs
- Coffee
- Tea
- Milk
- Chocolate
- Beef
- Corn

- Sugar
- Yeast
- Mushrooms
- Peas

These top triggers, listed in order of severity, were eliminated from the diets of the 60 patients. Fifteen of the patients who had hypertension (high blood pressure) no longer did after eliminating these foods. This shouldn't be a surprise to you. Healthy pipes in your body mean healthy pipes in your brain. A healthy weight loss was also observed. Again, you shouldn't be surprised that the "wheat belly" goes away without wheat. Migraines for the group dropped from 402 per month to just six per month.

That is phenomenal. Eighty-five percent of the patients became headache-free, and *all* of the patients significantly improved. In drug stats, that means it was 100% effective. This is seriously exciting—and I believe we can do better than that. By using the Headache Help Checklist in this book that combines everything we know today, we can beat the results of the 1979 diet.

The Strategy and Tactics of Food Eliminations

Since the 1930s, individual food allergens have been found to trigger migraines.[26] "How do we fix this allergy problem?" is the question that researchers have been trying to answer. In this chapter, you will learn the secret behind the migraine allergy.

Many studies have attempted to find the answer by following a very rudimentary approach. Food allergens trigger migraines in multiple studies, so we need to find what people are allergic to so they can eliminate those individual foods. This should eliminate the migraines, right? Well, the problem with this tactic is that it only addresses one piece of the inflammation puzzle. The studies need to be simpler.

The 1983 study said the same thing as the 1979 study: If people only eliminate their personal allergens, their reduction in headaches will be minimal. Yet the last 40 years of studies have failed to battle both chronic and allergenic food triggers. Still, in comparison to medications, recent food elimination studies have been successful. This makes food-allergen elimination diets a very important tactic in your overall strategy to become headache-free.

The words "strategy" and "tactics" were once reserved for the military. I became familiar with them from large fires and emergency incidents. Today, they are widely used in business and everyday language. A strategy is the larger overall plan that is comprised of smaller and less impactful tactics. Most "headache cures" are tactics and fail to acknowledge the entire problem, which is why most of them suck.

The 2010 IHS Study

Even though a tactic is less impactful, it is still an important part of your overall success. A 2010 food allergen study published by the International Headache Society took on the tactic of finding food allergens and eliminating them from participants' diets.[27] The study found a "significant reduction" in headaches and migraines when eliminating food allergens based on 266 food antigens. They basically poked people with 266 different foods (food antigens) and then waited to see if antibodies came to attack the food. On average, there were 24 reactions per patient.

The researchers kept it secret and gave half of the patients a diet with foods they were allergic to—that's not nice—and the other half of the patients were put on an elimination diet that removed their personal food triggers. After six weeks, the groups traded diets. The end result was a 30% reduction in migraines for those on the elimination diet. Some patients had over a 50% reduction in migraines. That's great, but that success rate is less than half that of the 1979 study. Furthermore, the elimination diets didn't eliminate *all* the major foods that are known to cause inflammation. So why do I mention it? This study is special because it acknowledges that individual headache triggers are only one part of a larger problem.

The study makes several references to those things that chronically raise inflammation and have been known to induce migraines. Obesity, stress, and poor diets are referenced as contributing factors in the rise of inflammatory cytokines. The study deems a food allergy test an important step in determining the foods we are allergic to on an individual level. It's also an integral part of the goal to reduce your overall inflammation. The study concludes that a more thorough approach to reducing all inflammation is needed to combat migraines, which gives us the go-ahead to get out there and start fighting inflammation. You may say, "Well, the 1979 study was still 100% successful with just eliminating the top inflammatory foods. Do I really need to get an allergy test?" The 1979 study significantly reduced migraines in all patients, but it didn't completely eliminate migraines for them. Today, we also have many more headache triggers. Just look at the list of ingredients in your pantry or even in your shampoo. We live with more headache triggers than we may even be able to guess.

You want to give yourself a 100% chance of reducing your headaches 100% of the time. Maybe the allergy approach with only a 30% success rate is not your cup of tea. This next study might change the way you think about allergies and headaches.

The 2007 Food Allergen Study

Welcome to Mexico, where dreams are made. At least, where dreams were made for 47 patients, 44 of whom stopped having migraines altogether. And it happened solely from an allergy elimination diet.

This study was completed in 2007 with 56 migraineurs and 56 nonmigraineurs in a control group.[28] How were the healthy patients in the control group different from the migraine patients? Did the migraine patients have more allergies? Yes, they did. Migraine patients had between six and 30 reactions to the 108 food allergens. The control group only had between zero and four reactions! Case closed: Food allergens are a problem for migraine sufferers.

Interestingly, patients with known allergies were turned away from the study, meaning that none of the people in the study were aware they had a food allergy problem. These migraine sufferers were between 35 and 56 years old, suffering for years without a hint that food was most likely their problem and solution.

These were the top triggers: eggs, cheese, milk, yeast, wheat, tomatoes, and beans. The top triggers for patients with allergies to the most foods (those with seven to 30 reactions) were: bananas, beans, cheese, eggs, milk from cows, mushrooms, sugar, yeast, and wheat. Trailing just behind the pack were shrimp, pork, nuts, rice, lemons, chocolate, oranges, corn, and chili peppers. The rest of the 108 allergens were scattered with just a few reactions for each food. For example, two people out of 56 had a reaction to cherries. You might as well take your chances eating cherries since every food may have reactions for a small number of people, and those reactions may not be significant enough to cause a headache.

Does this mean that the top triggers are definitely causing migraines? No. Even the healthy control group had reactions to some of the food allergens. The food triggers may only trigger a migraine in certain quantities or combinations. This study used an elimination diet based on individual reactions for six months, successfully treating 47 of the 56 patients. That's an 85% success rate, with 77% becoming completely migraine-free, making it one of the most successful migraine treatments in the last 30 years.

Why was it so successful? As far as allergies go, they used an IgG allergy test in combination with an IgE test, providing a broader scope. IgE antibodies are produced from immediate allergic reactions (think bee sting or peanut allergy). IgG antibodies provide long-term resistance to infections that can take from hours to days to initiate a reaction. In other words, they protect us from the allergens that we don't immediately feel. The test is so sensitive it is considered harmful by many doctors because it often shows positive allergies for foods that produce no physical symptoms of an allergic reaction.

A test that shows a two-day reaction from food raises an eyebrow at migraine triggers, especially at those triggers that don't cause allergic reactions. The IgG test that is "too sensitive" has also proved in the last few years to be an early indicator of IgE symptoms. One study showed that children with elevated IgG antibodies increased their risk of eventually becoming allergic to those foods.[29] Does this have anything to do with inflammation? Yes.

A 2008 study of 30 juveniles found that obese children have significantly higher levels of IgG antibodies and CRP (inflammatory cytokines), raising the possibility that the foods that hurt you can also make you fat. The results of this study showed a 99.99% chance that those foods that raise your IgG antibodies are correlated with an increased risk of obesity and inflammation.[30]

So was the IgG test the secret to the success of the 2007 food allergen study? No, not completely. The first study that checked for over 260 antibodies also used an IgG test, but it only had a 30% success rate. The first study was only six weeks, as opposed to the six-month-long 2007 study in Mexico. I don't believe that would change much. The most notable difference was that the American study allowed for the use of preventative and acute migraine medications. Acute medications can be dangerous and destructive. You'll learn in the chapter on drugs why the drugs that are meant to help you can become a crutch that's on fire.

I'm not concerned about the success of the 44 people who may never have another migraine or the three who greatly improved. I want to know why nine people couldn't be helped in the 2007

Mexico study. Those nine people were put on a diet that failed them. Let's say you're allergic to mushrooms and only mushrooms. You can't just eliminate mushrooms, sit on the couch, and continue to eat a whole slew of inflammatory wheats, oils, and other headache triggers. You won't feel good. This is a major flaw in most elimination diets.

So what have we learned since the 1970s? We've learned that taking an allergy test, specifically an IgG, can be useful in combination with your elimination diet. Hundreds of new studies are using the IgG test to treat all the major autoimmune conditions, such as celiac disease (gluten intolerance), inflammatory bowel syndrome, migraines, asthma, epilepsy, rheumatoid arthritis, and fatigue.

The limitation of the IgG test is that real food may produce slightly different results. The test may not bring up all the variations of modern wheat or different tomato strains. The American study pointed out that no allergy tests show all types of inflammation. The 2007 Mexico study concluded that cross-reactions may have been the problem for the unsuccessful nine and should be looked into for future elimination diets.

Cross-Reactions

Migraines are in the gut. Why? When you take studies of about 100,000 people with irritable bowel syndrome (IBS), or what I call "a beat-up gut," you find those with IBS are 40–80% more likely to have migraines, fibromyalgia, and depression.[31] When you look at the beat-up gut from the perspective of migraineurs, the migraineurs are twice as likely to have IBS. Young migraineurs—those under 30 years old—are more than three times as likely to have IBS. And the

The Strategy and Tactics of Food Eliminations

more migraines one suffers, the more likely he or she will have IBS.[32] So what?

We need to fix the gut, that's what.

We just read in the 2007 food allergen study that migraine sufferers are allergic to many more foods—they had from 50–3,000% more allergic reactions. This book explores why a beat-up gut triggers migraines. For now, we know it's a factor, and it's a factor that we can treat with successful food eliminations. In one migraine/IBS study, participants enjoyed a 44% drop in migraine attacks and a significant reduction in the length of their migraines after they eliminated the foods their tests showed they were allergic to.[33] Some see this as a success; I see it as a 56% failure rate. We know that chronic triggers will beat up the gut, and migraine studies are saying that it's about the inflammation, but where is that inflammation coming from?[34]

The Trouble with Gluten Sensitivity Testing

Here's the big problem: Most people don't understand what the problem is. Let's break it down with a summary of the wheat trigger, but keep your mind open, because we can apply this concept to any food trigger. This chapter isn't about wheat, but about how allergens form and why the problem persists after the allergen is gone. Most people identify a gluten problem with celiac disease with all of its glorious GI symptoms. However, even with some of the worst gluten problems, like celiac sprue, there may or may not be any GI symptoms. This is because it's an immune system problem that creates a unique immune system response in each person who has it.

You walk into the doctor's office and tell the doc that you may have a gluten problem with no stomach (GI) symptoms. The doctor may tell you that you don't have a problem. No symptoms, no problem. Dr. David J. Clark's video on YouTube called "Doctors just don't get it—gluten sensitivity" tells a different story. In fact, look at most of Dr. Clark's videos because he explains the gluten problem better than I ever could. He treats hundreds of headache patients and he delivers the answer to this complex problem in an incredibly simple way. In "Doctors just don't get it," he provides insight into why even some of the most brilliant doctors don't understand that most patients don't have stomach symptoms with gluten sensitivities.

Once you get a doctor to believe that you have a problem, he or she may administer a gluten test. The doctor will probably test you for antibodies to the protein alpha gliadin, which is one component of gluten (antibodies attack allergens). You may then test negative for celiac disease and continue to eat wheat because you think you don't have a gluten problem—but the test is flawed. This is a typical result for the extremely common and inaccurate testing of one component of gluten.

We now know that people can and do react to many other components of wheat and gluten, including multiple types of gliadin, glutenin, and transglutaminase.[35][36] These components can now be tested for by an innovative lab called Cyrex Laboratories. Many specialists will recommend this as your best bet for gluten-sensitivity testing. But I'm here to tell you that the cheapest and most effective way to test for a gluten problem is by eliminating it from your diet for three to 30 days and then evaluating how you feel.

Wheat testing comes with the same problem as any other food. Testing for a specific protein is not accurate when there are multiple strains and potencies of every type of food. A Korean study found that 50% of patients with atopic dermatitis had food allergies, but 95% of those patients were not IgE mediated, meaning that a typical allergy test would not identify their problems. Atopic dermatitis is inflammation of the skin, and as with acne, if you take the inflaming trigger away, the skin condition goes away, and it's the same with migraines.

The top food reactions for patients with atopic dermatitis were:[37]

- Eggs: 21.6%
- Milk: 20.9%
- Wheat: 11.8%
- Soybeans: 11.7%

The triggers of inflammation are the triggers of migraines, so eliminating these foods from your diet will help reduce your inflammation and migraines a great deal.

For the second part of this problem, let's say that you have come to the conclusion that you have an allergy problem, specifically with wheat. You completely eliminate wheat from your diet, which is a triumph considering it means you need to stop eating practically all processed foods. However, you don't feel better. You feel worse.

The problem is a cross-reaction, and the problem was first identified in the 1970s.[38] Your body sees similar proteins in other foods and attacks them in the same manner it attacks gluten. The most confusing part is that this problem can occur when a person stops eating wheat. If you're lucky, you'll have stomach symptoms or headaches to alert you to the problem. Either way, it was long established well before you'll experience any kind of symptoms.

Whether you have stomach symptoms or not, your body may attack these wheat proteins and damage your stomach lining. This inflammation can cause proteins to slip past the lining of the stomach and get into your bloodstream by way of your new "leaky gut." Stress can also cause or add to inflammation that destroys the gut, and it allows new proteins to enter the bloodstream.[39] Your body will then look at these proteins that were never a problem before and say, "Hey, you don't belong here. You're a problem. We need to create antibodies to attack you." This process happens more rapidly when the protein resembles something you already have antibodies for. Ultimately, you could become like one of those children who are allergic to everything and have to live in a bubble.

People who get off the wheat train make an immense effort to eat foods without a trace of gluten. The worst thing they could do is eat foods that have a high probability of cross-reaction and continue to damage their stomachs. What foods could these be? Unfortunately, as of the year 2012, there wasn't much solid information on what foods are likely to have a cross-reaction and ruin the rest of your life. Fortunately for you, it's not 2012.

An incredible study was published in *Food and Nutrition Sciences* in 2013 that sought the answer to why 30% of patients on a gluten-free diet do not improve.[40] The study noted that intestinal villi (the hair-like structures on the lining of the small intestine) returned to normal in only 8% of the patients, meaning 92% of the patients on a gluten-free diet did not fully heal their guts. The reason people are prescribed a 30-day gluten-free diet is to allow the stomach to self-repair. Why isn't this happening in the high majority of gluten-sensitive patients? The study took a handful of foods that multiple studies have suspected as cross-reactive foods but couldn't pinpoint why.

The new study looked at how those foods interacted with the antibodies that attack alpha-gliadin-33, the major peptide involved in celiac disease. You can think of cross-reaction foods as cross-fire. Soldiers will shoot at an enemy from all sides, and the crossfire may hit innocent bystanders or fellow soldiers. If the innocent bystanders and fellow soldiers are not distinguished from the enemy, there will be more casualties. In the gut, this means that the proteins that look similar to gluten proteins will be attacked and the crossfire will damage the gut. In other words, food proteins that resemble gluten will be attacked in the same way and cause the same damage.

The 10 biggest problem foods for gluten-sensitive people are:

- Milk products
- Yeast
- Oats
- Corn
- Millet
- Instant coffee (ground coffee had no reaction)
- Rice
- Potatoes
- Soy
- Eggs

These foods may be a problem while your stomach is damaged. Let's say you avoid gluten and double and triple up on these common gluten substitutes—that may be the tipping point for your stomach to become even more damaged. Ideally, you eliminate all of these foods and your stomach repairs itself within 30 days. You will then be able to reintroduce some of these foods into your diet.

Twenty years ago, Kurt Cobain didn't know about cross-reactions and elimination diets. In a TV interview only months before Cobain's death he said, "Most gastro-intestinal doctors don't know anything about stomach diseases. They just have PhDs, get paid a lot of money for pretending and prescribing drugs." Cobain was open about being suicidal for years as he struggled with what doctors generically called IBS. He turned to heroin for pain relief and ended his life at the age of 27. The new research on elimination diets, cross-reactions, and inflammatory diseases will give chronic sufferers options beyond drugs and suicide.

I actually first learned of one elimination diet while researching seizures in dogs. It may seem strange, but dogs are kind of like children in that we can easily manipulate their diets despite the smells of tempting foods. Well, we can at least have a little more discipline for a diet that will keep them safe, despite the beseeching puppy-dog eyes. We know seizures share autoimmune similarities to migraines—both often include auras, and both share drug and prevention efforts.

The veterinary site dogtorj.com has a large and astonishing list of testimonials from clients. "Kody, having 5 seizures in 15 days (now on what is called the Big Four diet) HAS NOT HAD A SINGLE SEIZURE SINCE!" was a response from one grateful dog owner. But all of this hit even closer to home when I read this from one of the other testimonials: "My epilepsy magically disappeared and my migraines are gone too." That wasn't a dog owner talking about a dog—it was a person talking about the same diet. Did a vet really have the answer for millions of humans?

The Big Four diet eliminates four large sources of glutamate: gluten, casein, corn, and soy. Obviously, they are all headache triggers, but this diet is what pointed me toward researching what happens when we experience a rise in glutamate and its byproduct—inflammation. A ton of research suggests that inflammation and glutamate play a role in migraines,[41] but this diet suggested that we can eliminate migraines by reducing our intake of headache triggers that raise glutamate and inflammation levels. It was like discovering a map to a lost city. Every study has perfectly aligned with this theory, and many of the enlightening comments regarding elimination diets have as well.

Enlightening is probably the wrong word for it. One comment from a headache and stomach sufferer changed the way I perceived modern medicine: "I had my surgery date set for a colostomy. I heard from a friend to try a gluten-free diet, even though I wasn't diagnosed with celiac disease. Within days it, worked."

While it's easy to point fingers at hospitals, they are working off limited information. There's still a great deal of confusion on how a variety of foods can trigger problems for gluten-sensitive people. Many recent studies have found coffee to be a problem for gluten intolerance. However, the new cross-reaction study found that this was due to gluten contamination found in most instant coffees, as there was no reaction from fresh ground coffee.

Rice is still an oddity. Rice is allergenic for a somewhat smaller number of people; however, the 2007 Mexico study found rice to be allergenic for a high number of migraine sufferers. It's known that people who are allergic to rice sometimes react to other foods of the same botanical family, such as barley, maize, wheat, oats, and rye, as well as foods like peaches and apples.[42] This is a conflict of interest for those headache sufferers who use rice as a comfort food. Andrew Levy, author of *A Brain Wider Than the Sky: A Migraine*

Diary, claims that this is one of the only foods he can keep down during his crippling migraines. So should we eat rice—or not?

The cross-reaction list combined with a gluten-free diet is extreme. You can't eat processed foods because it's almost guaranteed they will contain one of these 10 food products, aside from the already large task of eliminating gluten products. If you simply want to feel better, then reducing these processed foods is a good idea. If you have severe headaches, allergies, or stomach problems, then you may want to try a 30-day elimination diet that includes the cross-reaction list.

Is Gluten-Free Headache-Free?

"What is gluten?" That was the "pedestrian question" posed on an episode of *Jimmy Kimmel Live!* not long ago. He wanted to know if those people who were systematically depriving themselves of all things gluten knew the first thing about what they were doing. So a roving reporter asked several misinformed gluten-free joggers running in the park. The answers were 100% incorrect and truly hilarious. But Kimmel was right: "Gluten…is a mixture of two proteins found in wheat and some other natural grains, but here in LA, it's comparable to Satanism."[43]

I understand that many people will put this book down before they ever consider putting a slice of pizza down. I realize that going on a gluten-free diet is trendy beyond all reason, making it a distasteful proposition from the get-go. Maybe you don't even want to hang out with gluten-free people who have to spend 20 minutes online trying to find someplace where you can both eat. And if all of this is true, you definitely don't want to be the name that fills in the blank for this sentence: "We can't order pizza/have Italian/make that for dinner/go there to eat/do anything fun ever because _____ doesn't eat gluten."

I get it. But for the sake of your head, for the sake of your sanity, and for the hope of a life without headaches, don't put the book down yet. Instead, think of gluten simply as one of several possible triggers that could be causing your pain. And cross your fingers (tightly) that it's not one of your triggers if it makes you feel any better, but this chapter isn't going to teach you anything wonderful about gluten.

I don't have any interest in the gluten-free fad diets. I'm talking about gluten because it's a major headache trigger in the 1983 study and numerous other successful studies. In this chapter you'll learn what gluten and wheat are and how they contribute to making us fat, tired, and slow. You'll also read about a migraine study that was 100% successful at reducing migraines after participants eliminated wheat from their diets, laying the foundation for food triggers. While wheat is a major trigger, it is still part of a headache threshold, and it is just one of the many elimination options you can include on your personal checklist for migraine relief.

If you still want pizza—and cigarettes and booze—after reading this book, enjoy them. You'll learn that placebos are extremely powerful, and you need to believe in the parts of the Headache Help Checklist you choose to follow. And in actuality, it's important to enjoy the things that are likely to negatively affect your headache threshold as well. Elimination diets aren't intended to deprive you of what you love to eat; they're intended to teach you how what you eat affects you. Once you know that, you can do what you want with the information. After reading this chapter, however, you might not pick up another slice of pizza.

If you do cut gluten from your diet, I know you'll never look at bread the same way again—and hopefully your last headache will be *your last headache*. This food elimination is more likely to help you than any drug on earth. Are your fingers still crossed that it's not one of your triggers? Do you feel like finding me online so you can start a gluten argument with me? I mean, ancient Egyptians ate bread, so how bad could it be? Ancient Egyptians also had migraines, but that's not the point. And anyway, we're not talking about the same wheat—not by a long shot. Today's wheat is two and a half feet shorter and 10 times heavier than it used to be, and it has undergone severe hybridization. Forget the Egyptians; modern wheat is completely different—even from the wheat our grandparents ate.

Getting High on Gluten

Dr. William Davis, author of *Wheat Belly*, explains how we have created thousands of hybrids that contain new proteins with a higher quantity of genes associated with celiac disease. Despite these genetic alterations, wheat has never been thoroughly tested for its health risks. *Wheat Belly* is a best seller for a reason. Its findings are unbelievable—you really must check this book out.

According to Davis (and the glycemic index), two slices of wheat bread are equivalent to eating a candy bar or drinking a full can of Coke with 44 g of sugar. That's right, wheat creates more blood sugar than eating pure sugar. Of course this will make you fat, but the real detriment is in the unnatural spike in your blood glucose (sugar) level. With every up, there is a down. So when you eat wheat, your sugar goes through the roof—and just two hours later, it's gone, leaving you hungry, tired, and slow. As those neurons slow down, your mind may feel as shaky as your body.[44]

This is not good for migraines. While they are not just headaches, migraines are triggered by the same things that headaches are. Among the top triggers are the foods you eat and missing meals—so it's true that whether or not you get a headache or migraine has a lot to do with blood glucose. As firefighters, we administer a blood glucose test in the field for nearly all neurological medical calls. Why do we do that? Because it can give us quick insight into what's causing a person's headache-related discomfort.

In those situations, people often say, "But I'm not diabetic." These are often the people with low blood sugar. You've probably had a headache caused by low blood sugar yourself. Have you ever skipped a meal and a little later noticed a headache emerging? Then you ate something, which brought your blood glucose level up, and your headache went away. This affects your blood vessels and the ability to regulate nutrients and oxygen to the brain. Wheat simply speeds up this process. With an unnatural spike in blood sugar, your brain will need nutrients sooner. I know; we have been told that wheat is so good for us. We've been lied to.

The truth is that wheat can have long-term effects on headaches. Eating carbohydrates forms small, low-density lipoproteins (LDLs) that are responsible for plaque buildup, which raises your risk of heart attack and stroke. Your blood vessels are one system. If your pipes are not clean in your heart, they are also not clean in your brain. In rare cases, migraines have caused stroke-like symptoms. A stroke occurs when the blood supply to part of your brain is interrupted and your brain is deprived of oxygen and glucose—the 911 responders will be moving at full speed, because every second of delayed treatment is a second closer to death. Vascular health is essential in preventing strokes and headaches.

There is a clear correlation with headaches and blood vessels dilating (getting bigger) and constricting (getting smaller). When that happens, it may trigger a headache. It is also an integral part of the pain mechanism. That plaque buildup from wheat will make it difficult for your brain to properly regulate your blood vessels. As you read on, you'll find studies linking migraines with stroke, cardiovascular disease, obesity, and your overall plumbing. So stop eating wheat. Easy, right? Maybe not. According to the *Wheat Belly* author, once ingested, gluten is converted to polypeptides that can actually penetrate the blood-brain barrier, which separates the blood from the brain. Wheat polypeptides bind to the brain's morphine receptors in a similar way to opiates. In other words, you get high—maybe just a little bit high, compared to what you would feel on opiates, but you get high nonetheless.

When someone gets too high on heroin (opiates), we administer a drug called naloxone. This will take someone from near death to sober in just two minutes. The drug completely stops the opiates from binding to the morphine receptors. When the patient is awake—and alive—rather than being grateful or relieved, an addict is usually angry that we killed his or her "high." Studies show naloxone has the same reaction to wheat polypeptides—it stops the high. Have you felt it? That feeling you get from a bagel that tells you this is exactly what you want right now. Or, are you to the point where you only need *some* carbs to feel normal? Just a little bit. Just a taste. Just a little taste. That's what addicts call getting "well"—when they no longer get "high" and just need a "taste."

A drug company recently applied to the FDA for naltrexone, the oral version of naloxone. The drug works by taking away that euphoric feeling you get when you get high—or eat a little wheat—which, according to Dr. Davis—reduces your craving. They used this drug in clinical trials on participants who didn't need to withdraw from heroin or any other type of drug addiction, but rather on participants willing to shake their gluten habits. Patients lost 22 pounds in the first six months of clinical trials. Great, right? But before you get too excited about the weight loss, stop and think a minute about that: They used the same drug that helps people overcome heroin addiction to help people overcome "gluten addiction."[45]

Are you starting to see Kimmel's connection between gluten and Satanism? Maybe not, but you might be thinking it deserves a spot in the section of your brain where you store other evil things. But all demonic deductive reasoning aside, the fact is that we don't know whether wheat is killing us or not. The *Wheat Belly* theory was based on limited information, arguable information. Thousands of people have lost weight and regained their health by eliminating wheat, and count millions more in if you include those on the Paleo and ketogenic diets. But we don't really know why.

The first study on obesity and gluten-free diets was published in 2012, one year after *Wheat Belly* was published, and yes, it did find that gluten-free diets reduced weight gain, inflammation, and insulin resistance.[46] Even if Davis was flat-out wrong, the euphoric feeling we get from wheat is very real—you can feel it—and so is the sugar spike.

Studies show a link between wheat and schizophrenia. And interestingly, naloxone has been proven to reduce hallucinations in schizophrenic people. In the 1960s, the veterans' hospital in Philadelphia, Pennsylvania, removed wheat from the diet of schizophrenics. Hallucinations decreased. Wheat was reintroduced and hallucinations increased. Again, wheat was taken away and hallucinations were reduced. It was as if a light switch had turned the participants' schizophrenia on and off.[47] One schizophrenic patient at Duke University had experienced 53 years of delusions, hallucinations, and suicide attempts. Researchers observed the patient's complete relief in just eight days after removing wheat from her diet. Fifty-three years of pain eliminated in eight days. Clearly, wheat can have powerful effects on the human brain.[48]

Substances that bind to your morphine receptors are powerful and can vary in how they affect your brain. If the drug used to stop the negative effects of opiate-like drugs is pushed too fast, it will shut the doors to all those morphine receptors in just seconds. Sobriety in seconds can be deadly for a severe drug addict. Going cold turkey on wheat may not kill you, but you will know the oh-so-euphoric wheat is gone. Most people have "withdrawal" symptoms for several days. The science is limited on the morphine receptors of wheat, but the feeling we get from wheat, and from the loss of wheat, is very real. Once accustomed to wheat, these sugar spikes of euphoria are hard to go without.

So wheat basically turns us into fat, lethargic drug addicts? Maybe even Satanists? Not Satanists—but as for fat, lethargic addicts, yeah pretty much.

More Damning Evidence

Original gluten and migraine studies date back to the 1970s when wheat was identified as highly allergenic for migraine sufferers. But before it was deemed allergenic, it was part of a successful elimination diet back in 1952. The study found chocolate, milk, and wheat to be the largest contributors to migraines that, when removed, led to either complete or "almost complete" migraine elimination in 80% of migraine sufferers![49] And it's a study most people have never heard of.

A 2001 study published in the journal *Neurology* found that 10 patients with long histories of severe headaches were all sensitive to gluten. Of the 10, nine went on a gluten-free diet, and seven of them stopped having headaches completely. The seven patients should consider this a miracle. The participants' headaches included severe migraine symptoms such as aura, nausea, photophobia, phonophobia, confusion, unsteadiness, and white brain matter abnormalities consistent with chronic migraines. To be completely migraine-free is a huge triumph. The other two patients who were on a gluten-free diet experienced significant, but not complete, relief.[50]

These results mean that going on a gluten-free diet is 100% effective at reducing migraines. It nearly doubles the success rate of the most successful prescription drugs. This is jaw-dropping information. Now all we need is for someone to fund a large enough study for doctors to be able to confidently prescribe patients a gluten-free diet. But wait—that won't happen, will it? No one wants to help people find free cures. There's no money in free cures. (Satanists.)

Fact: A recent year-long study of over 500 people by Dr. Alexandra Dimitrova of Columbia University found that 56% of people with gluten sensitivity suffered from chronic headaches. Gluten-free diet, anyone?[51]

Until recently, doctors considered gluten sensitivity to be extremely rare. New evidence suggests that between 5% and 10% of all people may suffer from gluten sensitivity. About three million have celiac disease, and 97% of those are unaware of their condition.[52]

When people with celiac disease eat foods containing gluten, it damages the villi, those hair-like structures on the lining of the small intestine. Once damaged, the villi can no longer properly absorb nutrients and the body becomes malnourished, no matter how much you eat, which results in possible digestive problems, skin rashes, iron deficiency, cramps, a tingling sensation in the legs, HEADACHES, seizures, and more.[53]

Gluten sensitivity, on the other hand, may not show damage to the intestinal tract but may exhibit similar symptoms as celiac disease. Gluten sensitivity will have a prevalence of non-GI (i.e., stomach) symptoms, such as a headache, "foggy" mind, joint pain, and numbness in the legs, arms, or fingers. Recent studies have found that gluten-sensitive patients can have intestinal damage, and it's not just gluten, but a number of proteins in wheat.[54] Symptoms typically appear hours or days after wheat has been ingested, and this aligns with the typical two to three days it takes for other headache triggers to appear after elimination and reintroduction.

The Center for Celiac Research estimates that 18 million Americans have gluten sensitivity, which is six times higher than the number of people who have celiac disease.[55] Celiac disease is just one type of gluten sensitivity.

One day, after coming to grips with my own gluten sensitivity, I was at work, telling a fellow firefighter about it. He rolled his eyes and said, "You are from Santa Cruz! Do you know how many people are actually allergic to gluten? All of these people are on a gluten-free diet; I highly doubt they are all allergic. Whole grain bread is not that bad for you. Most of those people go and replace gluten with food that's worse for you."

Two years prior, I would have said the same thing he said. But because I'd done my research and tried it for myself, what he said sparked a conversation that was just as heated as any argument over politics or religion.

He was right about one thing: People do replace gluten with a lot of crazy foods. But I had to explain to him that, fad diets aside, "Eating bread gives you more blood sugar than eating pure sugar. Sugar spikes make me feel terrible. It's simple. As with eating any bad food—a greasy burger, a ton of fries, or both—you're not going to feel good shortly after. I get sleepy and angry. And whole grain bread is the same as dumping sugar all over lettuce. The sugar will make you tired and eventually fat."

Down with the Food Pyramid!

We have been lied to since we were little kids. The food pyramid shows grains, breads, and pasta as our largest sources of nutrition. According to the USDA's original food pyramid, we should be eating six to 11 servings a day, which is more than the serving suggestions for fruits and vegetables combined. Are they out of their minds? We're living in a country dying of obesity. Just about everything is processed, those processed foods are heavy in wheat, and people are feeling the effects.

If you added up all the yearly deaths from gun violence (31,000), vehicle accidents (36,000), and alcohol deaths (100,000) and doubled it, you would come marginally close to the 400,000 people, according to the CDC, who die each year from obesity.[56] Researchers are constantly debating about obesity deaths and whether or not the foods that cause obesity are the true "cause" of death in obese individuals.

The good old food pyramid *is* killing Americans. But when the USDA introduced a new food pyramid, it flopped after heavy criticism. The current food pyramid is now a plate that does not specify portions. While fruit and vegetables are increased, grains are still the largest category, making American consumers happy about overindulging in the most profitable food group.

With respect to gluten sensitivity, there is no official test. That means that the problem could be much larger than 18 million Americans. But as I said before, the best way to find out if you have a gluten sensitivity is to do a self-test. Stop eating gluten. If, in a few hours to three weeks later, you begin to feel great, you're sensitive to gluten. The first three days were rough for me. I broke down and ate two slices of pizza. Before my last bite, I already had pure regret.

After eating that pizza, I felt slow, tired, and sick with a dull pain in my head. After that, giving up gluten was much easier. It's the negative reinforcement effect. The first thing that enters my mind now when I smell delicious lasagna is not the euphoric feeling that comes from eating wheat, but the much stronger memory of being ill and having a headache. I wouldn't say I'm fully recovered, but I am aware and have a desire to eat much smaller portions. Moderation keeps me feeling good; elimination makes me feel great.

The Benefits of Being Gluten-Free

People who eliminate wheat from their diets typically report improved moods, fewer mood swings, improved concentration, and deeper sleep within just days of their last bites of gluten. Try it for three days. I personally noticed a large increase in energy and clarity. There is, of course, the weight loss as well.

And then there's a whole list of new studies linking wheat to irritable bowel syndrome, fibromyalgia, skin inflammation, neurological disorders, and depression. Want to avoid that stuff? Yeah. Me, too.

Many factors influence headaches. This information only suggests that wheat plays a role in headaches. Parma, Italy, consumes a lot of wheat and may have the highest rate of migraines, but it's just a correlation. Italy is well known for having a Mediterranean diet, pasta consumption, and a low adult obesity rate. However, things are changing. Heavily processed wheat substances are becoming widespread, and that is one factor that explains why 34% of girls and 36% of boys are obese or overweight in Italy. Italy is now second to Greece for having the world's fattest children.[57] This will influence the future migraine prevalence of Parma, much like an Olympian who breaks his or her own record.

Even if we discarded all of this, wheat is still a common migraine trigger. WebMD,[58] the National Headache Foundation,[59] UC Berkeley Health Services,[60] and many other top medical organizations list wheat products like pizza and bread as significant migraine triggers. The most successful study discussed in this book lists wheat as the top trigger.

Later, I'll break down the gluten protein to show you exactly what causes damage and why it's a confirmed headache trigger. But for now, be happy that you already know more than the gluten-free boneheads on Jimmy Kimmel's show.

So what's the answer to the question this chapter posed? Is gluten-free headache-free? Well, it's a top migraine trigger, and it's proven that it destroys your gut. It has a high likelihood of being a major problem for just about anyone. Going gluten-free could, actually, make you free of a lot of problems.

Men, Women, and Children

Men make up only one quarter of admitted migraine sufferers and are more likely to walk off an illness than admit there's a problem. Is it possible that men are so tough that they can just push through a condition that leaves the majority in paralysis? Unlikely. Men do not have the social intelligence that women do. It's certainly not to our benefit to repeatedly overlook emotional cues that help solve problems before they begin.

I distinctly remember the moments after my first fire with a female captain. I couldn't believe it when she said, "How are you guys feeling?" It's a question that many great captains fail to ask, one that can prevent fatal accidents. This very small question made a big difference in an industry that is better known for working until your heart says, "I quit."

Women have 10 times more white brain matter than men. This is the same brain matter used to interpret emotional behavior and excel in leadership, and the same brain matter that becomes damaged during a migraine. However, female migraine sufferers have more gray matter in two regions of the brain that make a painful difference: the insula, which is well known for pain processing, and the precuneus, which is now linked to migraines and may be the home of your conscious self.

What happens to these regions of the brain when women with migraines are in pain? Researchers thought that was a great question and put both male and female migraineurs through MRIs and blasted their hands with a 15-second burst of scorching heat. The two areas of thicker gray matter, which are only found in women with migraines, worked together to respond to pain and triggered an emotional network of pain that was not observed in the less emotionally intelligent. The lead author said, "In men, the pain comes in, and the brain says 'ouch,' in women, the brain says "OUCHHHHH!"[61]

Men, on the contrary, only had pain in one specific area of the brain—the area associated with reward and addiction. So, for the women who have been told, "It's all in your head," there is now scientific proof that it's true in a way that those who have never had a migraine will never fully understand. That's not to say men can't become debilitated too—just not as often—and very few seek medical attention.

Migraines and Female Hormones

A "thicker" amount of gray matter in the area that connects the mind and body may further explain how a seemingly unheard buzzing light bulb can translate to a vibration of torment in the female migraineur. But how is the pain triggered in the first place? Hormones, right? Hormones are just one factor, but they're a big one. Migraines may quietly vanish, and often do, after menopause (occurring at the age of 51 on average). On the dark side, some women don't have migraines until "around menopause," a transition called perimenopause that can last anywhere from four to 10 years. Perimenopause comes with wide fluctuations of estrogen and can start as early as age 35 and ends 12 months after the last day of the final menstrual cycle.[62]

Children

How many children actually have migraines? The numbers on leading medical websites vary greatly. One reason for this is that children are often misdiagnosed because their head pain may be less severe than other symptoms, such as nausea, vomiting, sinus pressure, abdominal pain, and dizziness. In addition, children often don't experience the telltale aura that may come with a typical migraine. Furthermore, children may recover in just an hour or two from a migraine or an "abdominal migraine." This is sometimes accomplished through sleep, which makes it easy to think the kid just needed a nap. But that's not necessarily the case, and not all children can sleep migraines away.

A child's migraine symptoms can be just as debilitating as an adult's. It's especially difficult for children to understand that having migraines doesn't mean they're crazy and doesn't mean they've contracted some rare, scary disease. To make it worse for them, many people, including their parents and teachers, have no clue what they're going through. Many children carry the condition into adulthood with secrecy because they fear that their unsympathetic teachers and parents without migraines will think they're lying about their pain. Unluckily, parents often understand the pain. If one parent has migraines, his or her child has a 40% chance of developing them, and if both parents have migraines, that chance could be as high as 90%.[63]

Boys, Girls, Migraines, and ADHD

Boys will suffer from migraines slightly more than girls until puberty. While both groups may experience more headaches at that point, girls become disproportionately affected by migraines, with the trend continuing into adulthood.[64] Medication use in children is the exact opposite of adults because boys are more disruptive, and for some people this is an obvious sign of ADHD. Nearly one in five teenage boys will be diagnosed with ADHD and about one out of 10 teenage girls.[65]

Emotional or behavioral medication is prescribed for 7.5% of American children ages six to 17 years old.[66] While boys are on more medications and have more migraines, later on, women are on more mind-altering medications (25% of US women use medication for depression, anxiety, ADHD, or another mental disorder) and have more migraines than men.[67][68] While these drugs are considered safe, they all come with side effects that may include headaches and migraines.

Drugs and Kids

Over-the-counter medications, such as acetaminophen (Tylenol), Ibuprofen (Advil), and Naproxen (Aleve), are used for children's migraines, but regular use is recommended under the direction of a doctor. Since 90% of children have stomach issues with migraines, it can be very difficult to use medications that may negatively affect the intestines.[69] And if you think the giant companies that make drugs care about your children, you're wrong. McNeil, maker of Infants' Tylenol, pleaded guilty in March of 2015 to producing baby bottles with visible metal particles several months after consumer complaints. Even the safest medications carry a risk that is aimed at profit.[70]

Aspirin is not recommended for children with migraines because of a higher risk of Reye's syndrome—a potentially fatal, but rare, disorder. Stomach bleeding may also be a concern for children with migraines if they're given too much medication.

Nausea, preventative, and acute medications are all used for children with migraines. If you decide to take the medication route for your child with migraines instead of using the natural methods that have been described in this book, finding a specialist is important. You want to work with a doctor who understands the condition, as well as the short- and long-term risks of the drugs he or she prescribes.

The First Migraine Gene

Recently, the International Headache Genetics Consortium made a breakthrough. It scanned the genomes (genes and DNA) of roughly 5,000 migraineurs and compared them to over 10,000 nonmigraineurs. That's a lot of people. The consortium discovered gene rs1835740 and determined it to be the first genetic migraine risk factor.[71]

This is an incredible discovery because that gene is located between two other genes in the area responsible for glutamate regulation: PGCP and MTDH/AEG-1. That's right—glutamate, as in glutamic acid, as in monosodium glutamate (MSG), as in a main element in gluten. If we can understand how to use this information, we will understand migraines and headaches.

The area where this gene is located is responsible for glutamate homeostasis, which basically means that the genes are responsible for providing the proper levels of glutamate in the brain. If there is too much, the genes get rid of the glutamate before it becomes toxic. They accomplish this goal by regulating the gene EAAT2/GLT1, the major glutamate transporter in the brain. Follow me on this. The gene EAAT2 is like a truck, and the glutamate is that big cargo box on the back. When the EAAT2 is not doing its job by moving forward, those glutamate boxes get stuck. In your body, that means glutamate gets stuck in between neurons in the synaptic gap.

The study suggests that this accumulation of excess glutamate may be the cause of a migraine. Glutamate is your largest neurotransmitter. Right now there are messages firing across your brain. With the help of glutamate, the messages jump from one neuron to the next like lightning. It's a small highway, and the truck's job (EAAT2) is to get the cargo boxes (glutamate) off the highway. If too many cargo boxes (glutamate) are on the highway, it will look like a traffic jam, and nothing will get through.

During this glutamate traffic jam in your brain, the glutamate accumulates until it breaks the headache threshold and causes a migraine. Glutamate has long been suspected of playing a key role in migraine pathophysiology. I came across this study while researching seizures and their relationship to migraines.

One of the largest similarities between seizures and migraines is that both conditions may share an aura. The aura often lets migraine sufferers know what is to come with the perception of visual distortions, confused thoughts, and/or heightened sensitivity. In some cases, the sufferer mixes up sensations and will see a smell, smell a color, or feel a taste. I'm still trying to wrap my head around this concept. What is it like to smell a color?

An excess of glutamate may contribute to all of this. "It's reasonable to speculate that this accumulation can increase susceptibility to migraine through increased sensitivity to the CSD, the likely mechanism for the migraine aura," according to the International Headache Genetics Consortium.[72] CSD, or cortical spreading depression, occurs during a migraine aura when increased electrical activity starts in one part of the brain (usually the occipital lobe) and spreads like a thunderstorm.[73] Migraine sufferers can literally see this electrical thunderstorm unfold with a small visual disturbance that often grows and can eventually obstruct their full vision.

The electrical thunderstorm of extra connections may explain why the brain may interconnect sights, smells, and sounds. It's possible that this all starts from that excess of glutamate blocking one synapse. It's like taking one light bulb off a string of Christmas tree lights, and I'm not talking about those new high-tech lights. I'm talking about the old Christmas tree lights: If one goes out, you need to spend an hour trying figure out which bulb is responsible for none of the bulbs working. That's your brain: a string of lights that needs all its bulbs plugged in.

Supporting this glutamate theory is the fact that mice lacking the EAAT2 gene (responsible for getting rid of that glutamate) suffer from lethal spontaneous epileptic seizures. The buildup of glutamate actually kills them.[74] Interestingly enough, some seizure medications work by inhibiting the release of glutamate. Here's what will blow your mind: The exact same seizure medication that reduces glutamate is also used to prevent migraines. Wow, wow, wow! This suggests that taking natural measures to avoid a buildup of glutamate could be the answer to ending migraines.

Are you still with me? I hope so, because that was the beginning of ending migraines for good. So what do we know now? We know that migraines may have something to do with glutamate. We also know that migraines can be triggered by monosodium glutamate (MSG). If our friends in the food industry are correct, MSG is just glutamate. And if MSG is a migraine trigger, then so is an excess of glutamate. Wheat has gluten, gluten contains glutamate, and excessive glutamate is linked to migraines. These connections are about to add up. We're finally getting some answers.

The Glutamate/Estrogen Factor

If you're a woman with migraines, you probably already know from experience that the fluctuation of estrogen can trigger migraines. To understand why that happens, we need to understand what happens to glutamate and estrogen during a woman's monthly cycle. Why hasn't your doctor brought this up? It could be because this advancement in neurological research just happened in 2010, and it wasn't for migraine research.[75] As the study notes, it's well established that high concentrations of glutamate result in brain damage after acute events, like a stroke, or during chronic conditions, like Alzheimer's or rheumatoid arthritis. Estrogen is known to regulate glutamate, so if we can begin to understand a single month, we can begin to understand how to prevent the damage of glutamate excitotoxicity that takes place during headaches.

Estrogen begins to rise on day one of the menstrual cycle and peaks around day 12. A woman's fertility window is likely to be around days 12 to 17, so know that if you're a woman trying to get pregnant—and *really* know that if you're not! Estrogen levels out until the next cycle when it drops back down. These aren't subtle changes. We're talking about estrogen levels starting at 50, skyrocketing to 386, and plunging back down to 50 at the beginning of the next cycle.

The glutamate levels were exactly the opposite of the estrogen, just as predicted by the authors. Glutamate levels started high while estrogen was low and then dropped nearly in half as estrogen rose, only to shoot back up for the next cycle. When do women often get migraines? Before or during a period, when estrogen levels are low and glutamate levels are high.

What Can You Do?

Aleve is a favorite anti-inflammatory among female migraineurs that is often taken as a preventative several days before and during menstruation. Aleve will reduce inflammation and glutamate buildup. However, reducing all headache triggers several days prior to menstruation will be the most powerful way to reduce glutamate and menstrual migraines—especially reducing foods with high glutamate levels. (Check out the lists of foods with high glutamate levels in the section titled **A Magical Fat Sprinkle by Any Other Name…**)

This would seem to explain the entire problem: high glutamate levels from low estrogen equals a migraine. Up to 70% of women say they have migraines related to their menstrual cycles. Many women only have migraine symptoms during their cycles, making it extremely easy to become misdiagnosed.

What this study lacks, as it urges for future research, is the exact mechanism by which glutamate causes damage. The answer will be very complex. Men consistently have higher levels of glutamate, but they also have higher levels of enzymes that convert glutamate. The study found that the women's enzymes did not rise to combat higher levels of glutamate. The real problem of glutamate, based on seizure research, stems from too much glutamate between those neurons.

Estrogen has been shown to enhance astrocyte glutamate transporters, which could provide neuroprotection. Astrocytes were the transporters picking up all of those boxes (glutamate) off the road (the synaptic gap) to prevent a traffic jam (an aura or depolarization).[76] But if estrogen prevents migraines, why do migraines go away after menopause? Well, the migraines don't always go away, nor does estrogen completely disappear. The human body continues to produce estrogen with less fluctuation. There are also numerous other factors that come into play with aging. For example, most people experience cognitive decline as they age. Many of these lost thoughts were once the rapid firing of glutamate, the primary neurotransmitter. Less thoughts running may be attributed to less glutamate becoming stuck in those synapses.

What About Bumping Up the Estrogen?

In theory, birth control pills that provide constant estrogen for several months at a time would reduce the menstrual cycles per year and migraines per year. This may actually work for some, but there isn't enough research to know for sure. The problem is not so easily solved for most.

Birth control, for one, may come with an increased risk of stroke, and so does the female migraine with an aura. Both risks are low, however it's not recommended to combine the risks.

Even without risks, we're still leaving out the role of progesterone. Progesterone, another important hormone, shows a similar rising trend to estrogen during the menstrual cycle. However, instead of lowering overall glutamate levels, progesterone is associated with an increase in glutamate transporters, thereby picking up those glutamate boxes off the highway and offering neuroprotection.[77]

Remember that it's not all about high glutamate levels. If it were, men would have more migraines than women. Progesterone's ability to help mop up glutamate between the synaptic gap could offer an explanation as to why low progesterone levels are associated with migraines and seizures.

Again, we wonder if female migraineurs can just take a pill or get one of those multiyear progesterone implants used for highly effective contraception. The implant does work to reduce migraines for some, and new research is being conducted on efficacy. However, just like with estrogen, progesterone contraceptives have a variety of side effects that include headaches.[78]

Where does that leave us? Estrogen and progesterone can both trigger and prevent migraines in different clinical settings. Estrogen, progesterone, and glutamate transporter levels are low just before and during menstruation, while glutamate levels are sky high. This means you have a glutamate traffic jam in the brain—too many cargo boxes on the road and not enough trucks to pick them up.

If you're interested in this type of solution, talk to your doctor about birth control that can raise progesterone levels throughout the month. Some doctors are prescribing progesterone just for migraine relief. There is also cream, like the popular Emerita Pro-Gest cream, which you can find on Amazon for about $25. Some migraineurs swear by this cream. One reviewer writes, "My migraines are nonexistent, 10/10 in my book." Another reviewer writes, "I have been migraine-free for a whole month...miracle."

Pregnancy

Many pregnant women find a reduction in allergies and migraines after a 500-fold increase in DAO during the second trimester. Researchers believe that because DAO breaks down histamine, it's likely to limit unwanted inflammation.

Pregnancy would rival any migraine drug on the market. A small study found that migraines improved in 46.8% of women during the first trimester, 83% in the second, and 87% during the third trimester. Nearly 80% of the women had complete remission from migraines. So we must ask, what's up with the progesterone and estrogen levels?

Estrogen and progesterone begin to slowly rise near the end of the first trimester. By the third trimester, estrogen levels are 30 to 40 times higher and progesterone levels are 20 times higher than the peak levels of a normal month.[79] There are a number of chemical changes going on, but it's clear that estrogen and progesterone have some preventative benefit to migraines.

Migraines per Pound

You probably already know what the Center for Disease Control says about obesity: that it raises the risk of insulin production and that insulin resistance is associated with the leading causes of preventable death in the United States.[80] We know obesity may increase migraine risk, but where is the hard evidence? Sure, rural Tanzanians have few migraines and few jelly bellies, but what's the connection?

As you would assume from a disease that is just as often misdiagnosed as diagnosed, the numbers from past studies on large populations are not consistent. However, two provocative studies will change the way you perceive both obesity and migraines.

The Bariatric Surgery Study

The results—and methods—of the first study are extreme. Eighty-one morbidly obese patients with migraines underwent bariatric surgery. This extreme procedure is a last resort to cut down on fat by slicing out a piece of the stomach. Within six months, 89% of patients reported significant improvement in migraine headaches, and 57 of 81 patients reported complete resolution.[81]

These are mind-numbing statistics that had previously only been associated with elimination diets. However, after the surgery, most patients could not stomach more than a Hot Pocket's worth of headache triggers. The weight loss takes care of the majority of the insulin problems, while the excessive intake of all those biogenic amines is no longer possible. Bariatric patients are typically assigned a nutritionist for a plan to obtain the proper levels of nutrients. This includes water and minerals, giving them a significant advantage over the normal migraine patient assigned medications with no hope for the future.

But there's got to be another way, right? Right.

Hara Hachi Bu

Hara hachi bu translates to "eight parts out of 10." *The Okinawa Diet Plan* by Dr. Brad Wilcox explains that the country with the lowest obesity rate in the developed world, Japan, at a mere 3.5%, takes pride in the cessation of eating when 80% full. I typically stop eating when I say, "Oh no, I've done it again! I somehow ate too much for the millionth time in my life." Simply eating slower, limiting our headache triggers, and stopping before we are full will give the body the time it needs to process those at-risk foods. And you won't need to cut a piece of your stomach out.

So why did the extreme surgical procedure fail 11% of migraine patients? Unfortunately, many bariatric surgery patients fill their Hot Pocket–sized stomachs with exactly that type of processed food. Go on YouTube and find "Jim Gaffigan – Beyond the Pale – Hot Pockets." Hot Pockets have nearly 90 ingredients—many of them are headache triggers—and Jim describes how terrible they make us feel.

Tanzanians, who don't eat Hot Pockets or anything like them, may successfully practice *hara hachi bu* out of a lack of food, but that's not the goal of *hara hachi bu* or successful weight loss. The goal of any weight loss attempt should be satisfaction. The ketogenic diet promotes weight loss while suppressing hunger. Whether you try bariatric surgery, *hara hachi bu*, or any diet, you should lower the amount of migraine triggers you ingest while eating food that provides nutrients and satisfaction. Otherwise, your body will be in constant war with your thoughts, and the body, at some point or another, will win. Why fight with hunger when you can eliminate it? *Hara hachi bu* eliminates hunger within just a few minutes of patience and self-control.

The Johns Hopkins Study

The second study was accomplished by researchers from the John Hopkins University School of Medicine and found that obese individuals under the age of 50 were 86% more likely to have migraines. [82] Interestingly, this correlation between obesity and migraines was only observed in women under the age of 50.

What happens to women after age 50? Migraines may quietly vanish, and often do, after menopause (occurring at the age of 51, on average). [83] As you already know, stable levels of estrogen and progesterone after menopause may decrease glutamate levels and migraine frequency. That doesn't explain why the study found no correlation between obesity and migraines in men. For now, it's clear there is a substantial correlation between migraines and obesity in women. This is a good thing, because it opens up one more option for treatment.

One Pound, One Trigger at a Time

Obesity doesn't happen overnight; it's a slow buildup from pound to pound. What's wrong with packing on the pounds? The human body identifies excess fat as exactly what it is: a problem. The body then attacks that problem in the same way it attacks other problems: with inflammation.[84]

Why would your body treat one of the top killers in America any differently? IL-6 cytokines are inflammatory markers that are 50% greater in the blood concentration of obese individuals.[85] This is profound because the body is not just identifying a problem in belly fat; it's spreading the message throughout the entire system.

IL-6 marker levels are shown to be elevated during a migraine attack and have been labeled a contributing factor in the "cause" of migraines.[86] We know that the headache threshold is an accumulation, and so is getting fat. Inflammation is part of this accumulation. The body is saying, "Hey, whatever you're eating is killing us. The only way I can attack this is with inflammation. Hopefully, you get a headache that makes you not want to eat that stuff, because you're about to kill us."

But migraine sufferers come in all shapes and sizes, right?

The pounds aren't the problem; they just help the problem. As we put on pounds, we're decreasing our threshold of insulin, inflammation, and glutamate. The cup is getting smaller and the headache triggers are still pouring in. A skinny man can eat his excess of omega-6 fats, MSG, and biogenic amines to create virtually the same headache result of an obese woman's insulin problems combined with her fluctuating hormone levels. It's as shocking as learning of a slim 40-year-old who unexpectedly suffers a heart attack from the hidden buildup of heavy foods.

Many doctors and patients still believe that if skinny patients have migraines, it can't be an obesity problem. What about the obese migraineur who loses weight but not the migraines? Some people even develop migraines for the first time after they lose the obesity title. This type of thinking doesn't acknowledge that there is a migraine threshold that's affected by multiple factors. Excessive fat is now one of those factors.

Hey, that doesn't explain why males have no increased risk of migraines from an increase in obesity problems. The researchers agree and mention that further research is needed to determine the link between obesity and migraines in men. The smaller occurrence of migraines in men and the outside factors that have not been studied deliver no real answer. This doesn't leave men off the hook from eating a healthy diet; it just means we know obesity is a problem and don't yet have answers for the male migraineur.

Let's Talk About Poop

The human body contains 10 times more bacteria cells than human cells.[87] There are more than 3,000 species living within you, and nowhere is that more apparent than in your gut.[88]

Doctors recently used a fecal matter transplant to treat a slim, 33-year-old woman with a chronically inflamed gut. They took the stool from a "healthy" woman and put it in the colon of the sick woman, and poof—her gut was repaired by these healthy bacteria.

The "healthy" woman was obese, and 16 months later, the slim woman who received her transplant was also obese. Coincidence? The woman who was cured of the gut infection and who had never been obese, was put on a medically supervised liquid diet and exercise program. Exercising and removing food should work for anyone, yet she became obese.[89] Her case report may lead to the exclusion of obese individuals for fecal transplant donations.

Is it possible that obesity could result from bacteria in the gut?

That theory has been well supported by animal studies where the transfer of gut bacteria from obese mice to slim mice results in weight gain. Anthony Bourdain strengthened his distaste for vegetarians in *Kitchen Confidential* by referencing a study that showed vegetarians had species growing in their guts that the average carnivore didn't. The general public thinks bacteria is disgusting. The general public and Anthony Bourdain are wrong.

A recent study found that the "gut community in lean humans was like a rain forest brimming with many species but that the community in obese people was less diverse, more like a nutrient-overloaded pond where relatively few species dominate." The lean individuals had more bacteria that break down nutrients. So if you want to be fat and unhealthy, stay away from a variety of vegetables and nutrients that create a diverse and healthy gut with "disgusting bacteria."

Researchers took this theory a step further: They took the rainforest-like bacteria of lean individuals and the less diverse species from obese guts and put them up the rear ends of mice. As expected, mice that received the obese bacteria gained weight, while mice that received the lean bacteria had guts that created an efficient energy-producing cycle similar to that of a rainforest, and they remained lean.[90]

The gut is now being referred to by some as "the second brain." Some gut bacteria can convert glutamate into GABA, which inhibits excitotoxicity, meaning an obese individual may be stuck with excessive amounts of migraine-triggering glutamate, while a slim individual may convert the glutamate into migraine-preventing GABA. Of course, anyone with migraines and a damaged gut will be at risk of lacking these healthy bacteria that produce the right neurotransmitters in the right portions. This is just one of the many studies that have determined that the gut produces thought- and emotion-carrying neurotransmitters.[91]

Will a Probiotic Drink Help Heal the Gut?

Adding a probiotic drink into this equation would be the equivalent of introducing thousands of Tasmanian devils to the Bahamas. Would they kill all of the native species? No one knows. Would they be dead on arrival? We don't know that either. The FDA does not properly regulate probiotics, so you don't know whether they're dead or not. And you don't know if that probiotic of one species will help your gut or end up creating an overloaded pond with few species.

Fun fact: Splenda was found to decrease good fecal bacteria, negatively changing the gut's pH levels, which is known to limit the bioavailability of orally administered drugs. This means that, if you use Splenda, the drugs you paid for won't have the same kick, nor will the nutrients you ingest, leaving you hungry for more.[92]

How Do You Take Care of Your Gut?

Nearly everything you'll learn by reading this book is about taking care of your gut, because when it comes to healing headaches, it seems to be the last place many sufferers look as the source of their pain—and it is most likely the biggest source of their pain. But in general, to take care of your gut, there are a few simple, overarching guidelines:

- Stay away from inflammatory foods and processed foods.

- Avoid taking antibiotics unless you absolutely have to, because they will kill everything in the gut's biome, including the Tasmanian devils.

- Eat natural, whole foods as often as possible. Many natural foods are prebiotics—foods that feed good bacteria—and produce butyrate,[93] which is a natural immune system builder. Butyrate also improves insulin sensitivity and increases energy.[94]

- Try *hara hachi bu*.

Headache Triggers

The Heavy-Hitting Headache Triggers

All of the headache triggers listed here have the ability to break your headache threshold. Those listed in this chapter are some of the biggest heavy hitters—more migraineurs have trouble with these foods and additives than any others.

What's important to remember as you read on is that it's all about balance. The heaviest migraine triggers are from a combination of biogenic amines and amino acids. Single ingredients rarely break the headache threshold in isolation. Spinach becomes even more confusing because it is listed as a food high in histamine, higher than nearly all other fruits and vegetables. Histamine is one of those biogenic amines that specifically add up to break the migraine threshold. So why isn't spinach a huge migraine trigger?

The reason is because the headache threshold is about balance. There are fibers and numerous nutrients in spinach, such as magnesium, that will lower the ability of the biogenic amines to raise glutamate and inflammation in the brain. This is similar to how the glutamate found in fruit is not going to trigger a headache like the excessive concentration of glutamate in MSG: We're not comparing apples and oranges here. Fruits and vegetables will take care of whatever they produce in your body—MSG won't.

This doesn't mean that you can't have an allergic reaction to spinach that will break your headache threshold. It hasn't been proven in any studies, and there certainly aren't a lot of people claiming spinach is a headache trigger, but it is possible. We need to look at foods as a whole.

The Heavy-Hitting Headache Triggers

Luckily for us, the headache threshold is like a cup and is based on multiple ingredients that can raise the contents of that cup or lower them. We want to turn that cup into a giant jug so your headache triggers never reach the top and spill over. To do this, we need to know exactly how the cup is manipulated, so what you read in this part of the book will help you understand all of the headache triggers, those that are chronic and those that are not, more effectively. Then, you can use the Headache Help Checklist to guide you through your own elimination process to find out, specifically, what shrinks *your* threshold or overcomes it.

Heavy Hitting Trigger #1: Foods that Inflame

Eliminate the foods that inflame from your diet and you have a 100% chance of reducing your headaches. When you see the chronic headache triggers in the next chapter, you'll see one thing they all have in common: The top headache triggers are all common allergens. This section will link all of the headache triggers together. And once you understand the trigger, you'll be able to take your finger off it.

All of the top 10 food triggers from the 1979 study were common allergens that, when removed, created a 100% success rate. The allergens most likely to cause an inflammatory response are also most likely to give you a splitting headache. In fact, one study found that people with allergic rhinitis, "allergies," are four times as likely to have migraines.[95] So migraines, then, are an inflammation problem, right? Does that seem far-fetched? Aren't there too many headache triggers for the answer to be that simple? What about MSG?

MSG studies do, in fact, show an acute (fast) inflammation response. More recent studies show that MSG is responsible for chronic inflammation that leads to a variety of diseases. This isn't a maybe; this is confirmed in 100% of MSG-treated mice.[96] MSG is allergenic, but all the food triggers are possible allergens. For unknown reasons, a select few migraine sufferers have the headache triggers of bananas, avocados, and latex. A quick Google search will let you know they all contain similar allergen proteins. If your body doesn't like latex, it probably won't like bananas or avocados.

We have an inflammatory link between all food triggers that doesn't explain the link between headaches and many other diseases. What about diabetes, rheumatoid arthritis, depression, heart diseases, stroke, and Alzheimer's? All of these diseases have been linked to migraines, and all of them have one common denominator: inflammation.

Within the last 10 years, obesity has been added to this list.[97] Obese individuals show higher expressions of a whole list of proinflammatory proteins. An increase in these inflammation-causing proteins may lead to insulin resistance and the promotion of atherosclerotic buildup in blood vessels. It's all linked together. This is all bad for your pipes.

The inflammation from diabetes, rheumatoid arthritis, and migraines will even inflame the median nerve in the wrist. Do your hands ever feel numb, tingly, or just weak? Migraine sufferers are 2.7 times more likely to have carpal tunnel syndrome.[98] Multiple sclerosis (MS) is an inflammatory disease of unknown cause that uses the immune system to attack the nerves in the brain and spinal cord. Migraine prevalence is threefold higher in those with MS.[99] So why is all of this inflammation happening in the first place?

Inflammation: The Reason You Shouldn't Play "Waspball"

"Help! Help! It's in my ear!" the man yelled while trying to shake his swollen ear open with one hand and holding a crack pipe with the other. We walked straight past him to his friend on the ground who was lying there after a game of "waspball" with a hornet's nest. He was going to die from multiple wasp stings. We didn't have time to deal with the live wasp in the other man's ear—we had to try to reduce this man's severe inflammation.

Inflammation is very complex, but the overall picture is easy to understand. Let's take the example of a wasp flying around and landing on your arm. The wasp stings you and your immune system immediately kicks in. Your mast cells release histamine to rapidly inflame the broken skin. You already know what histamine is. Anytime you have cold, symptoms like a stuffy or runny nose, histamine is responsible, and you might take an antihistamine to get through the day. Foods high in histamine can also be migraine triggers—more on that later.

In the case of the wasp sting, histamine does more than just cause swelling, redness, itching, and annoying pain. The inflammation spreads to the capillaries lining your blood vessels. These capillaries are like bricks, and when they puff up, they allow certain cells to go through and attack invaders. The attacking cells are known as antibodies, or immunoglobulin E, and they attack and destroy the wasp venom. That's it. In a perfect world, the venom is attacked and your problem goes away.

Unfortunately, the world is not all perfect, and everyone has his or her own immune system response to foreign substances. Remember the 1991 film *My Girl* in which Macaulay Culkin steps on a hornet's nest? This classic family movie took a dark turn when Macaulay's character was overcome by hornets and died from a severe allergic reaction. Not a happy moment in a movie you watch with your kids. It drives the point home, however, because wasps live close to most American homes and can be deadly for many of the Americans in those homes, including those smoking crack while playing waspball. As firefighters, we take allergic reactions of any kind very seriously.

A severe allergic reaction can start in one place, such as where a person was stung by a wasp, and spread throughout the skin, respiratory tract, stomach, heart, and brain. Your immune system is not independent. One of our primary concerns on a medical emergency like this is making sure the patient has a good airway. That annoying histamine, no matter where you were stung, can rapidly inflame your throat and entire respiratory tract. This is exactly what happened to that man who was lying on the ground about to die.

These were the times that I felt very lucky to be on a fire engine that provided advanced life support, because we could push drugs. Benadryl is an anti-inflammatory drug we carried, and for extremely severe reactions, we used the more powerful vasoconstrictor epinephrine (adrenaline) to fight the inflammatory response. And yes, it just so happens that Benadryl is often part of a migraineur's personal over-the-counter "cocktail" of preferred headache drugs.

But don't get excited about adrenaline as a headache treatment. It's not. A shot of adrenalin is over the top as a headache reliever. It makes sleep difficult because it basically turns you into the Hulk, so instead of resting off your headache, you instead feel the need to throw cars into the air. Adrenalin stimulates the flight-or-fight response. This is what we administered to the waspball player with a constricting airway, and it probably saved his life. It gave us just enough time to put an endotracheal tube in his throat before it became swollen shut. But if you're not about to die, you want Benadryl, the safe, over-the-counter anti-inflammatory that will help you sleep and reduces headaches.

Inflammation: Also the Reason to Avoid Food Allergens

How does that man's wasp-related inflammation relate to foods? It's exactly the same thing. Think peanut allergy. A number of foods can cause a severe allergic reaction, including milk, eggs, peanuts, tree nuts, seafood, shellfish, soy, and wheat.[100] Hmmm. If any of these top food allergens sound familiar, that's because many of them are also headache triggers.

There's a lot that can happen between getting an upset stomach from something you ate and dying. And you may have a food allergy that causes no upset stomach at all, which is what makes figuring all of this out so difficult to begin with. Ninety-seven percent of people with celiac disease don't know what's wrong with them, and many do not have noticeable stomach symptoms. Celiac disease may ultimately damage the lining of your intestinal tract, but make no mistake: It's an autoimmune disease.

Celiac is just one type of gluten sensitivity. Your immune system also has a problem with gluten, because your body sees it as an invader and wants to kill it. This causes an inflammatory response, and because your pipes are all connected, it can make your entire body feel like crap. And as it turns out, your brain doesn't like this any more than the rest of your body.

Inflammation and Migraines

This is a great inflammation theory, but inflammation doesn't explain why glutamate is a problem—or maybe it does. We know from the largest migraine study of genome sequences that there's a link between migraines and the regulation of glutamate. We know that "monosodium glutamate" can terrorize this regulation and build up an excess of glutamate, which is toxic to our brains. Yes, toxic. Don't forget about the mice that couldn't regulate glutamate—they all died from seizures. We know that the answer has something to do with glutamate from the hundreds of migraine-related glutamate studies. So how on earth can we say migraines are an inflammation problem?

Well, thank goodness for our pill-popping country. The drug companies that make medication to treat depression are hard at work on this problem and have been for some time. I originally looked for this answer in the underfunded area of migraine research. Silly me. There are dozens of studies on depression that I believe answer the migraine question.

Inflammatory cytokines are the answer. Cytokines are just "markers" that identify, in this case, inflammation in the brain. If you have an inflammatory cytokine in the brain, it's just like a check mark that states, "Yep, there's inflammation here." Multiple studies have found that people with depression have more inflammatory cytokines.[101]

Researchers look into glutamate when they're studying depression because excess glutamate can cause overexcitement in the glutamate receptors and lead to clinical depression (and a whole list of other problems). The more inflammatory cytokines you have, the more glutamate you have. Those inflammatory cytokines interfere with astrocytes, which clean up the glutamate stuck in the synaptic space.

It's back to the theory that your brain is like a highway and there are little packages of glutamate all over the highway. If nothing picks those glutamate packages up, they are going to wreak havoc on your brain. You can't just jam up a highway in your brain. You get angry when you have to sit in traffic. But your brain? Your brain has a full meltdown from glutamate traffic.[102]

Michigan State University researchers evaluated the glutamate levels and inflammatory responses in 100 suicidal patients. Those with the strongest desire to kill themselves (two-thirds actually tried) had the highest levels of glutamate. The patients who were no longer suicidal returned to normal levels of inflammation and glutamate within six months.[103]

Depression is more prevalent in migraine sufferers, but here's where it gets interesting. In 2011, a small study was published on 64 newly diagnosed migraine sufferers.[104] The results were no different than those for depression, obesity, diabetes, cardiovascular disease, and dementia. Migraine patients had significantly higher levels of inflammatory markers and lower levels of anti-inflammatory markers. If the same theory holds true, just as it has in dozens of non-migraine-related studies, these migraine patients will also have high levels of glutamate. Now in order to find this answer, you would need to geek out hard and run a search for "serum cytokine and pro-brain natriuretic peptide (BNP) levels in patients with migraine." Then get your medical dictionary out, and don't forget your biology books. Or skip all the research and simply know this: The bottom line is that inflammation is a major factor in a migraine.

I believe inflammation is the answer. Things our bodies don't like cause inflammation. As you read on, you will find that *every* headache trigger is associated with inflammation, not just the food triggers. Inflammation raises glutamate traffic in our brains. Excess glutamate is toxic and causes the worst headaches. It's that simple, and we're about to uncover how perfect this theory is with every headache trigger backing up the "new" inflammation theory.[105]

Foods that Cause Inflammation

Let's take it back to foods that cause inflammation in the first place. When I eat an excessive amount of dried mangos, it hurts me. How do I know this? I love them. I can eat an entire bag of dried mangos in one sitting. But then, just 12 hours or so after eating them, my neck starts to break out in hives, and I get a stomachache. It's not as bad as it sounds. It's just a little redness, and my throat feels a little swollen.

Now you may be like most of my friends and say, "Why would you do that?" I'll give you the same response I give them: "I love mangos." I've learned the hard way that the green mango is not my friend. My reaction to green mangos is much worse than my reaction to orange mangos. The hives are terrible, and I don't get just a puffy throat, but also shortness of breath. However, I don't get a stomachache when I eat green mangos.

When I was a kid, I never had a problem with mangos. As an adult, I don't eat green mangos, and I will no longer eat an entire bag of dried mangos. But I do, occasionally, fall off of my mango wagon. While on vacation recently, I ate a couple of slices of Chile Spiced Mangos from Trader Joe's. Because I was on vacation, I was eating and drinking whatever I felt like, and those spiced mangos are delicious. Two days later, I had a headache with sinus pressure. It wasn't painful, but it lasted for three straight days. According to the last decade of research, "over 90% of self-diagnosed and doctor-diagnosed sinus headaches meet the criteria for migraine."[106] The sinus headache may account for the largest misdiagnosis and mistreatment of migraines, such as the harmful use of senseless antibiotics. My problem was not a sinus infection; it was most likely the inflammation caused from the food I ate—the food I know hurts me.

So how should I have treated that headache? Benadryl (an antihistamine) or aspirin (an anti-inflammatory) would have been just the thing to take care of this food-inflammation problem. In fact, studies show that 1000 mg of aspirin, when taken in a timely manner, is just as effective as the strongest and most expensive migraine medications.[107] It's a handy tip, but really—I knew what the mangos would do to me, so the better fix for the headache would have been not to eat what I knew would cause it.

Poison Oak, Mangos, and Fire

It was a nice, sunny day in the San Francisco Bay when we got the call to respond to a wildland fire on the top of San Bruno Mountain, the mountain that separates San Francisco from, well, the rest of the world. It was one of my first calls as a professional firefighter, but I knew this mountain very well since I grew up in a part of San Francisco shaded by it. The fire was making a downhill run toward some houses, one of which happened to be owned by a good friend of mine.

This was a dirty burn, meaning there was a lot of brush that didn't fully burn. We made a downhill attack on the fire, hoping to reach the homes in time. We crawled through mounds of half-burnt poison oak as we laid hose. I wasn't worried; I'd crawled in poison oak as a kid and never had a reaction. Plus, my buddy's house was about to catch on fire. We ended up hooking the head of the fire, and we were home by nightfall. My friend's house was still standing, and the fire was out. When we got back to the firehouse, several of the guys immediately broke out the Tecnu.

I said, "What's Tecnu?"

One firefighter responded, "You better use it if you are even slightly allergic to poison oak." Tecnu, I learned, removes the oil from poison oak.

I said, "I don't get poison oak."

What do you think happened? Two days later, I had poison oak everywhere, and I do mean *everywhere*. The red, itchy, pulsating, throbbing, can't-sleep-at-night feeling lasted for three weeks. The firefighter who told me to use the Tecnu ended up in the hospital. Brushing up against poison oak is one thing; rolling around in its smoke and ash is a different story.

What changed in my immune system? The intense exposure gave my body a chance to identify urushiol, the oil found in poison oak, ivy, and sumac, as bad stuff. Since the poison oak fire, I have developed antibodies that are now on the hunt for this urushiol. When they find it, they can tell my immune system to send more troops for a full immune-system attack.

At the time, I thought, "Hey, what doesn't kill you only makes you stronger." That's not always the case. Now I can't even touch something that has been exposed to poison oak. Those antibodies remember that urushiol, and here is the kicker: Urushiol is found in the skin of mangos. While eating the juicy fruit inside should be OK, exposure to the mango skin can be just as painful as poison oak. Dried mangos may be processed with this oil. The green mango, my enemy, carries the most urushiol.

This story exemplifies the problem of inflammation from start to finish. It took two days for the poison oak to really affect me. Two days was the average time it took for a food trigger to cause a migraine in the 1983 study. The Chile mangos from my three-day headache, also a two-day reaction time, were accompanied by a lot of other headache triggers.

The best way to *get* a headache is to combine multiple inflammatory foods to break that headache threshold. It took three weeks for me to get rid of the most severe poison oak exposure. Removing migraine triggers is likely to eliminate migraines within a few days, but toxins may remain for up to three weeks. The 1979 study showed most patients were headache-free after two to three days of eliminating triggers. It shouldn't come as a surprise that it's possible to be headache-free in the same amount of time it takes most food triggers to set off a migraine.

It's not a venom problem, a poison oak problem, or a mango problem. This is an immune system problem. Your body is saying, "No," and inflammation accompanies that "No." Are mangos a top headache trigger? No, they are my individual headache trigger. Some headache triggers, like allergies, are individualized.

I did other bad things while on vacation as well. I had a Labor Day party. I drank beer and ate mangos and pizza—my weakness. That delicious pizza wasn't a temptation until a couple of beers became involved. I didn't exercise, and I didn't eat the things that reduce inflammation, such as vegetables.

So was it the pizza, the mangos, or the beer that broke my threshold?

It was all of them. However, it is important to realize that my severe headache wouldn't have happened without the pizza and beer. While true allergies can produce headaches and horrible symptoms, they're usually a small part of a big headache threshold. Inflammation is an accumulation, just as the headache threshold is an accumulation. The chapter in this book on chronic headache triggers will show you how reducing those heavy triggers will make a personal trigger, like mangos, a very small problem.

But wait. Is there a pill that fixes the entire problem?

Well, there is one. It's called ketamine, and it's a horse tranquilizer. This drug goes straight to the problem and mops up the glutamate before it builds up and causes an inflammatory response, which is exactly what we need to prevent a migraine.

Also, it instantly (and temporarily) ceases depression. You won't even remember why you were depressed. It puts you in such a dreamlike state, you may not remember anything at all. But, here's the thing: Ketamine, aside from being sold as a horse tranquilizer, is sold on the black market as a date-rape drug. Don't try this one at home, kids.

Besides, you can't just splash a bucket of drugs in the brain and expect everything to be OK. Mop up glutamate? What's wrong with us? Glutamate is our primary neurotransmitter. It's how we think. It's who we are. Cleaning it up is not an option. Mopping up glutamate creates problems.

This is exactly what drug companies are working on, but it's not in my personal plan to use it. Even the anti-inflammatory pills that people take every day are controversial. High levels of inflammation may hurt the body, but inflammation is also how the body fights off infections. It's not a good idea to start thinking, "My body's natural response to fight off infection is annoying, so I'm going to suppress this entire process." Maybe your body is fighting for a reason. Small amounts of inflammation can even be healthy, but building up chronic levels of inflammation can be deadly.

Heavy-Hitting Trigger #2: MSG

Search online for "MSG rat" and you'll find some images of rats before and after they ingested MSG. They became obese—morbidly obese. Seriously, these rats are fat. No strain of rats is naturally obese. In order to create obese rats, scientists feed them MSG or inject them with it. These animals are referred to as "MSG-treated rats." You can find hundreds of studies on PubMed that use MSG-treated rats to study obesity and a number of diseases.[108] MSG increases insulin levels, which regulates the absorption of sugar (glucose) by the body's cells.[109]

Glucose that your cells do not use turns into fat. So eating foods with MSG increases your fat and lowers the level of glucose in your blood stream. Your brain won't be happy about this and may punish you with a headache. Your brain needs glucose to survive. That is, unless you know how to burn ketones by following a ketogenic diet

In one of many studies, MSG-obese rats developed insulin resistance.[110] This is exactly what it sounds like: The cells resist insulin, so the pancreas produces more. This produces more glucose in the blood stream than your cells are able to use. High blood sugar, or hyperglycemia, is toxic to your body. If untreated, this will turn into type 2 diabetes, which is no surprise to researchers. MSG-treated rats will develop type 2 diabetes in about 60 weeks.[111]

Insulin resistance symptoms may include the following: "brain fogginess" and an inability to focus, bloating, sleepiness, increased blood pressure, depression, atherosclerosis (hardening of the arteries), weight gain, and difficulty losing weight.[112] This is all bad. If your blood vessels are hard, how do you think this will affect your ability to control blood flow to your brain? Even worse, this leaves people helpless in the weight control battle. One study of more than 750 Chinese men showed that users of MSG were nearly three times as likely to be obese.[113]

You already know that obesity will drastically increase the likelihood of many conditions, including migraines. But the effects of MSG on a headache are much more prompt than they are with those other conditions. Most large medical resources list MSG itself as a top migraine trigger. Other resources will use words like "preservatives" or "additives" instead of "MSG." MSG is one of the most common "preservatives" listed under the category of "food additives,"[114] although MSG is better categorized as a flavor enhancer.

Not only does MSG trick your brain into thinking food tastes better, MSG causes leptin resistance. When you eat too much food, the leptin hormone lets your hypothalamus know you're full so it's time to start burning fat. When you eat MSG, the hypothalamus doesn't receive the leptin hormone message and you remain hungry.[115] So, when you're eating food with MSG, you're eating foods that make you hungry. This is great for companies that want to sell you more food, which explains why up to 80% of all flavored foods contain MSG.

Leptin resistance may also play a significant role in many chronic illnesses, such as heart disease, obesity, diabetes, osteoporosis, autoimmune diseases, reproductive disorders, and it may increase the rate of aging as well. Each ailment listed is triggered by the high levels of hormones that come from eating the stuff Americans most commonly eat: sugar, refined grains, and processed foods that contain MSG.[116]

The FDA has received many reports of adverse reactions to MSG, including headaches, facial pressure, numbness, heart palpitations, nausea, and general weakness. For this reason, the FDA requires MSG to be on the label of all food products that contain it. Many researchers label MSG as an excitotoxin that damages your brain cells. However, researchers have not found definitive evidence on that, and MSG is "generally recognized as safe," according to the FDA.[117]

So MSG is safe, "generally," but is that enough? Isn't that just a better way of saying "It *looks* safe—mostly—but not all of us agree"? What's behind that rhetoric? No matter what the *true* meaning is there, it's important to remember that simply because something is "safe to eat" doesn't mean it's healthy. MSG is *not* healthy.

Researchers feed rats pellets of MSG to study obesity. And food companies feed it to us in so many things. You'll find these magical fat sprinkles in flavored potato and corn chips, in fast food, salad dressing—the list goes on and on. Some people working to lose their excess weight go on low-calorie diets, but if their diets still contain MSG, it's as if they're tossing their healthy green salads with lard for dressing.

When I was a firefighter, we often responded to nonemergency calls called public assists. A common public assist firefighters face is for fall victims who can't lift their body weight. The victims are usually embarrassed and apologetic about the situation. It's very sad to see people in a condition that they don't know how to change. Cutting MSG would make a huge difference to anyone struggling with weight loss.

Those "Natural Flavors"

There is the argument that glutamate is naturally occurring in protein found in meat and vegetables. MSG was originally developed from seaweed and, later, from vegetables like corn and soy, which are common migraine triggers. Keep that in mind as you make connections between migraine triggers. Today, MSG is produced by a fermentation process and will contain unwanted byproducts or impurities. Most manufacturers do not fully disclose the process and may use genetic modification and chemicals. MSG also contains sodium and L-glutamic acid, but unprocessed protein does not.[118]

So MSG is not naturally occurring, but even if it were, MSG gives the body an unnatural amount of glutamate. Glucose is also naturally occurring in the human body. You wouldn't say that just because sugar is found in nature that it's perfectly healthy to eat as much as you can. That doesn't make any sense. Cocaine is derived from the natural coca leaf, but isolated in large quantities, it becomes a different story, a *Scarface* story.

It's the same with MSG. The protein becomes isolated from its normal chemical structure and is also referred to as "free glutamic acid." The process allows your body to take in enormous—and unhealthy—amounts of glutamic acid. Glutamic acid interacts with biogenic amines, like those found in Parmesan cheese and Parma ham. When glutamic acid is "free," it is free to wreak havoc. At the end of the day, MSG is derived from natural ingredients, though what it does to your body is not natural. And top medical authorities list MSG as a major migraine trigger, so let's avoid it.

A Magical Fat Sprinkle by Any Other Name...

Let's talk more about MSG on food labels. The FDA only requires MSG to appear on the label if it fits the exact definition in the Food Chemicals Codex. Any variation containing MSG is required to be identified by names other than "monosodium glutamate." Crazy, right? During the Vietnam War, 58,286 US soldiers died. People poured gasoline on themselves and lit it on fire to protest this war. Last year, 400,000 Americans died from obesity, which MSG directly influences. And so far, I don't see any big rallies against it. A product can have multiple forms of MSG in it that add up to toxic levels, and it does not need MSG on the label. In fact, a product like that is not allowed to have MSG on the label. Nor is the food company required to tell you that anything that contains free glutamic acid will give you the same reaction as MSG—no matter what they call it. So read the lists below so you'll know what you're looking for when you're checking food labels.

Ingredients that contain processed free glutamic acid:

- Glutamic acid (E620)
- Glutamate (E620)
- Monosodium glutamate (E621)
- Monopotassium glutamate (E622)
- Calcium glutamate (E623)
- Monoammonium glutamate (E624)
- Magnesium glutamate (E625)
- Natrium glutamate
- Anything "hydrolyzed"
- Calcium caseinate, sodium caseinate
- Yeast extract, torula yeast, yeast food, yeast nutrient, autolyzed yeast

The Heavy-Hitting Headache Triggers

- Gelatin
- Ajinomoto products
- Textured protein
- Whey protein, whey protein concentrate, whey protein isolate
- Soy protein, soy protein concentrate, soy protein isolate
- Anything "protein fortified"
- Soy sauce
- Soy sauce extract
- Protease
- Anything "enzyme modified"
- Anything containing enzymes
- Anything fermented
- Vetsin
- Umami

Ingredients that *often* contain free glutamic acid:

- Carrageenan (E407)
- Bouillon and broth
- Stock
- Maltodextrin
- Citric acid, citrate (E330)
- Anything ultra-pasteurized
- Barley malt
- Pectin (E440)
- Malt extract
- Anything listed as "flavors," "flavoring," or "seasonings" (You sneaky food people!)

Foods and additives that may cause an **MSG** reaction in some people:

- Cornstarch
- Corn syrup
- Modified food starch
- Lipolyzed butter fat
- Dextrose
- Rice syrup
- Brown rice syrup
- Milk powder
- Reduced-fat milk (skim, 1%, 2%)
- Most low-fat or no-fat foods
- Anything enriched
- Anything vitamin enriched
- Anything pasteurized
- Annatto
- Vinegar
- Balsamic vinegar
- Certain amino acid chelates (Citrate, aspartate, and glutamate are used as chelating agents with mineral supplements.)[119]

As you can see, we're all screwed. MSG is in nearly everything processed. In order to avoid it, you need to limit your intake of processed foods. That's right—*limit* your intake of those foods. You don't have to become maniacal about avoiding them or swear that you'll never eat any of them ever again. The key here is awareness and consumption control.

I used to cook and eat at my firehouse; it's a second home for firefighters, and cooking was a large part of what brought us together. A lot of teamwork can develop from cooking. We used food that contained MSG all the time, so eating it was hard to avoid, especially if I was not the one cooking the main dish. I often made large salads and side dishes for that very reason. Then I would fill up on the healthy stuff so I didn't want to eat as much of the unhealthy stuff. It's actually that simple.

Hidden Evils: Food Additives in General

The 2010 study with 266 tested antigens found food additives to be a top immune system trigger—listed above the combined groups of 26 vegetables, 37 fruits, and 19 milk products. With respect to headache trigger strength, this labels food preservatives and additives as comparable to the foods they are combined with. Trying to eliminate single food triggers while continuing to eat processed foods is a great plan—if you enjoy paddling up river. Why would you attempt to eliminate one fruit while eating preservatives that cause more problems than all 37 fruits combined?

The 1983 study had a single food preservative (benzoic acid) as the sixth top migraine trigger. There are a number of aspartame and MSG headache studies and complaints, but we know very little about headaches from our combined food preservatives. Pick up any box or can in your pantry and read the ingredients. What kinds of additives does it have? Do you see words such as "maize," "soy," "wheat," "sorbic acid," "pectin," "tartrazine," and "glutamate" or words you can't pronounce?

Do you know what all of these do in combination? No, no one does! Tartrazine was the ninth migraine trigger in the 1983 study. Tartrazine, also known as yellow dye number 5, is a common dye for foods that want a little more yellow or green swank. Harvard Medical School also lists yellow dye number 6 as a well-documented trigger—found in Mountain Dew, Doritos, Peeps, and a million other foods.[120]

Food additives are very powerful in small amounts. It's easy to pick up a bag of Doritos and think that eating just a few chips won't cause a headache. A handful of chips has just a few pinches of food additives, after all. Look how small and light they are. How bad could these delicious chips be? What if I gave you just a tiny little pill and said that I don't know what's in it, but it will give you immediate gratification? There's not a lot of difference between that handful of chips and the tiny little pill. Many food additives are drugs made by drug companies. We eat these drugs in combination and don't even ask what they are, and these food additives and preservatives are among the most powerful headache triggers. There are multiple food additives linked to brain damage, cancers, obesity, and more.[121] So start getting serious about reading the labels on the food you buy. The fewer ingredients you see there, the better, and no doubt about it, the more ingredients that are identifiable as actual food, the better. And remember—you can't believe everything you read there.

Heavy-Hitting Trigger #3: Gluten, Glutamate, Glutamine, and MSG

The largest connection to headaches is here, and it's extremely complex, like open-up-that-chemistry-book complex and keep-a-medical-dictionary-handy complex. But don't fret; I've broken down the confusion to make a headache's worse culprits easy to understand.

What's Gluten?

Gluten is a protein found in wheat, barley, rye, and thousands of processed foods. Gluten is about 25% glutamic acid (glutamate) by weight.[122] Products with gluten typically contain high levels of glutamic acid. For example, a 100-gram serving of sourdough bread has 3,287 mg of glutamic acid, and that's a lot (yes, sourdough is a top migraine trigger). To give you an idea of what this means, a peach has 31 mg of glutamic acid. Carrots or lettuce have 100 mg of glutamic acid.

The food with the highest concentration of glutamic acid is wheat gluten (in powdered form) with 29,000 mg (yeah, that's 29 g).[123] An old study published in the *Journal of Neuropathology & Experimental Neurology* found that infant monkeys fed 1 mg doses of MSG developed brain lesions proportionate to the amount of glutamate ingested.[124] You are no baby monkey, but this is a huge concern because migraine sufferers have an increased risk of brain lesions proportionate to their attack frequency and years of suffering, according to a study published in 2010 by the International Headache Society.[125]

So don't go eating gluten powder. That's not a joke. Protein supplements often contain enormously high amounts of glutamic acid. The whey protein Body Fortress proudly shows 6,208 mg of glutamic acid for its recommended serving of a protein shake.[126]

How Does MSG Relate to Gluten?

Monosodium glutamate is the fermented sodium salt of glutamic acid and contains a small number of impurities.[127] The impurities are due to the fermentation process, which always produces unwanted byproducts. Yes, that's the same fermentation used to make beer, but we'll get to that later. The glutamic acid found in naturally occurring protein does not contain sodium or impurities.

MSG is a free glutamic acid, meaning that it is freed of other amino acids. In nature, glutamic acid is usually bound to long chains of amino acids. No big deal. What harm could a little chemistry do? Let's go ahead with the notion that our friends in the multibillion-dollar food industry are right and MSG is just an abundance of natural glutamate. That would make this headache problem easy. MSG is a migraine trigger; therefore, glutamate in large quantities is the "cause" of migraines. If only it were that simple. It's not.

MSG makes food taste good. It's not exactly sweet, sour, bitter, or salty. It's umami, the other of our five basic tastes. I'm not making this up. I've never said something tastes "umami," but apparently this "brothy" or "meaty" taste is responsible for the mouthwatering craving that people get from foods like bacon. Here in Santa Cruz, California, we have chocolate covered bacon, bacon ice cream, and other weird bacon-fetish foods. Bacon being pumped with MSG may be the reason that some people have an uncontrollable "love" for bacon. It may be why Shaneka Monique

Torres shot up a McDonald's in 2015 after they forgot the bacon on her bacon cheeseburger—twice.[128] True story. People love bacon.

What's Glutamate?

Glutamate is essentially glutamic acid. The suffix "-ate" means that it's an acid that's lost a hydrogen atom. Glutamic acid is usually found in the body without that hydrogen atom and is thus called glutamate. There is so little difference between glutamate and glutamic acid that you will find the terms used interchangeably in medical writing and in this book. "Free" glutamic acid in high concentrations has the same effects on gluten-sensitive people as MSG.

Glutamate is generally acknowledged as the most important neurotransmitter for normal brain function. It's responsible for sending signals between nerve cells and, under normal conditions, plays an important role in learning and memory. Glutamate makes it possible for you to read this sentence. However, in high concentrations, glutamate results in overexcitation of nerve cells, which eventually leads to cell death.

Look up the "excitotoxicity theory" for more on the toxic effects of glutamate. It can destroy your brain.[129] Glutamate can also be used by the body as fuel, just like burning any amino acids for cellular energy, which may explain why working out is so effective at raising the migraine threshold; working out burns glutamate and supports healthy blood flow for getting rid of toxins.

What's Glutamine?

If glutamate were the devil on one of your shoulders, glutamine would be the angel on the other. Glutamine and glutamate are both amino acids of the "glutamate family." They are both found abundantly in plants and animals. However, they play very different roles. One of the places that the body converts glutamate into glutamine is in the cells lining the intestinal tract (the villi). Glutamine is then used for a number of things, including protecting the lining of the intestinal tract (villi) and removing body waste (ammonia), and we need it for normal brain function.[130]

Glutamine protects the villi, the very thing that makes glutamine. With damaged villi, you may have an excess of glutamate (not good) and not enough glutamine for normal brain function (very bad). Glutamine rapidly removes ammonia in the liver before it builds up to toxic amounts.

The body then excretes the large amounts of ammonia by way of urination. Yeah, you pee it out. But, your brain doesn't operate this effectively and cannot excrete large amounts of ammonia. Excess ammonia in your brain causes progressive drowsiness, seizures, brain injury, intellectual impairment, and cerebral edema, and it can even be fatal.[131]

A rise in brain ammonia will also increase glutamate accumulation and lower the main glutamate transporter in the brain. Those transporters are responsible for removing excess glutamate in the synaptic gap.[132] This all goes back to the theory that an excess of glutamate between neurons will cause a migraine.

Remember the truck and cargo box analogy? Well, here it is again. Those cargo boxes (glutamate) are accumulating on the road because of the increased ammonia and have no trucks (glutamate transporters) to take them out of your synaptic gap. Ammonia helps the glutamate build up a traffic jam. Glutamine gets rid of ammonia before that happens. Glutamine is good. Ammonia is bad.

The Heavy-Hitting Headache Triggers

So why not just take glutamine supplements to reduce ammonia, thereby reducing glutamate levels? You're pretty quick if you already thought about that. Pro athletes do this for muscle repair. Glutamine has even been used to treat AIDS, liver damage from alcoholism, and a number of other diseases. But neurological disorders are trickier than that.

Your body can create glutamate from glutamine and vice versa. It's called the glutamate-glutamine cycle. Studies show intricate rises and falls of glutamate and glutamine in interaction with ammonia.[133] Taking glutamine supplements may actually raise your glutamate levels. This complex symphony of glutamate/glutamine conversion may be why there is no consensus on glutamate and migraines in the medical community.

There are too many factors that influence glutamate and glutamine. The focus should be on creating a natural conversion of glutamine in the villi. Remember what celiac disease is? When people with celiac disease eat gluten, their immune systems form antibodies that attack the intestinal tract and damage the villi. It's like taking care of a problem in your gut with a grenade.

Nutrients will no longer be properly absorbed, no matter how much you eat. Celiac disease leads to a deficiency in calcium, iron, magnesium, vitamin D, vitamin B9, and vitamin B12.[134] All of these vitamins and nutrients prevent migraines. In some cases, people are "cured" of migraines from taking these vitamins and nutrients alone. However, vitamins are a Band-Aid solution to the problem. If you stop hurting yourself, you won't need the Band-Aid. Take care of those villi. A happy gut means more glutamine, less ammonia, and less glutamate, and that adds up to no headaches.

We know that free glutamic acid (MSG) is a migraine trigger. Thus, all migraine triggers are probably high in glutamic acid, right? Nope, not really. The chart below shows several possible migraine triggers and the amounts of glutamic acid each contains.[135]

Food	Glutamic Acid (mg)	Portion
Anchovies	4,312	100 g
Bacon	5,642	100 g
Beans, garbanzo	866	100 g
Beans, lima	3,038	100 g
Beer	47	100 g
Bologna	2,296	100 g
Cheese, Cheddar	6,092	100 g
Cheese, Parmesan	8,208	100 g
Cheese, Mozzarella	4,458	100 g
Chicken broth	285	100 g
Chocolate	586	100 g
Corn	636	100 g
Eggs	1,676	100 g
Figs	72	100 g
Ham	1,934	100 g
Milk, whole	1,581	8 oz.
Milk, reduced fat	1,901	8 oz.
Nuts	4,506	100 g
Overripe avocado	287	100 g
Overripe bananas	152	100 g
Oranges	94	100 g

The Heavy-Hitting Headache Triggers

Papayas	33	100 g
Pasta	4,022	100 g
Pickles	177	100 g
Pizza (cheese)	3,536	100 g
Pork loin	3,231	100 g
Sauerkraut	209	100 g
Snow peas	4,196	100 g
Sourdough	3,287	100 g
Soy sauce	2,411	100 g
Soybeans (seeds)	7,875	100 g
Wheat	5,016	100 g
Yeast	5,651	100 g

So, you see, not all of these possible headache triggers are high in glutamic acid. Does this prove the glutamate theory is false? No. "Free glutamic acid" is a known migraine trigger. The glutamic acid in the foods listed in the chart above may include free glutamic acid. There are many triggers to migraines. It's not the amount of glutamic acid in your food, but how your body (or the food industry) processes this glutamic acid. However, reducing this trigger will most likely raise your threshold to a point where other triggers do not affect you. Let's break all of this down with the help of that 1983 study. Remember, this study was 93% effective at reducing or eliminating migraines.

1983 Study Findings

Finding #1: Milk

Milk from cows provoked adverse symptoms (that often included migraines) in 27 patients. In fact, in this study, milk was the largest migraine trigger. You won't find studies like this backed by the food industry. All migraine-provoking foods from the study were processed into powdered form. Milk has 1,581 mg of glutamic acid, while reduced-fat milk contains 1,901 mg of glutamic acid. Reduced-fat milk is made from powdered milk. This process only adds a few hundred milligrams of glutamic acid, but much of the glutamic acid is converted to free glutamic acid. And by now, I probably don't have to tell you—that's bad. Milk powder, reduced-fat milk, and "pasteurized" and "enriched" products are triggers for people highly sensitive to MSG or glutamic acid. Get off the milk; get rid of the headaches.

Finding #2: Eggs

Eggs provoked adverse symptoms in 24 patients. Eggs? Isn't that nature's perfect food with an abundance of good stuff? "Abundance" is the key word. The glutamic acid in 2 eggs amounts to 1,676 mg, but it's made for a baby chicken to absorb fast and easy. Are you a baby chicken? No, you are not a baby chicken. Easily absorbing glutamic acid may not be a good thing. Stop eating baby chicken food!

Finding #3: Chocolate

No one likes hearing bad things about chocolate but it came in third, provoking adverse symptoms in 22 patients in this study.

Chocolate only has 586 mg of glutamate. Online resources don't mention that most studies suggest milk chocolate is the culprit, not pure chocolate. The free glutamic acid from chocolate milk powder can be quickly absorbed due to high levels of sugar and the stimulant caffeine. Chocolate is one of the most widely known migraine triggers. It is also a myth. Before this cognitive dissonance starts giving you a headache, put this information on hold until you get to the chapter dedicated to chocolate. It truly does have a strange effect on headache sufferers.

Finding #4: Wheat

Wheat caused 21 patient reactions. Wheat has 5,016 mg of processed glutamic acid. Wheat protein is high in free glutamic acid. Wheat products in general are high in free glutamic acid because they are processed. For the patients in this study, wheat was introduced in small amounts in powdered form. Though it came in fourth here, it takes the gold medal for the worst headache trigger in other studies.

Notable takeaways from the 1983 study were that preservatives "appear to be an important cause of migraine," and "processing a food may affect its ability to provoke symptoms."[136] Some patients reacted to bacon, but not other types of pork. Stop what you are doing right now, go to YouTube, and search "how bacon is made." Watch as giant needles come down and repeatedly inject the bacon with "flavoring," better known as MSG.

If you're one of those people who love bacon like it's a drug, your love makes sense—it is, in fact, loaded with a drug. Labeling bacon as "pork" doesn't mean much to migraine sufferers. Pumping bacon up with MSG puts this meat in a dangerous category. Thankfully, high-quality non-MSG bacon does exist.

Chicken broth only has 285 mg of glutamic acid per 100 g. That's nothing. However, if you look at the glutamic acid per calorie, chicken broth has 14,250 mg per 200 calories.[137] This puts chicken broth in the number one spot for foods highest in glutamic acid. And I'm referring to chicken broth from a box or can, not the chicken broth from real homemade chicken soup.

It's no surprise that chicken broth is a top migraine trigger, even though you would never consume 200 calories of chicken broth. That's over 22 cups. This trigger is powerful in small doses because, per calorie, it is potent. Little amounts of food triggers can affect us in a big way when they are processed in high concentration. Top Ramen is on the list of the top 10 worst things to eat for a reason. Remember, it's processed, so it's full of free glutamic acid.

Your body won't process the glutamic acid in vegetables and meat as fast as it will with already-processed foods, such as pizza or chicken broth. Take that meat and tenderize it or inject it with crap and you will get more of a reaction, just like with corn that's dumped into a can with MSG. The more processed the food, the more likely it is to give you a headache. It's not the glutamic acid; it's the buildup of glutamate in our bodies. Free glutamic acid begins to work immediately on our taste buds and causes neurological changes that increase our appetites in just 30 minutes.[138]

This speed and rate of ingestion will put your threshold into hyperdrive. One study showed that a threshold of 2.5 g of free glutamic acid can cause adverse reactions, including headaches.[139] I could make a great counter argument about how there are no definitive studies stating health risks to MSG. But there is no argument to the fact that MSG and free glutamic acid are contributing to American obesity, which costs the country $147 billion annually.[140] That's just the medical costs. Add in the fat pants, workout gimmicks, and extra food consumption, and you have one heavy price tag.

While obesity does affect headaches, the real detriment of free glutamic acid is when it's combined with other headache triggers. In other words, free glutamic acid fills up the headache threshold and makes all other headache triggers more dangerous.

Heavy Hitting Trigger #4: GMOs

In a 2014 Washington State University and New Castle University meta-study of 343 peer-reviewed studies, it was found that organic crops had 18–69% more antioxidants than conventional crops.[141] You didn't need a study to tell you that the overgrown vegetables that taste like cardboard have fewer nutrients. For this reason alone, I recommend eating organic crops that have more of the nutrients that prevent headaches and migraines.

There's also a risk from ingesting poison that is designed to kill insects by obliterating their stomachs. A peer-reviewed study actually found that pigs fed genetically modified (GM) corn and soy had higher rates of severe stomach inflammation compared to 125 non-GM-fed pigs.[142] Corn and soy are top genetically modified foods and also happen to be top migraine triggers. This added risk of inflammation could jeopardize a migraineur's ability to process both food triggers and nutrients, creating a genetically modified migraine.

But GMOs may cause more than debilitating headaches. According to Dr. Don Huber, an expert in the toxicity of genetically modified foods, genetically modified plants are developed by Monsanto to withstand the poison glyphosate. You probably have used glyphosate to kill weeds under its marketed name of Roundup. Dr. Huber explains that glyphosate becomes systemic in the plants: You can't wash it off. Not only does this result in lower levels of nutrients, the intent to kill living organisms also breaks down enzymes in the plant that help with digestion. This means that the human body may have a hard time digesting the already low levels of nutrients.[143]

Nutrient deficiencies are a major health concern—and, frankly, so is poison. Glyphosate may be safe in small amounts, but we don't know what will happen when GMO foods like corn and soy are concentrated into powder and then mixed in processed food with numerous other headache triggers.

GMOs and Tumors

A 2012 French study published in the journal *Food and Chemical Toxicology* found that mice fed Roundup-tolerant GMO corn had much higher mortality and tumor rates.[144] Tumors in males were up to four times more likely in GMO-fed rats, and they were massive, accounting for 25% of the rat's body weight. Most studies that deem GMOs safe have lasted less than 90 days. The French study found appalling side effects during a study that lasted two years. This was the longest running study on the health effects of GMOs.

Dr. Huber points out that studies like this are rare because GMOs have patents to prevent researchers from studying them. Shortly after the study was published, the prestigious peer-reviewed journal was bullied into retracting the study for allegations of fraud. After review, the journal found no evidence of fraud and stated that the study was retracted for having a small sample size of Sprague-Dawley rats.[145]

The study used a small number of Sprague-Dawley rats to be consistent with the 90-day tests submitted to gain regulatory authorization of GMOs.[146] Sprague-Dawley rats are used in countless studies because they are about as prone to developing tumors as humans living in industrialized countries.[147] Essentially, the critics are saying that the sample size is enough to prove GMOs are safe, but not enough to prove that they are dangerous.[148]

How Did We Turn into Guinea Pigs?

We've been eating genetically modified food long before anyone started making a stink about it—maybe long before you knew anything about it at all. But get this: Corporations are able to give huge sums of money to politicians in the form of campaign financing—some countries refer to this as bribery. Companies use campaign financing to influence government. Section 735 of the bill HR 933, also known as the "Monsanto Protection Act," was written with representatives from Monsanto and essentially stripped the federal government's rights to roadblock the sale or cultivation of genetically modified foods, despite future health and environmental concerns.[149][150][151] You know, concerns like giant tumors in rats.

We should be concerned, because around 90% of our soybeans, corn, canola, cottonseed oil, and sugar beets are genetically engineered. The Oscar-nominated documentary *Food, Inc.* explains exactly how Monsanto was able to patent "life" in the form of corn seeds and held the rights to widely distributed GMO corn. Farmers can still grow organic corn, but it's only a matter of time before cross-pollination happens and the GMO makes its way into the local farmer's field.

According to the film, Monsanto has a team of 75 employees dedicated to investigating and prosecuting farmers for patent infringement. This model has made a few companies very successful in controlling the market share—successful enough to have the funds to influence government policies.

What our guinea pig future holds, based on a few recent studies:

- In a Russian study, all first-generation GMO-fed hamsters emerged A-OK from eating GMO foods. Second-generation

GMO-fed hamsters had an infant mortality rate that was fivefold higher, and they had a slower growth rate. If the second-generation babies die, doesn't that mean that something was wrong with the first-generation GMO hamsters? Nearly all of the third-generation GMO-fed hamsters became sterile, and some had the rare phenomenon of hair growing inside their mouths. Russia has banned many GMOs.[152]

- A European study reviewed 19 GMO studies that indicated kidney and liver problems but noted that the 90-day tests were insufficient to evaluate chronic toxicity. There are no minimal lengths for testing GMOs, and this is "socially unacceptable in terms of consumer health protection."[153] This is huge. Don't read past this accumulation of 19 harmful studies without thinking about the harmful possibilities in your grocery aisle.

- In a government-sponsored study in Italy, mice that were fed Monsanto's Bt (Bacillus thuringiensis, a pesticide) corn showed a number of immune system responses that are consistent with a damaged gut, including elevated IgE and IgG antibodies, increased inflammation markers, and elevated T cells. We already know that corn and soy are inflammatory. The added inflammation from BT toxins could prove to be harmful for autoimmune conditions, such as gluten sensitivity and migraines.[154]

A number of studies report that risk assessment for GM food has not been standardized. There are no guidelines for testing the safety of GM foods. As a result, no studies have successfully proven that GMOs are safe.[155]

How do you like them apples? GMOs are designed to destroy the stomachs of insects and have not been thoroughly tested for the safety of humans. We're the first generation of guinea pigs, and we'll soon find out if GMOs are safe.

Want to Learn More?

- www.mercola.com – For Dr. Huber's interview, along with over 30 other negative GMO studies
- www.gmoseralini.org, "Ten things you need to know about the Séralini study"– A well-referenced article that could end your doubts about the safety of GMOs
- "Robyn O'Brien at TEDxAustin 2011," YouTube– Describes the GMO threat to Robyn's family and to the nation

Heavy Hitting Trigger #5: OJ, the Killer

Oranges are good for you. No, they're great for you. They're packed with vitamin C and nutrients. We've been told our whole lives that oranges keep us healthy, and they do. So why am I calling orange juice a murderer? Because, unfortunately, oranges are one of the most common migraine triggers. Oranges are on just about every migraine trigger list. The 1983 study had oranges tied for fourth place on its top trigger list. The 1979 study had oranges at number two, with 65% of patients reacting.

As far as fruit consumption is concerned, oranges are consumed in the largest quantity. But many people are sensitive to citrus, including lemons, limes, and grapefruit. A little squeeze of lime, a lemon wedge in your drink, or a once-in-a-blue-moon grapefruit for breakfast is probably not going to burst your headache threshold. But when you take a pile of oranges that you are sensitive to or even hypersensitive (allergic) to and concentrate all of them into one little cup, that's a dangerously potent little cup.

Orange juice that's commercially squeezed with the rind contains synephrine, a vasoconstrictor. Does synephrine sound like something familiar? Remember ephedrine, the weight-loss stimulant taken off the market for heavy side effects? Ephedrine is chemically similar to synephrine, and both can cause a whole list of inflammatory side effects.

Anything that plays with the size of your blood vessels may cause a headache. In this case, synephrine makes your pipes smaller, increases blood pressure, and may increase other biogenic amine levels.[156] Blood pressure medications are often given to migraine sufferers to prevent this type of added stress.

Orange juice is acidic and can cause an upset stomach in the same way coffee can. Think about when your stomach hurts. Do you feel like drinking orange juice? No. Acidic juice can be a large problem for those who already have stomach inflammation, which can also be stress induced. If your stomach is upset, there's inflammation present.

Alka-Seltzer feels good when you have a tummy ache. The aspirin in it helps to control the inflammation, and the sodium bicarbonate (baking soda) neutralizes the acidic foods that are giving your belly a rumble. Your body makes sodium bicarbonate naturally, so why then does it feel good to get more of that baking soda?

When you eat a whole orange, your body uses sodium bicarbonate to slowly neutralize the acidity as it breaks down the minerals, vitamins, and fiber. What would happen if your body didn't neutralize the acid? Human blood has a pH of around 7.4,[157] and it needs to stay that way. If your blood were to lower to a pH of 6.9, you would likely fall into a coma and not wake up.[158]

Oranges have a pH of around 3 and lemons have a pH of around 2, while battery acid is at a pH of zero. A pH of 7 is neutral. On the alkaline end of the spectrum is baking soda with a pH of 8.3, ammonia with a pH of 11, and the drain cleaner sodium hydroxide with a pH of 14. You might be thinking, like I did when I first learned this, that lemons and oranges are acidic enough to kill you. It doesn't work like that.

The pH of a lemon or orange has almost nothing to do with the pH of your blood. "The human body has an amazing ability to maintain a steady pH in the blood,"[159] according to an article in the *Journal of Environmental and Public Health*. In fact, most acidic fruits are considered "alkaline foods" because the stomach neutralizes them and uses their high levels of mineral content. Minerals or electrolytes, such as sodium bicarbonate, are used to stabilize the pH level of the blood and keep your cells hydrated.

This brings us to the tummy ache. Drinking a blender full of orange juice is going to tax your ability to produce sodium bicarbonate. Your intestines will freak out and say, "Are you crazy? I can't let that much acidity enter the bloodstream! I'm going to produce a belly ache of inflammation to slow things down." An inflamed stomach has a hard time processing the proper levels of minerals and amino acids, so the sodium bicarbonate you now desperately need can't effectively enter your bloodstream.

So why not just help the stomach out and drink some baking soda? The stomach is acidic, just like our skin. The body does this to kill outside germs. You wouldn't go swimming in a bacteria-infested pond when you have open cuts, would you? Well, that's what we do. We say, "I don't like this acidic digestion process that kills diseases and makes nutrients available. I'll just dump some baking soda down there to fix the issue."[160]

You want a stomach that naturally regulates acid. A stomach that is inflamed may let proteins into the blood that would have normally been filtered out. This is a leading theory regarding why people with high stress levels tend to have more allergic reactions—and that gets really interesting when we look into allergies and migraine sufferers.[161]

Recent studies question if citrus-triggered migraines are caused by an allergic reaction. We eat the citrus fruit, and our body reacts with an inflammatory response. Your face might not puff up, but your blood vessels will.[162] Who knows if this is from an actual allergic reaction or the fact that your stomach pH balance is off and you can't properly regulate nutrients. This problem may go away completely when your stress levels go down and you eliminate other problematic foods that stress the stomach.

If you have "outdoor allergies," specifically if you have a grass allergy, you should avoid oranges altogether. People who don't like grass pollen often don't like the proteins in oranges, which basically means that oranges bring on headache season.[163]

Let's say you're not sensitive to oranges. This is pretty much impossible to know for sure due to the lack of accuracy of allergy tests. And if you have a "low" sensitivity to oranges, you'll never know it from a simple blood test. Headache triggers can take two to three days to have an impact, and oranges can be part of that headache threshold for up to three weeks. But for fun, let's just say you know that oranges are not a trigger for you. Oranges will still bombard your brain.

Let's take it back to any neurological medical emergency firefighters respond to. If your head hurts, we want to know why. What's your blood sugar looking like? Is it low? We actually carry an orange drink in our drug box for this very reason. Diabetics with low blood sugar know all too well that orange juice is their friend.

Diabetics who are hyperglycemic (have high blood sugar) know that orange juice can make them feel terrible. Orange juice works very well at raising blood sugar. Our brains need sugar for survival, but too much sugar is not good.

Studies show that fructose, the fancy Latin name for fruit sugar, is a large accomplice for the worldwide increase in obesity. It's not funny that one of the very things responsible for diabetes is the same thing keeping many diabetics alive. Technically, it's the sucrose (table sugar) in orange juice that rapidly increases blood sugar, but it

The Heavy-Hitting Headache Triggers

comes with the impact of fructose. Fructose has a low impact on blood sugar, but it rapidly produces body fat—especially around the belly. Rodents fed high-fructose diets develop insulin resistance, obesity, diabetes, and high blood pressure.[164] Later, you'll read about how fructose and sucrose can make us fat yet have little to negative impact on weight gain when paired with certain foods.

Some orange juices have 50 g of sugar per 16 ounces. That's about the same as a Coke. For some people, that's enough sugar to cause an inflamed stomach. This is on top of the acidic nature of both soda and orange juice. It's not surprising that the risk of gout (itchy red inflammation) goes up considerably with both OJ and soda.[165]

A 22-year study of women and gout was completed in 2010. One orange juice a day was associated with a 41% increased risk of gout! Two OJs per day brought that increased risk up to 242%, surpassing the 239% increased risk of two sodas per day! Commercially squeezed OJ that's stripped of the oranges' natural fiber and nutrients does not resemble oranges anymore.

Have you ever wondered why every glass of store-bought OJ tastes exactly the same? It's science. Many nutrients and nearly all the flavors are destroyed when the OJ is removed from oxygen so that it can be stored for long periods of time in giant vats required for the millions of gallons of weekly American consumption. To get flavor back in, an artificial process is used to add in an orange's oils and essence; however, the ingredients are technically from an orange, so they're "all natural" and won't be on the label.

What's the end result of drinking too much of this so-called natural fruit juice? A 2008 study that followed 71,346 female nurses for 18 years found that green, leafy vegetables and whole fruits were associated with the lowest potential to cause diabetes, while fruit juice was associated with an 18% higher potential of causing diabetes.[166] This is to say nothing of how bad it is for a migraine.

This brings us all the way back to acidic blood, or acidosis. While oranges have very little effect, if any at all, on the pH of the blood, diabetes can. The inability to properly burn sugar may release ketones (acetone) in the blood. This is perfectly healthy for most people, but it becomes toxic if your body has a sugar-related insulin shortage. The medical term is "diabetic ketoacidosis" (DKA), and it can make your blood acidic while your breath begins to smell of nail-polish remover or "acetone."

This is a condition that can result in coma or death. A problem that most police officers don't understand is that high blood sugar and the fruity smell of "acetone" breath can mimic alcohol intoxication. It can even trick the breathalyzer, leaving a diabetic emergency to go unnoticed in the back of a cop car.

Can acidosis negatively impact your health? Yes. Acidity is a well-known factor associated with cancer, and sugary drinks are found to have a large impact, while fruits and vegetables have a negative association with cancer.[167] In 2013, for the first time in history, a large study found that dietary acid load was positively associated with the risk of type 2 diabetes. This was after adjusting for the high-risk foods that cause diabetes.[168] Processed foods have few nutrients, minerals, and vitamins. According to the study's author, "Even lemons and oranges actually reduce dietary acid load once the body has processed them."

The body can't regulate pH without minerals. Processed OJ may deplete minerals required to prevent migraines. The researchers recommend natural foods and state, "Most importantly from a blood-sugar control perspective, increasing acidosis can reduce the ability of insulin to bind at appropriate receptors in the body, and reduce insulin sensitivity." This is fantastic. It means that eating more fruits and vegetables (with all the terrible foods we will inevitably eat) can lower our risk of diabetes and weight gain. In this case, eating more may actually help us lose weight.

Oranges have over 170 phytonutrients. Well, that's before the OJ kills the phytonutrients because of their bitter taste. Phytonutrients are yet another reason to limit processed foods.[169] Phytonutrients not only reduce cancer risks, they also are one of the extremely rare substances that fight cancer. Many phytonutrients are anti-inflammatory, antitumor, anti–blood clotting, and powerful antioxidants. Because of these phytonutrients, oranges, not orange juice, sound like the perfect antimigraine drug, but only in moderation and only after an elimination period to ensure you are not allergic. OJ, on the other hand, is too much and should be locked away.

The Chronic Headache Triggers

Chronic headache triggers are those foods that give you chronic inflammation. These are foods that may not give you an immediate headache, but they will chronically lower your threshold over time to a level that makes it incredibly easy to break. Eliminating the chronic headache triggers will make you feel better—and happier!

Each of these chronic triggers is a heavy hitter on its own. Together, these triggers make a combination that is more likely than not to give you an unshakable headache. They slowly fill your headache cup to dangerous levels.

Remember: The headache threshold is like an individual cup that each of us fills at our own pace. I don't drink soda, so soda is more likely to fill my cup a lot faster than a daily Big Gulp drinker. But over time, that Big Gulp drinker will have a cup that's consistently full. The headache triggers are all relevant to how much and how often we consume them.

You may have other chronic headache triggers as well—things that aren't listed in this book. And those triggers will do exactly the same thing as one of these big headache triggers. And they can be anything—*anything*—that makes you feel bad: teas, cigarettes, perfumes, oranges, dried fruit, nuts, fermented foods and drinks, chronic pain (e.g., neck injury), weather, pollen, and just about anything that may affect you on a personal level. I have dried mangos on my list. You may have bananas, avocados, shellfish, or who knows what else.

The great part is that eliminating the big triggers will make those little triggers irrelevant for most people. Life is about moderation. It's also important to avoid overdosing on the things that are good for us. Olive oil is a great anti-inflammatory that will likely raise your headache threshold, but consumed in large quantities, olive oil is quickly stored as fat. When your body stores too much fat, it starts an inflammatory response that will cause chronic inflammation. Moderation is the key.

Likewise, eating fish several times a week may be a great way to lower inflammation, but consuming too much fish may present a problem from the rising levels of mercury in our polluted waters—not to mention radioactive spills. Many people are OK with small amounts of shellfish, but they run into trouble when they consume large amounts.

It doesn't matter if you consume a lot of one trigger or small amounts of multiple triggers. Pizza is the best example of this equation. Pizza is listed as a major headache trigger on most medical resources, but that doesn't narrow much down for us. These websites added pizza as a headache trigger and gave no information on why it's such a major headache trigger.

You can't be allergic to pizza. That's like saying I'm allergic to sandwiches or burritos. It's the combination of headache triggers in pizza that make it such a whale of a headache trigger. Many people do not have a reaction to the individual ingredients. They can eat bread, tomatoes, and cheese without a problem. This is why medical resources get confused and simply list pizza as the headache culprit without a good explanation of the problem. But we can't help ourselves if we don't know what the problem is.

Pizza may contain the following: aged cheese, bread, tomato sauce, herbs, processed meats, and maybe a sprinkle of delicious MSG. These are *all* headache triggers. Even the tomato sauce may seem innocent, but it's preserved, processed, removed of fiber, and loaded with amino acids and processed glutamate. All of these ingredients on their own may not be a problem, but together they represent a top headache trigger.

Remember, the most successful studies completely eliminate multiple foods that are likely to cause migraines. However, they reintroduce certain foods after health is restored. Obviously, some foods, such as milk or wheat, may become strikingly intolerable after a successful elimination, and that's great. Foods that present immediate problems clear the confusion. With other foods, you may be able to moderate, so having a sundae only on Sundays may be fine according to your personal headache threshold. Lowering your number of chronic triggers expands your threshold so eating the foods you love (that is, eating the headache triggers you love) in moderation becomes less of a headache risk.

Chronic Trigger #1: Cooking Oils

Sunflower, soybean, corn, sesame, cottonseed, grapeseed, and other cooking oils are omega-6 heavy hitters. We need omega-6, but not in large quantities. Cooking oil is up to 70% pro-inflammatory omega-6 fatty acid and may contain no anti-inflammatory omega-3 fatty acids. Can you say gut bomb? Walnuts, almonds, cashews, and peanuts contain high natural amounts of omega-6 but are accompanied by the anti-inflammatory omega-3. A good balance makes obesity and inflammation less likely. Cooking oil is pure inflammation.

Alternative: Olive Oil

Olive oil breaks the rules a little bit. It has a high ratio of omega-6 to omega-3: about nine parts omega-6 to one part omega-3.[170] This doesn't make sense because anybody who is anybody will tell you to replace your cooking oil with olive oil. And those people are right. While some vegetable oils are 70% omega-6, olive oil is only around 9% omega-6. That's way less omega-6, despite the ratio.

We need omega-6, just not in super large quantities. Olive oil's nine to one ratio of omega-6 to omega-3 is looking pretty good in comparison to something with 70% omega-6 and no omega-3. While you probably don't want too much of any oil, olive oil has shown benefits when paired with the Mediterranean diet.

Recently, a study followed 7,000 people for nearly five years and found that participants on a Mediterranean diet benefited from the addition of olive oil or nuts with significantly fewer cardiovascular events.[171] The control group was allowed to use olive oil or vegetable oil with a balanced low-fat diet with the recommended portions of processed carbs. They didn't fare as well. Olive oil is healthy when balanced with foods like vegetables, fruits, seafood, white meats, nuts, and legumes.

What to Look Out For

You probably already know that virgin olive oil is better than regular olive oil. But you may not know that there are extra virgin olive oils that have as little as 3% omega-6 and others that go beyond 20%.[172] The olive oil companies aren't lying to you—they don't have to tell you if the olive oil has a great omega-6 to omega-3 ratio or not. You must make sure you're buying high-quality olive oil.

In 2010, the University of Davis called bull on 69% of the imported olive oils in the United States.[173] The high majority of extra virgin olive oils failed to meet the minimum international standard because of poor quality and oxidation issues—which will equate to inflammation. Many contained oils that were not olive oil. They were fake. However, none of the Australian and Californian samples failed, and a very low rate of premium Italian brands failed.

Remember: The food industry is designed to make money, not to make you healthy. Given that, read the ingredients before you buy your food and look for whole foods. Look for 100% olive oil.

Alternative: Coconut Oil

Coconut oil is only 2% omega-6 fat. It doesn't contain omega-3, so you will need to combine it with some omega-3 from other foods to offset its very small amount of omega-6.

Alternative: Grass-Fed Butter

Grass-fed butter has an incredible omega-3 to omega-6 ratio of one to one.[174] Grass-fed butter has a very small amount of milk protein and most people, even those with milk problems, have no trouble digesting it. All the milk protein can easily be strained out with a cheesecloth, or you can purchase already-strained butter, which is called ghee or "clarified butter."

Chronic Trigger #2: Trans Fats

At least one type of trans fats won't be a problem here in the United States for long, because the FDA has just labeled partially hydrogenated oils unsafe and has implemented a ban of use in food starting June 18, 2018.[175] The decision may prevent millions of deaths and lower our risk of headaches and migraines. Until then, however, we all need to monitor our intake of these bad, bad fats.

Trans fats are anything with the words "hydrogenated" or "partially hydrogenated" on the label. The words "trans fat" *will not* be on a package label until a product contains over 0.49 g per serving. The American Heart Association recommends that you limit your daily intake of trans fat to less than 1% of your total calories. That's only 2 g! Let's see—if I eat a whole bag of chips (16 servings) with "0 trans fats," I may have just eaten over 7 g of trans fat.

Here is the worst part: Small amounts of trans fats occur naturally in meats and dairy products that the American Heart Association says "you probably eat every day." They go on to say that "this leaves virtually no room at all for industrially manufactured trans fats."[176]

How bad can trans fat be? One study shows that a 2% increase in trans fat is associated with a 23% increase in cardiovascular disease. That's some powerful fat. Two percent of daily consumption is roughly 4 g of trans fat or half a bag of FDA-regulated chips with "0 trans fats."[177] If you're not able to eat half a bag of chips in a day, you could also go for a baked apple pie from McDonald's with 4 g of trans fat or Burger King hash browns, also with 4 g of trans fat.[178] These are old measures of trans fats; even the fast food industry is limiting this deadly product. Ten years ago, I could have easily eaten four or five of those hash browns, amounting to 20 g of trans fat. If I did that every day, I would increase my risk of cardiovascular disease to 115%.

Denmark is already on board. They practically made trans fat illegal by restricting any ingredients that are "hydrogenated" or "partially hydrogenated," meaning natural foods may contain small amounts of trans fat, but companies can't add it in. Not even a little 0.49 g that no one needs to know about. That lowered Denmark's average daily intake from 6 g of trans fat to less than 1 gram per day. Some hypothesize that this is responsible for a 50% decrease in national deaths in Denmark from ischemic heart disease.[179] Denmark has less than a third of the United States' obesity rate.[180]

Trans fats make you fat—really fat. A six-year study on monkeys showed a 7.2% weight gain for monkeys fed trans fats versus a 1.8% weight gain for those fed monounsaturated fats. Trans fat also disproportionately increased abdominal fat, and the monkeys eating trans fat showed evidence of insulin resistance.[181]

This means increased inflammation and a multitude of problems, including headaches and migraines. Trans fats are poison, and when you start reading food labels, you are going to be shocked at the number of products with the word "hydrogenated" in the ingredients. You may even be compelled to give up coffee creamer, ice cream, pancakes, popcorn, cookies, canned chili, fries, and just about everything that comes in a package. The trans fats from these foods will increase the same inflammatory markers responsible for heart attacks and headaches alike.

Chronic Trigger #3: Sugar

We all know that processed sugar makes you fat, but did you know it makes you age? Advanced glycation end products (AGEs) are complex groups of compounds formed when sugar reacts with amino acids. The acronym fits well because AGEs cause inflammation, which leads to disease, aging, and eventually death. AGEs link sugar to cardiovascular disease, Alzheimer's, and diabetes. Studies show that reducing AGEs in animals may lead to an increased lifespan and lower inflammation markers.[182]

Sugar molecules can be dangerous. One of the most common medical emergencies for responding firefighters is a hypoglycemic (low blood sugar) emergency. What's the fix to low blood sugar? We put sugar straight into the bloodstream. Here is where it gets tricky. Sugar in the bloodstream may be safe, but pour one of those Pixy Stix straight onto muscle and it will die. Sugar is much more powerful than we give it credit for. If a patient has an internal brain bleed, the sugar administered for hypoglycemia could be deadly. This is especially difficult to know because someone with low blood sugar is often in an altered state and can't tell you if they bumped their head.

If you want to move to rural Tanzania, you won't eat much refined sugar, and you won't have many migraines. Sugar is a pro-inflammatory with a "mild inflammatory" rating of -14. High-fructose corn syrup, which is found in soda, is insanely inflammatory with a "strongly inflammatory" rating of -1,022.[183] The average American diet is composed of over 10% fructose, which, sadly, amounts to 54.7 g of fructose per day. A very small amount of this fructose is from natural fruit. We Americans get our fructose predominantly from processed foods that contain high-fructose corn syrup.[184]

Why is fructose the bad sugar? Fructose is processed almost completely by the liver, unlike glucose. Glucose can be quickly absorbed by all of the cells and stimulates insulin, unlike fructose. That's not exactly a plus for glucose, but at least with the insulin spike comes the leptin—the hormone that tells your brain that your belly is full. Fructose does not stimulate leptin.[185] Have you ever wondered how you could drink a 64-ounce Big Gulp in one sitting? Your brain on fructose has one speed: *Go*. The leptin stop sign will not turn on with fructose. A 64-ounce Big Gulp has 170 g of predominantly high-fructose corn syrup with 620 calories.

Warren Buffet will twist the idea that high-fructose corn syrup is bad. Buffet drinks five cans of Coke per day. Sure, he owns 9% of Coca-Cola, and he's no specimen of health, but that's impressive.[186] There is also a 104-year-old woman who drinks three cans of Dr. Pepper every day and has outlived the doctors who said Dr. Pepper would kill her. These examples do not represent the big picture. Everyone is different. There are multiple factors of health, and you could be the outlier that survives this bad stuff.[187]

A Big Gulp could amount to a lot of pure fat, probably in your midsection. Although these numbers are not completely accurate, it's said that consuming 3,500 calories amounts to 1 pound of fat. Based on the math, drinking one 64-ounce Big Gulp per day would lead to 64 pounds of fat per year. You're probably not going to gain 64 pounds, but it gives you an idea of how easy it is to go overboard in sugar calories. A childhood-obesity study showed that just one 12-ounce soda per day will increase the risk of obesity by 60%.[188] I remember going to the vending machine every day in high school for a 20-ounce soda. Come to think of it, just a couple of years ago I went to our firehouse soda machine every day.

New studies are coming out every year that show soda is worse than we thought it was the previous year. Don't forget about the in-depth, 22-year study of more than 80,000 women that showed a can of soda a day gives you a 75% higher risk for gout.[189] Gout is a clear sign of inflammation—technically an itchy red sign—and may be a warning sign that your headache threshold is ready to overflow.

The fact that fructose is terrible doesn't change the fact that all sugar can be harmful. The average American eats 2.5 pounds of sugar every week. When we eat this much sugar, our bodies develop lots of AGEs. This kicks up your immune system so it says, "There are too many AGEs! I don't want to get old, so release the RAGEs!" Those receptors of AGEs, known as RAGEs, cause raging inflammation and scar tissue known as plaque. Put two and two together here and you have a recipe for heart attacks—and for headaches.[190]

Have you seen a child eat too much candy and turn into a little monster? The sugar rush puts a kid's little body into a warp-speed roller coaster ride of emotions. For every up there is a down. After the "high" wears off, a child may become exhausted, cranky, and tired. Adults can have the same roller coaster ride ending in fatigue, the inability to concentrate, and a headache. These short-terms effects are minimal compared to the chronic inflammation that accompanies excessive sugar intake. Sugar is one of the most underestimated headache triggers.

Chronic Trigger #4: Refined Grains

An abundance of refined grains come from wheat. People have had wheat allergies at least since the Roman times when slaves handling flour were required to wear masks for what is now called baker's asthma, one of the leading causes of occupational asthma. Baker's asthma (a chronic inflammatory disorder) has been brought to light due to recent cases that may have been developed from the new innovations in cereal allergens that are now added while baking, specifically wheat Tri a25.[191]

Interestingly, the problem may start before we add anything to dough. A wide range of new wheat proteins have been developed through hybridization and have been shown to react with our immune systems. These new plants are referred to as "modern wheat" and represent the high majority of wheat fields. Some are skeptical that overconsumption of wheat has led to the increase in wheat-allergy reports, while others think that people are lying—or wrong—about having a wheat allergy. Some researchers state that an increased awareness is responsible for the growing number of wheat allergies. It doesn't matter what we theorize; wheat is recognized as one of the top eight allergens, which together account for 90% of allergic-inflammatory responses.[192]

There are a variety of allergic responses from multiple wheat proteins and enzymes. Over a hundred years ago, breeders began to make wheat "dwarfs" that not only produced higher yields, but also were stronger against climate changes. They were disease resistant as well. Breeding has resulted in thousands of different "wheat dwarf" varieties, and these numbers are growing due to the recent use of synthetic wheat for their disease-resistant properties.[193]

How do these stronger dwarfs inflame our population? A 2010 study set out to find that answer by evaluating 36 modern wheat strains with 50 kinds that were grown over a century ago.[194] The results were simple. The protein in modern wheat contained more Glia-a9. Glia-a9 is associated with the inflammatory disorder celiac disease, which causes diarrhea, bowel pain, headaches, growth retardation, osteoporosis, infertility, lymphoma, etc. The immune system of a person with gluten sensitivity may identify Glia-a9 (among other proteins) as an invader and then attack it with a long list of post-inflammatory problems. A ripping headache is just one casualty of this biological war.

In war, you never want to hear that the enemy is increasing in numbers. Between 1839 and 2009, wheat output increased 26-fold in the United States.[195] Wheat cereal was the world's second-most produced cereal in 2009, surpassing rice cereal.[196] How has this really affected the United States? Let's look into something you really can't fake: death. During the last 50 years, the prevalence of undiagnosed celiac disease has increased dramatically and was associated with a nearly fourfold increase in death.[197] Unfortunately, wheat gluten is increasingly applied as an additive to the growing market of processed foods, and most people don't balk at this because at some point we learned to identify wheat as healthy.

It's unlikely that improved detection and early recognition are responsible for this increase in celiac disease. Finland doubled its celiac disease rate in just the last two decades, which "definitely could not be ascribed to improved detection only."[198] We know that the "Western diet" is spreading like a disease and creating a worldwide health problem. Glia-a9 is associated with gluten sensitivity, and wheat now has more Glia-a9. Common sense tells us that this is a problem and that we are increasing our consumption of this problem, but the hard facts are still not clear.

Let's look at figuring out the problem for just one person. Many celiac tests simply are not accurate. One study showed that antibody tests taken from stool show a "specificity" of 58%, meaning that the test may misdiagnose 42% of healthy people.[199] You may as well flip a coin at that point. Blood tests can be up to 90% accurate if you *do* have celiac disease. However, that means that one in 10 healthy people are wrongly diagnosed with a disease they *do not* have.[200]

The flaw with all of the tests is that you must be eating gluten in order for the test to work. If you don't eat the inflammatory food, you won't produce the antibodies that attack them. If the antibodies are not attacking, the test won't show damage to your villi.

You don't go from completely healthy to immediately having a destroyed intestinal tract that can no longer process foods. Between these two things, there are varying levels of gluten sensitivity that are not accurately diagnosed. About 40–50% of gluten-sensitive patients produce measurable gluten antibodies, "anti-gliadin antibodies." However, "healthy people" may produce antibodies close to these levels (30–40%), which means you are more likely to test negative for gluten sensitivity if you have a gluten problem, and there's still a good chance that you will test positive if you *do not* have gluten sensitivity.[201]

This all makes testing for gluten sensitivity almost useless. Don't even look for ballpark numbers of gluten-sensitivity misdiagnoses; you won't find them. Without accurate testing, we won't know how many people are diagnosed or misdiagnosed.

Dr. Fasano made the estimate that 18 million people suffer from gluten sensitivity, which is six times higher than the number of people who suffer from celiac disease. Dr. Fasano was once criticized for the belief that celiac disease was a problem. He founded the University of Maryland Center for Celiac Research and began studying antibodies that are found after the inflammatory destruction of the intestines takes place. After screening 13,000 people in 32 states for antibodies with follow-ups of small bowel biopsies, he found his answer. One in 133 people in the United States has celiac disease.[202] His work shook the medical community and is currently the most reliable statistic of celiac disease. This breakthrough happened in 2003.

Just a few years ago, no one believed gluten could be a problem. Dr. Fasano believes that there are varying degrees of gluten sensitivity, and villous atrophy (intestinal damage) is just one sign of this autoimmune disease. Dr. Ford, author of *The Gluten Syndrome*, explains that there is a potential that 30–50% of the population may have one form or another of gluten sensitivity.[203]

White bread, wheat bread, gluten products, and processed grains all increase blood sugar more than sugar itself. In terms of sugar spikes, they are all pretty much the same. However, in terms of inflammation, refined grains take the cake as one of the most damaging inflammatory foods. Refined grains lose many of their anti-inflammatory benefits by processing out vitamins (like vitamin E) and fiber. Vitamins and fiber can reduce the inflammatory effects of a sugar spike or any inflammatory problem.[204] It's no surprise that studies show super high levels of inflammatory markers with refined grains.[205]

Alternative: Whole Grains

Whole grains in their natural form are healthiest. I am referring to a bowl of brown rice, quinoa, or oats. If you chop it up and keep 100% of the original kernel—all of the bran, germ, and endosperm—it's still considered whole grain, but eating it that way is more likely to cause a sugar spike than eating the grain in its whole form, and it's not as healthy. Refined grains are significantly modified from their natural states, and the refining process generally involves removing the bran, germ, and many nutrients. Further refining may include mixing in additives and bleaching.

Bleach is a migraine trigger. This may be because it blocks iodine. Iodine deficiency is the most common cause of hypothyroidism and hypothyroidism increases your risk of getting migraines.[206][207] Soy is commonly added to refined grains and also has been known to block thyroid function and may increase migraine risk.[208]

This is all extremely confusing because processed foods that are labeled as "whole grain" may also be significantly modified, bleached, and contain numerous migraine triggers. This is why I make it clear that whole grains in their whole form—like a bowl of quinoa—are much healthier than processed grains. And of course, vegetables are healthier than any grain, because grains come with sugar spikes and have fewer nutrients for migraine prevention than vegetables do.

What to Look Out For

It's easy to say wheat is healthy when you compare it to processed foods. Seriously, cardiovascular disease is killing Americans faster than anything else. So on the one hand, we have death, and on the other hand, we have "whole grain foods." But the food companies don't tell us what's hidden in "whole grain foods." I would expect a "whole grain food" to contain whole grains. In 2006, the FDA adopted this as the definition of a whole grain: "any mixture of bran, endosperm, and germ one would expect to see in an intact grain." There is nothing "whole" about processing foods and putting them back together. You can't cut a living thing up, mix it with some other stuff, cook it, and put it back together and then say it's whole again, as it was when you started. That's like making a meatloaf and calling it a cow. When you do this to grains, they are lower in fiber and nutrients.

It's not a matter of reading labels on packaged foods—the false advertising is built in to the packaging. For a product to be considered a "whole grain food," the FDA requires that it contain only 51% or more whole grain ingredients by weight.[209] What's in the other 49%? More sugar, calories, and refined grains we don't want? According to a recent Harvard study, yes.[210]

But we see it all over the grocery store: Whole grain! Multi-grain! Wheat! A healthy source of whole grain! Lucky Charms with "Whole Grain Guaranteed"! Lucky Charms must be healthy; it basically says so on the FDA-approved package. But that little leprechaun is very misleading. There is a big difference between a bowl of Lucky Charms and actual organic whole grains like wheat, oat, barley, quinoa, and brown rice. When we genetically modify it, use hybridization, overprocess and overheat it, add a bucket of sugar, and then put it all back together, it becomes a different product. Wheat, even in its natural form, is a headache risk, and destroying its nutritional benefits does not help the problem.

Chronic Trigger #5: Milk

Milk is made for baby cows, not you. Baby cows stop drinking milk anywhere from six months to one year of age because they begin to lose their ability to produce lactase.[211] Seventy-five percent of adults lose their ability to produce lactase usually between ages five and seven.[212] This is because milk truly is for babies. It would be weird to see an eight-year-old breast-feeding, because it's just not normal in nature. But many of us have developed lactase persistence, which is the continued ability to produce the enzyme that digests lactose in milk. According to the Physicians Committee for Responsible Medicine, those once called "lactose intolerant" are now referred to as "normal."

If everybody had lactase persistence, scientists would probably just call it lactase production. We would also think of lactose intolerance as a disease or allergy. But lactose intolerance is far from an allergy. It's actually normal. An allergy starts with your body's immune system identifying a foreign object as an invader and attacking it. In "normal" people, the human body doesn't really care about the toxic sugar molecule called lactose. We just let lactose mosey on down to the last stop of our digestive system, the colon. Here the lactose sugar begins to ferment and produce gas. This is where your body says, "I don't like gas, and I'm going to start attacking everything with inflammation," which may result in cramping, nausea, flatulence, diarrhea, and headaches.

Individual regions where people have produced milk for thousands of years, like Switzerland and Sweden, have developed lactase persistence in over 90% of their populations. Conversely, regions in Europe just a few miles away range in lactase persistence from 6–36% due to a lack of milk consumption, so the people in those regions will have trouble with gas when they consume milk.[213]

The problem is that even if you come from a long line of milk drinkers, there is still a 10% chance that you will be lactose intolerant. And let's get real: Having lactase persistence does not mean that you will fully digest milk. It's still true that most people rapidly lose much of this ability in childhood. This means that some of the milk you drink will rot in your stomach—not all of it, only some. How do you think your mind and body will feel with something rotting in your stomach? Headache, maybe?

Self-diagnosis of a milk allergy is tenfold higher than clinically proven incidence.[214] Milk allergies have close symptoms to common lactose intolerance. Because of this, we will never know how large the problem actually is. The inflammatory response for milk allergies can be severe and, in rare circumstances, cause anaphylactic shock. However, the secondary inflammation produced from the rotting effects of lactose intolerance can be an equally powerful headache trigger. But that's not the worst of it: Multiple studies show milk is a contributing factor in cancerous tumor growth as well.[215,216,217] In fact, headaches are often a late sign that cancer is taking a toll on your entire body.

Other studies show great health benefits from milk, but I can't buy all of that.[218] There are too many studies that show that dairy is too deadly to risk consuming large amounts of it. One study took a number of asthmatics and migraine patients and put them on a six-month elimination diet. The 22 asthmatics previously averaged hospitalization at least once per month. The 26 migraineurs had required bed rest once every other week. The sole elimination of milk resulted in zero hospital visits for 15 of 22 asthmatics and the complete absence of migraines for 18 of 26 migraineurs.

The nearly 70% of migraineurs "cured" from a single milk elimination raised a question: What would happen if we gave them milk after six months of complete relief? Nine were brave enough to help answer this question, and all nine suffered a classic migraine within two to three days after consuming milk, with one patient requiring sedation and hospitalization.[219] If I had a little more will power, I'd eliminate it altogether, although studies seem to suggest that moderation is the key to survival.

As for low-fat milk, it's highly processed. They pasteurize it, turn it into powder, and then add water. You want 1% milk? Let's add a little more water. That's like asking for water with your doughnut to make it healthy. The glutamate is unbound from its chain of amino acids and becomes free glutamate. This could be why a 2005 study published in *The Journal of the American Medical Association* (*JAMA*) found that low-fat milk is associated with the most significant weight gain in children.[220]

So yes, low-fat milk may make you fat and give you more headaches. Harvard researchers found in 2015 that female health professionals who experience frequent migraines—weekly or more—consumed significantly less wine and low-fat milk than average women. If health professionals with the same problems are avoiding these things, they probably have the right idea.[221]

There is one way to tell if milk is increasing your inflammation levels: acne. Acne, by definition, is an inflammatory disease of the skin marked by embarrassing pimples and blemishes. It's also absent from large populations that don't consume milk[222] and, according to research published in the *Journal of the American Academy of Dermatology*, teenagers were up to 44% more likely to have acne if they consumed low-fat milk or skim milk, while whole milk drinkers were in the clear.[223] The study suggested that highly processed milk contains more factors that influence hormone levels.[224] That makes sense. If you pump a cow full of steroids and turn its milk into a powder of chemicals and then drink it, it's likely to play with your own hormone levels.

The bottom line: Low-fat milk causes both chronic and acute inflammation that can inflame your face in the same manner that it may inflame a headache or a migraine. Up to 75% of people worldwide cannot properly digest milk. When we don't feel good, we get headaches. The 1979 study had milk as the sixth top headache trigger, and the 1983 study positioned milk from cows as the number one headache trigger. Numerous other headache studies from the past 60 years show that milk is a common headache trigger, and patients show significant relief when milk is eliminated.[225]

Chronic Trigger #6: Artificial Sweeteners

A morbidly obese woman walks into a fast-food joint and orders a supersized meal with a big burger, big fries, and a big soda. What kind of 30-ounce soda does she order? She orders a diet soda. It's more likely that she is a she, because women are more health conscious and likely to stay away from high-fructose corn syrup. So she knows how bad this meal is for her. Somehow, she thinks, this diet soda will offset the damage that the fast food is about to inflict on her body. After all, doesn't it seem like a better choice to go with a diet soda? It's not.

Diet soda makes us just as fat as regular soda, and it gives us all the chronic inflammatory problems that regular soda gives us as well. There are no studies that show long-term weight loss from replacing regular soda with diet soda.[226] In 2005, the University of Texas analyzed a 25-year heart study and found the more diet soda a person drinks, the greater the chance that he or she will become overweight or obese. In fact, the study suggested that diet soda was more likely to cause obesity than regular soda.[227]

This is just breathtaking after we consider how fat regular soda makes us. Most of us just assume that "diet" refers to products that will help us lose weight. The FDA allows "diet" on a soda label because the Latin translation of "diet" means you will literally "die" from "et." That's not actually true—I just made it up. I have no clue why the FDA allows "diet" on products that significantly increase our weight. It doesn't make any sense. But if artificial sweeteners truly helped people lose weight, there would be hundreds of studies sponsored by Coca-Cola and Pepsi that prove it.

In the last few decades, the explosion of artificial sweeteners has paralleled the rise in obesity. Think about the last time you were not hungry and had the tiniest little candy. You probably wanted another. Studies show that sweet foods stimulate appetite, and artificial sweeteners are so sweet. Aspartame is 200 times sweeter than sugar, which means you don't need much.[228]

Foods and drinks with artificial sweeteners have been studied for years. The results aren't good. They can lead to obesity, type 2 diabetes[229], slow metabolism[230], migraines, depression[231], and a whole spectrum of inflammatory problems. Aspartame contains methanol (what you know as "wood alcohol" or "grain alcohol"), which is bad enough before your body converts it into formaldehyde.[232] Long-term, low-level exposure to formaldehyde may cause headaches, sleeping disturbances, irritability, memory loss, depression, cancer, and asthma. Even acute exposure to minimal amounts of formaldehyde may result in an inflammatory response of the nose, throat, chest, and respiratory tract. It's bad stuff.[233] Artificial sweeteners are one "food" you can easily move over into a category of pure evil.

Aspartame, the most common artificial sweetener, is responsible for over 10,000 complaints filed with the FDA.[234] Headaches, migraines, and memory loss are at the top of the FDA's list of aspartame complaints. In addition to the thousands of recognized complaints, the FDA documents that there may be millions of people who suffer but don't make a connection between their malaise and aspartame. This is because most don't realize what's causing the problem until they stop using aspartame, as in this documented FDA case: "I have suffered from migraines for years. As soon as I gave up NutraSweet my migraines disappeared. All those Cat Scans, MRIs...for nothing."[235]

Aspartame is aspartic acid (40%) and phenylalanine (50%), with a methyl ester bond that includes methanol (10%). Aspartic acid and phenylalanine are amino acids that are each found in natural foods at 4–5%, but they are bound to other natural amino acids.[236] The methyl ester bond is broken shortly after aspartame is ingested and deadly methanol is released into the bloodstream.[237] Simply put, aspartame is a colossal amount of two unnaturally isolated amino acids, bonded together by poison.

The aspartic acid found in aspartame is unbound or free from other amino acids. Ingesting free aspartic acid raises the levels of aspartate and glutamate in your blood. Both glutamate and aspartate are neurotransmitters that are considered excitotoxins.[238] Too much of either of these neurotransmitters will "excite" the cells in the brain to death. They kill neurons in the brain with an influx of calcium.

Going back to CSD (the start of a migraine), the glutamate theory holds calcium as partially responsible for the detonation of a migraine. Glutamate is considered the gun, and calcium is the bullet. As glutamate initially triggers excitotoxic injury, calcium continues into the neuron like a bullet, followed by depolarization and neural death, marking the beginning of a meltdown.[239] It seems that aspartame may operate in the same fashion. This causes the same inflammatory problems that come from MSG. Your brain takes a beating.

The History of Aspartame

The largest and most comprehensive study on aspartame gathered information on 10% of the US population for over 22 years and found that, in comparison to all other factors, aspartame is a "promising candidate" for explaining the large increase in malignant brain tumors.[240]

Dr. Walton of Northeastern Ohio University did an analysis of the 166 studies published from 1980 to 1985. There were 74 industry-funded studies, and all 74 showed that aspartame was safe. Of the remaining 92 independently funded studies, 84 identified adverse reactions.[241] This isn't a coincidence. Companies pay for studies that will show their products are ready to hit consumers. Many of the worst health concerns were found before the FDA approved aspartame.

Were the toxic side effects of aspartame hidden from the FDA? You can find this answer on the FDA's website. The answer was originally a response written by the Aspartame Toxicity Information Center, and it begins a story you won't believe. The research done for the aspartame industry by G.D. Searle, a research-based pharmaceutical company, was labeled as "abysmal," and the preapproval research was described as "even worse." The document goes on to say, "Despite this fact, FDA officials essentially 'sold out' to the manufacturer and approved the junk." The 2002 document reviews years of horrific findings by the FDA task force investigating Searle's research for its unreliability, misleading nature, and inaccurate reporting to the FDA.[242]

The FDA found that Searle had removed tumors from live animals and conveniently left out this critical information when submitting its studies to the FDA. Instead of performing autopsies on monkeys that suffered seizures, the company financed a new testing methodology that showed no problems. Normally, a company would want to look into why its product is causing deadly seizures before selling it to the public. Animals that were reported as dead were later reported with normal vital signs and vice versa.

The Searle employee responsible for reviewing most of these studies was hired with only one year of experience from the Illinois wildlife service where he studied populations of rabbits. You don't go from studying rabbits to senior research assistant on a multimillion-dollar project. His title should have been "the fall guy." The list goes on and on about the discrepancies, lies, and misconduct found in all of the studies investigated by the FDA. The FDA task force recommended that Searle should face a grand jury for what was obviously criminal activity. Well, jail time doesn't sound good to any millionaire, and the stockholders weren't exactly happy about being lied to.

In 1975, the stockholders filed a class action lawsuit against Searle for concealing information regarding the quality of its animal research. When your shareholders sue their own company, it's a sign that the ship is about to sink. So, as its next move, the company hired Donald Rumsfeld in 1977 as its new president and CEO. Yes, the same Donald Rumsfeld who would later serve as secretary of defense in the Bush administration and who had served as secretary of defense in the Ford administration. In the same year, US Attorney Samuel Skinner was requested by the FDA to investigate whether Searle's actions were criminal. Shortly after a meeting with Searle's lawyers, Skinner resigned his position as US attorney. He was then hired by Searle's law firm.

Oh, it gets better. US Attorney William Conlon was assigned to take over the case. Despite complaints from the Justice Department, Conlon sat on the case until he too joined Searle's law firm in 1979. The FDA established a public board that ruled that aspartame should not be approved pending further investigation of brain tumors in animals. Jump forward to 1981 and a new commissioner was appointed to the FDA. FDA Commissioner Arthur Hayes backed off Searle and stated that there was sufficient evidence that aspartame did not cause tumors in rats. This went against everything the FDA task force had submitted.

Why would Arthur Hayes blindside his FDA task force? President Reagan appointed Arthur Hayes to the FDA. At the time, Rumsfeld was both the CEO of Searle and part of Reagan's transition team as the new president of the United States. Now, a conspiracy is a secret plan to do something harmful, but this was done in broad daylight for the entire world to see. Arthur Hayes was hired by the Reagan administration that included Searle's CEO, Donald Rumsfeld. In 1981, Arthur Hayes ignored the FDA public board, the internal scientists, and the FDA task force. Aspartame was approved for use as a tabletop sugar, and in 1983 it was approved for use in soft drinks.

In the summer of 1983, Commissioner Hayes resigned from the FDA after much criticism. A suit was filed with the FDA objecting to the numerous safety issues of aspartame. Hayes quickly found a new job with Burson-Marsteller. Burson-Marsteller happened to be Searle's public relations firm. There you have it. This was how a deadly product made it onto the shelves of nearly every store in America. Aspartame went on to become the best-selling artificial sweetener.[243]

The list of health concerns related to aspartame is too long to reprint here. The most common reported side effects are migraines and headaches. The excitotoxic effects of aspartame will give the same rise of inflammatory markers that MSG will. Depression and obesity will raise inflammatory markers and leave us prone to headaches. The tumors, seizures, and cancer should scare you. If the industry knows we may develop tumors from that stuff, do you think they care about our headaches?

Chronic Trigger #7: Inflammatory Meats

N-Glycolylneuraminic acid (Neu5Gc) is in the spotlight for cancer research because there is proof that it's found in human tumors. This is odd because humans do not produce Neu5Gc. But other animals do. Are we getting this cancer-linked molecule from eating animal products? To test this theory, researchers from the University of California went vegan for two days to clear their systems of Neu5Gc by eliminating all meat products. Then they drank a glass of porcine mucin, which is basically diluted pig mucus. Tasty! Within days, Neu5Gc was found seeping from their bodies in their saliva, urine, and hair clippings.[244]

Further research shows that, after the molecule is ingested, it incorporates itself into human cells. This process of digesting Neu5Gc itself causes inflammation for many people. The body then creates antibodies to attack the Neu5Gc, which causes an immune system response that can spread a secondary inflammation throughout the body. Tumors contain more Neu5Gc; therefore, "Neu5Gc must somehow benefit tumors," according to Dr. Varki, one of the lead researchers from the San Diego Neu5Gc study.[245]

It's pretty simple. Neu5Gc causes inflammation, and inflammation is known to promote cancer. So what do you think the researchers used to treat their mice with Neu5Gc tumors? The same medication that is among the most effective at treating your inflammation-caused headaches. That's right, they used nonsteroidal anti-inflammatory drugs (NSAIDs)—like aspirin—to effectively block the inflammation. The treatment caused the tumors to shrink. Obviously, eliminating meat would eliminate the need for aspirin. In fact, studies show that a vegetarian diet actually lowers the risk of cancer and heart disease.[246,247]

The popular belief—although an arguable one—is that the increased risk of cancer and heart attack from an animal-based diet comes from large amounts of saturated fat.[248] But that theory is disproved by the ketogenic diet, which is very high in fat. Neu5Gc could be another reason patients with autoimmune diseases like rheumatoid arthritis (RA) experience relief in just weeks after they eliminate animal products from their diets.[249] RA is very common in humans and has not yet been reported in vegetarian apes in captivity. It's possible that Neu5Gc could be inflaming the tissue of arthritic joints, potentially aggravating the arthritis process.[250]

Is All Meat Bad?

Despite this compelling new research, I don't condemn meat. We've been eating meat for more than a few years. Apes don't have rheumatoid arthritis, and they also don't consume our most inflammatory foods. The rise in chronic diseases have come with a rise in meat consumption and, more significantly, with a rise in food that contains completely unnatural additives. A corn-fed, steroid-pumped pig that we inject with MSG is not the same pork our ancestors ate. This new research is just that—new.

A study in 2007 by the University of Western Australia confirmed that not all meat is terrible. The study found that a moderate amount of lean red meat does not influence the inflammatory precursors of heart disease.[251] We may find that unnatural amounts of Neu5Gc are bad for us, but that goes with anything in life. It's all about moderation.

Why are today's meats inflammatory? Meat should have a good balance of omega-6 to omega-3 fats. The ratio should be between the ranges of 2 to 1 and 4 to 1 (two parts omega-6 to one part omega-3 and four parts omega-6 to one part omega-3), but many health educators advocate lower rates of omega-6. The Mediterranean diet shows many health benefits from an emphasis on foods that are rich in omega-3 fatty acids. Fresh fruits, vegetables, fish, and garlic are anti-inflammatory, with high levels of omega-3 fatty acids.

The typical American diet is not rich in omega-3 fatty acids. Instead of an omega-6/omega-3 ratio of 2 to 1, our diet is more like 25 to 1. That's 25 parts inflammatory and one part anti-inflammatory. We are what we eat. If we're eating too many inflammatory foods, we'll become inflamed.[252] But the big question is: Will they give you a headache? Go eat a huge, greasy burger and find out. Too much omega-6 fat makes us feel yucky.

Meat allergies are uncommon, but they are on many migraine trigger lists. Bacon, sausage, hot dogs, lunch meats, pepperoni, cured meats, canned meats, and any meats with food additives like MSG or nitrates are common headache triggers. Highly processed meats are more likely to be injected with hormones, and they're more likely to be corn fed. They're also more likely to contain fewer vitamins and have high inflammatory factors. Search online for "foods highest in omega-6," and you will find processed meats with a disgusting ratio of omega-6 to omega-3. This is no longer meat. We're creating the perfect headache trigger. Eating a salami sandwich is just asking for a headache.

Alternative: Natural Animal Products

Grain-fed cows eat pro-inflammatory grain. In turn, they have more omega-6 fat. A 2010 study looked into the ratio of omega-6 to omega-3 for grass-fed beef versus grain-fed beef. The averages were 1.53 to 1 for grass-fed beef and 7.65 to 1 for grain-fed beef.[253] Smaller studies show grain-fed beef ratios that exceed inflammatory ratios of 20 to 1. You can also see this stupefying 20 to 1 ratio in supermarket eggs, but free-range eggs are closer to 1.5 to 1.[254] It's safe to say natural animal products are less inflammatory.

Alternative: Fish Oil

Rather than calling fish oil an alternative, I might do it more justice by calling it an antidote to eating inflammatory meats. A 2002 study out of Rhode Island found that we can reduce migraines by increasing our omega-3 intake with fish oil. While the study showed a significant reduction in migraines, from 15 episodes down to two per month, the study also showed a huge benefit to the placebo effect.[255] The placebo effect will always be powerful in headache studies, but the fact still holds true: Omega-3 is anti-inflammatory and has the same anti-inflammatory benefits as NSAIDs without the side effects.

Many studies show that omega-3 lowers the risk for high blood pressure, heart disease, and rheumatoid arthritis. Omega-3 may, in fact, work better at controlling pain than medications. A study from the University of Pittsburgh Medical Center had 59% of back- and neck-pain patients discontinue their use of NSAIDs in preference of fish oil.[256] NSAIDs may come with side effects, but they work. It speaks wonders that a majority of people preferred fish oil.

According to Oregon State University, six out of seven studies on patients with RA who were treated with omega-3 showed positive results: Patients demonstrated a reduced requirement for anti-inflammatory medications.[257] Luckily, you don't need to choose between the two; you can use both until you decide that you no longer need the medication.

Chronic Trigger #8: Alcohol

Looking a little rosy after a couple of drinks? One reason for this redness is an accumulation of acetaldehyde, a nasty byproduct of alcohol. Appearing "toasty" after a couple of drinks means that you are more likely to suffer from the inflammatory response of acetaldehyde. This type of blushing is also known as Asian flush syndrome and may result in headaches, nausea, and vomiting. You don't need to be Asian to feel this way—this inflammatory response goes along with anyone's typical hangover.

The problem with Asian flush syndrome is that acetaldehyde is converted much faster, and a person can start feeling hung over before becoming even slightly drunk. Some five minutes after consuming alcohol, a patient may experience rosy cheeks, nausea, vomiting, a throbbing headache, visual disturbances, and confusion.

According to a 2010 study published in *BMC Evolutionary Biology*, the gene responsible for the syndrome coincides with the cultivation of rice in certain areas of China. Over 50% of Chinese people have this genetic mutation, hence its name.[258] Those unfortunate people are also less likely to become alcoholics, because who wants an immediate hangover?

I'll tell you who wants an immediate hangover: a committed alcoholic. Normally, our livers filter acetaldehyde into harmless acetic acid, which allows us to drink copious amounts of alcohol, although most recent headache studies show that, even when we convert acetaldehyde into "harmless" acetic acid, it may still cause headaches for migraine sufferers.[259] Ever notice the drowsy effects of alcohol you get the day after a night of drinking? Some of the worst headaches go hand in hand with the foggy days following the wear and tear of boozing. But even when you don't notice a hangover, it doesn't mean you've escaped the inflammatory response of acetaldehyde.

A flushed face and acetaldehyde have been linked to inflammation in the throat, stomach, skin, and liver. A flushed face and headache may be the least of your trouble. High blood pressure, cancer, and Alzheimer's disease have recently been added to the blushing list of acetaldehyde side effects. Whether you blush or not, the headache you get from acetaldehyde is yet another example of your body telling you that something is wrong.[260][261][262]

Most people who blush or feel ill from drinking notice it only from some drinks, but not from others. Those people are more likely suffering from allergens within the alcohol, such as barley, hops, brewer's yeast, glutamic acid, rye, wheat, gluten, histamines, sulfites, and hundreds of other ingredients. The more you drink, the more exposure you have to your specific allergy. Unfortunately, this will cause a snowball effect due to the rise in your inflammatory markers from alcohol itself.

But really, Asian flush syndrome is only part of the problem with alcohol. It's a numbers game of known allergens. The more allergens you consume, the greater your odds are of finding a personal headache recipe. Alcohol speeds up the infection process with systemic inflammation throughout your entire body. We know that heavy alcohol consumption causes chronic inflammation in the liver, gut, brain, lungs, and more. This inflammation results in the body's compromised immunity and increased risk of infectious disease. Alcohol's rotten history is well documented with hundreds of thousands of alcohol-related deaths that are often aided by a pummeled immune system.[263]

Alcohol's effect on your gut is very simple and much like any inflammatory food. In this immune system response, your body attacks the threat, and the lining of your gut ends up with collateral damage. This results in a leaky gut, better known as "increased gut permeability," making your gut an open door to outside invaders.[264]

Drinking too much for too long will result in a catastrophic failure of your immune system. The inflammation in your brain and liver affect your body's central nervous system and its ability to detoxify potential invaders. Those herbs, along with the brewer's yeast, the refined sugars, the wine byproducts, and the once healthy nutrients, may now sneak by your gut, enter the bloodstream, and create an immune system response that affects your entire body, including your noggin.

Here are a few other things we know about alcohol:[265]

- Alcohol is a diuretic. You drink one cup and pee up to four cups.
- Alcohol causes inflammation of the stomach lining.
- Severe drunkenness causes low blood sugar.
- Drinking alcohol disrupts sleep and biological rhythms.
- Clear liquor induces fewer hangovers.
- Alcohol eventually depletes vitamins.

Gonna Drink Anyway? Read On.

OK, OK, OK. We all know that too much alcohol is deadly, and we really don't care. We're going to drink anyway. If you are much stronger than I am, you can skip the rest of this section. For those of us who will stubbornly drink anyway, we need to know how alcohol gives us headaches and how to avoid them.

Actually, we need to kill the hangover. In spite of over 10,000 years of drinking, we have yet to discover a true hangover cure, although many argue this fact with their own remedies. Killing a hangover is especially difficult because we don't know exactly what it is. But drinking is like anything else that might break your headache threshold, so here are some ways you can avoid that and keep drinking.

Drinking Rule #1: Moderate

Alcohol falls into what researchers call a U-shaped association. We've heard that a drink a day may keep the doctor away and may even reduce your risk of heart attack. Studies are showing that inflammatory markers like IL-6 and CRP first go down with a small amount of alcohol consumption and then begin to rise when people have more than one drink per day. So you have a drink, and your risk of heart disease, diabetes, autoimmune diseases, and migraines goes down. More than two drinks a day and your risk of disease goes up exponentially. "U" get the pattern? It's clear that alcohol in moderation is an anti-inflammatory, but when we drink too much, it becomes a pro-inflammatory.[266]

RA and gout are great examples of the U-shaped association with alcohol. People with these conditions can feel and even see the positive effects of a small amount of alcohol. But too much alcohol and that roller coaster ride slingshots back up with swollen red-hot inflammatory pain. The same IL-6 markers begin to lower with a minimal amount of alcohol and then rise when one drink leads to another.[267] However, don't think that drinking in moderation will keep everyone in the clear.

Drinking Rule #2: Choose Simple Booze

Ever had Fernet? When I was studying Spanish at the University of Buenos Aires, I learned about this popular Argentinean drink. I was living in a house with twenty other young travelers who all had one thing in common: Fernet and Coke. Of course, we had to try the local drink on our first night out there. And the next morning, most of us found out just how ill Fernet made us feel—not just ill, but deathly ill.

And there is no reason why it shouldn't. Fernet is made with a secret recipe of over 30 different herbs and spices. This is a shotgun blast of allergens at your stomach. Maybe you survive the first shotgun slug. Fire a couple more shells at your immune system, and you're bound to find an herb that doesn't jibe with your body. I learned that my magic number was four Fernet and Cokes. This was a sufficient amount of unknown herbs, alcohol, and sugar to effectively produce genuine inflammation and multiple trips to the baño in the morning.

In general, people with RA and gout, headache sufferers, and drinkers are more likely to have reactions from complex alcohol, such as beer and wine, than from alcohol with simpler ingredients, such as gin and vodka.

Beer and wine contain brewer's yeast. Brewer's yeast is extremely high in glutamic acid. And as with the fermentation process of MSG, the fermenting process of beer and wine creates unwanted byproducts. Histamine is one of those unwanted byproducts, which is fine when it's combined with fibers and other healthy nutrients that prevent its ill effects. But you're probably not thinking about fiber and nutrients while you're tossing back a few. As such, the histamine is readily available to attack your stomach and immune system. So here's what I'm saying: Avoid drinking beer and wine. I know that's a sad sentence. I'm sorry.

Histamine has the same issue as tannins and sulfites, which you'll read about later: Histamine may be a headache trigger when combined with other amino acids and biogenic amines, yet it may be harmless when found in small quantities and/or in isolation. It's all about the headache threshold. It's an accumulation of headache triggers that's the problem.

Drinking Rule #3: Stop Drinking Cheap Crap

The "champagne headache" is usually not from actual "champagne." Champagne is typically very high in quality and from the region of Champagne in France. What most people are drinking is cheap sparkling wine.

The cheaper the alcohol, the more likely it is to have a bunch of nasty byproducts. From higher methanol content to problematic ferments, cheap liquor companies put your health last. Cheap liquor means that time is money. Wine and beer may come with many ingredients like egg whites, milk, fish oils, plastics, gelatins, herbs, wheat products, and a long list of chemicals. Just read the ingredients on the bottle—wait, there's nothing there. The FDA wanted to let you know that they don't care if you drink plastic and there is no need for ingredients to be listed on alcohol.[268]

The precision of high-end wine makers doesn't come cheaply. The oak barrels are not treated with cheap and poisonous chemicals. The tannins are from just the right part of the grape, eliminating the very bitter taste of the grape stem. They don't just dump a bucket of chemicals in at the end. They don't throw in the bottom-of-the-barrel ingredients that may have mold and high amounts of pesticides. They don't need to add a bucket of sugar to make their wine flavorful.

The same holds true for other cheap alcoholic beverages. While I was in Thailand, many people claimed the local poor man's beer, Chang, would give them immediate headaches. Rumor had it that formaldehyde was added to the beer. The rumor was printed in a 2005 issue of a Beijing newspaper where Chang is also brewed. The investigative report stated that this was a cheap way to prevent sediment from forming during storage. China's beer industry quickly came back to say, "Consumers need to know that formaldehyde in beer is different from that in household chemicals."[269] Sure, China, sure.

Cheap drinks are cheaply made. Don Tadeo is high-quality tequila from Puerto Vallarta, Mexico. The owner claims that it is impossible to get a hangover from his tequila because of the purity of his fermentation process. I took his test and had 15 shots of tequila. The result: no perceived hangover. Give me cheap vodka from the United States, and I will feel terrible after just a few drinks.

Vodka, in general, has fewer congeners than dark liquor. Acetaldehyde is known as a congener, and congeners are believed to be responsible for hangovers. Congeners are produced along with ethanol during the fermentation process. The more congeners, the more likely your hangover is. Gin and vodka have few congeners, while whiskey, brandy, and red wine contain significantly more. Methanol is one of the most serious congeners, because it can be metabolized into formaldehyde. Cheap dark liquors and even cheaper wines are more likely to contain higher methanol levels, which can cause a headache and, in some cases, blindness or death.

A study by Italian migraine researchers found that bourbon has 37 times as many congeners as vodka, resulting in more severe headaches during hangovers.[270] But that doesn't mean cheap vodka is good. Bourbon has more congeners, because it is usually distilled once; scotch is often distilled twice; and most good whiskey is triple distilled. Good vodka can be distilled six times!

Distilling is essentially filtering out bad byproducts. Cheap vodka may be distilled just once, leaving the worst congeners in your drink. It doesn't matter where the liquor is from or the type of liquor. Cheap alcohol, in general, is less filtered, less precise, and likely to contain *more* headache triggers. Stop drinking cheap crap.

Drinking Rule #4: Hydrate

Hydrate, hydrate, hydrate! Alcohol dehydrates the heck out of you. Alcohol inhibits an antidiuretic hormone that prevents the kidneys from retaining water. It's almost like magic. You drink one part alcohol, and two to four parts water come out. The more you drink, the more severely dehydrated you will become.

I've had people ask me, "How much can I drink without getting a headache?" Dehydration is a major headache trigger. You're probably already dehydrated before you consume alcohol. According to media reports, 75% of people are severely dehydrated and don't get those eight glasses of water per day. The medical community itself hasn't put a number on the hydration problem, but it agrees that most people don't get enough of this vital nutrient.

Weakness, cottonmouth, low blood pressure, a rapid pulse, dizziness, lightheadedness, and headaches all come with dehydration and hangovers. Before you get to the point of feeling like someone hit you repeatedly all over your entire body with a bat, drink some water. Hydrate before a night of drinking. Hydrate between drinks. Hydrate in the middle of the night. Hydrate in the morning after drinking.

It's simple. If certain drinks give you headaches, stop drinking those certain drinks. But if you are going to have them anyway, ensure that you're hydrated when you do.

In addition to all of that, alcohol tears up your stomach. All types of alcohol will metabolize into acetaldehyde, which, in excess, will inflame your stomach. Drinking water helps dilute the acetaldehyde in the blood and helps flush it out before it makes its way to the bloodstream.

Drinking Rule #5: Choose When to Drink

This one is so simple there's not much to say about it: Drink when you can afford the hangover. As a firefighter, I never drank the night before I went to work, not even a little. I could feel the difference in the morning, and I couldn't do the work of a firefighter without feeling 100%. Some people can do this without the slightest issue; I am not one of those people. Besides, that job required razor-sharp thinking and, occasionally, saving people's lives.

Drinking Rule #6: Sleep Hard

Have you ever awakened after a night of drinking and felt reality hit you like a freight train, without even a touch of the dreamy, surreal calm the night usually brings? That's because alcohol disrupts your REM (rapid eye movement) dream state. Alcohol also disrupts the 24-hour rhythm of your body's temperature—your temp is lower while drunk and higher during a hangover, which may partially account for the nausea and sweating you experience before the previous night's drinks begin to come back up.

Because of this, allow plenty of time after drinking for adequate sleep. Normal sleep patterns are essential to reduce the chance of a headache, but sleep may also play a large factor in inflammation. Several studies have found that a lack of sleep raises inflammatory markers (CRP), although the physiological reasons are still unclear.[271]

One reason that alcohol withdrawal results in poor sleep quality may be because of the noticeable rise in glutamate it causes. Just as the studies of MSG noted that a rise in glutamate is excitotoxic, the bump in glutamate from alcohol may keep your brain awake because your cells are "excited to death." While studies are not conclusive, they do show a clear spike in glutamate followed by a rise of inflammatory markers.[272]

Sleep is more important than we understand, so don't sacrifice sleep, especially after drinking.

Drinking Rule #7: Limit Sugar

Refined sugar is a pro-inflammatory and will help beat up your stomach, so avoid the sugary drinks. As with any sugar spike, a night of drinking will eventually end with low blood sugar in the morning. This is the time to replenish glucose. Drinking sugary beverages with no nutritional value in combination with large amounts of alcohol will only bring on more inflammation—along with the hangover. Drink mixers are often full of sugar. As for alcohol mixed with OJ—don't get me started.

Drinking Rule #8: Keep Your Threshold in Mind

Remember, your headache threshold breaks due to an accumulation of your headache triggers, and since alcohol can give *anyone* a headache, not just those who get chronic headaches, it's already taking up a lot of room in your cup of headache triggers. This means, have the wine—but don't have the cheese. Have the beer, but don't eat the bread. The tannins, sulfites, brewer's yeast, sugars, glutamic acid, and all the other headache triggers need to be avoided. Everything in moderation!

Drinking Rule #9: Don't Take Tylenol

Tylenol, better known as acetaminophen, especially in combination with alcohol, can kill you. Alcohol beats up your liver, and so does acetaminophen. This typically happens to severe alcoholics or athletes who are heavy users of Tylenol. However, just one night of drinking followed by Tylenol may land you in the hospital for good. Acetaminophen has a narrow safety margin, meaning just a little more than the recommended dose can cause liver damage. Alcohol accelerates this process.[273]

Acetaminophen is the leading cause of acute liver failure (ALF). Failure! Your liver is your filter, and without it you will die. What does it really take to damage your liver? Liver damage has been reported from less than 2.5 g of acetaminophen consumed per day (about five extra-strength Tylenol). This is serious business.[274]

We're talking about something deadly. If you bring it back to a headache, of course a deadly mix of alcohol and Tylenol can give you a headache. It could be just a couple of drinks and two Tylenol that does it. When you combine them, you increase your headache odds. But really, it's a little hard to care about headaches when you're talking about a combination this deadly. Just don't drink and take Tylenol—ever.

Hangover Help

If you accumulated too many triggers and you wind up with a hangover anyway, here are a couple of things you can do about it. Having a little hair of the dog isn't one of them. Drinking to fix the ill effects of drinking is only a temporary relief that prolongs the inflammatory effects of alcohol. The help listed here falls on opposite ends of the spectrum: One is pretty simple, cheap, and doesn't require anyone else's help. The other one, not so much.

IV Cocktails

There is a company in Las Vegas called Hangover Heaven where you can either drag yourself in or someone will come right to your hotel room door and, for as low as $100, they'll hook you up to an IV bag of "Myers' cocktail," consisting of B vitamins, vitamin C, magnesium, calcium, and, most importantly, fluid. You will be back up and running in under 30 minutes.

Does it work? Yes. There are multiple reviews across the internet of people stumbling and puking on their way into this place and walking out 30 minutes later as if nothing had happened.

Coconut Water

If you don't want to go through the trouble of getting hooked up to an IV bag, you can try nature's isotonic beverage: coconut water. Isotonic beverages contain salts and minerals that are similar to a human cell. Coconut water has even been used as a successful IV fluid during shortages of medical supplies.

Coconut water is the new electrolyte drink of choice for many athletes. I've recently seen coconut water distributed for hydrating firefighters during larger California wildfires. It hydrates, replenishes electrolytes, and is packed with minerals and vitamins, including potassium, calcium, magnesium, iron, zinc, and vitamins C, B1, B2, B6, B9, and E.[275]

Coconut is actually very similar to Hangover Heaven's Myers' cocktail. Alcohol can deplete the following vitamins and minerals: B1, B2, B6, B9, C, E, magnesium, zinc, calcium, and iron.[276][277] One of the only successful hangover studies used vitamin B6 to reduce hangover symptoms by 50%.[278] Post-2000 studies have begun to identify the deficiency of vitamin B6 as a sign of chronic inflammation and therefore a risk of hypertension, diabetes, stroke, and heart disease.[279]

Vitamins E and C are major antioxidants. Magnesium, iron, and zinc—also found in coconut water—have antioxidant properties.[280] Insufficient levels of these antioxidants cause oxidative stress and damages cells, resulting in chronic inflammation. Since alcohol depletes antioxidants, you need to replenish them.

When you think of oxidative stress, think rust. Rust is one of the most widely known forms of oxidation. In a beach town like mine, you'll see metals exposed to the sea air rust as oxidation slowly eats through old cars and lawn ornaments. To prevent this from happening to your body, consume foods with antioxidants.

During a two-week study in 2005 involving 28 people with high blood pressure, researchers found that coconut water significantly reduced the blood pressure of 71% of the participants. So there you go: Alcohol in excess eventually raises blood pressure, and coconut water eventually brings it down.[281]

Coconut water seems to be the perfect hangover drink with an abundance of vitamins, minerals, sugar, and electrolytes. But don't overdo it. Coconut allergies are rare, but they do exist. Coconuts are also on a couple of migraine trigger lists, but there are no reliable studies regarding coconut as a headache trigger. Coconut is only used as a temporary IV source of fluid because it has high levels of potassium, a concern for anyone on heart medications. In the case of a hangover, replenishing potassium is a good thing.

There is not enough evidence to recommend coconut water as a hangover cure or headache remedy. In fact, there isn't enough clinical data to recommend *anything* for a hangover. Thousands of hangover remedies across the internet just don't have studies with large enough sample sizes to back them up, according to science.[282] Coconut water has the nutrients that dehydration takes away. That's a simple enough answer for me.

Chronic Trigger #9: Corn

Is corn a vegetable or fruit? Neither. Corn is a grain. Corn gluten meal is used as an herbicide to kill plants. Your body may also have a reaction to the toxic effects of corn. A study published in the medical journal *Pediatric Research* found that corn oil increases villous atrophy and also increases the production of inflammatory chemicals.[283] It hurts your intestines and, at the same time, releases inflammatory chemicals that can trigger headaches.

Have you ever wondered why corn doesn't pass through your system very well? You know exactly what I'm talking about. I don't trust any food that looks exactly the same coming out as it did going in. As a top genetically modified food, corn is built to withstand destruction.

All corn is very similar to wheat gluten. Corn contains an amino acid sequence that resembles wheat gluten peptides. As you know, wheat peptides bind to the brain's morphine receptors in a similar way to opiates (you get high) and may play a role in migraines and schizophrenia.

Antibodies are formed to attack gluten (specifically, alpha-gliadin 33-mer) in people with celiac disease because the body identifies gluten as a foreign invader. And, as you learned in the section on cross-reactions, because corn is similar to gluten, the antibodies attack corn in a similar way. So even without eating gluten, people with celiac disease may get the same inflammatory response from their immune systems when they eat corn.[284]

Now here is the terrible part. Corn is a common "gluten substitute" for hundreds of gluten-free products. This may explain why so many people on gluten-free diets never get better. In many cases, they get worse.[285] How frustrating would that be? The inflammation may be similar to MSG since the high levels of glutamate in corn were once used to create MSG. Processed corn products will contain high levels of free glutamic acid, and you know that's bad. A study out of Milano, Italy says the use of corn for gluten-sensitive people must be reevaluated.[286] I couldn't agree more.

French fries are not recommended for gluten-sensitive people—even from potatoes that aren't sprinkled with gluten—because potatoes are generally fried in corn oil. Don't think that you'll avoid corn oil by frying up "vegetable oil." The food industry labels corn oil as a vegetable oil, even though corn is not a vegetable. What kind of poppycock is that? People are exposed to the harmful effects of processed corn and don't even think about it. Doesn't vegetable oil sound healthy? Like it might even contain vegetables?

High-Fructose Corn Syrup

We've known since the 1970s that high-fructose corn syrup is bad stuff—horrifyingly bad stuff. Even so, the use of high-fructose corn syrup increased 1,000% from 1970 to 1990 and now represents 40% of the sweeteners added to food. It mimics MSG by not stimulating leptin production (that thing that tells you to stop eating or you will need to buy a new pair of fat pants) and is a well-known factor in our rise in obesity.[287] Processed corn contains high levels of free glutamic acid. People gain weight, stay hungry, and experience huge sugar spikes. Everyone knows corn syrup is bad, but maybe people don't know just how bad it truly is—or how pervasive it is.

Hidden Corn

Corn is hidden in all kinds of ingredients, and that hidden corn increases our insulin production to a point of changing our body chemistry so we retain more and more fat. And that makes it harder and harder to lose weight. Meanwhile, most people believe that fat people are simply fat because they're lazy. Look at this long list of ingredients that may contain corn, and it becomes easy to spot how people are spinning their wheels in the opposite direction of weight loss.

Ingredients that may contain corn/corn allergen list:[288]

Acetic acid
Alcohol
Alpha-tocopherol
Artificial flavorings
Artificial sweeteners
  (aspartame, saccharin,
  Splenda, sucralose, etc.)
Ascorbates
Ascorbic acid
Astaxanthin
Baking powder
Barley malt (generally OK,
  but it can be contaminated)
Bleached flour
Blended sugar (sugar
  dextrose)
Brown sugar (generally OK
  if no caramel color)
Calcium citrate
Calcium fumarate
Calcium gluconate
Calcium lactate
Calcium magnesium acetate
  (CMA)
Calcium stearate
Calcium stearoyl lactylate
Caramel and caramel color

Carboxymethylcellulose
  sodium
Cellulose, powdered
Cetearyl glucoside
Choline chloride
Citric acid
Citrus cloud emulsion (CCS)
Cocoglycerides
Confectioners' sugar
  /powdered sugar
Corn alcohol, corn gluten
Corn extract
Corn flour
Corn oil, corn oil margarine
Corn starch
Corn sweetener, corn sugar
Corn syrup, corn syrup
  solids
Corn, popcorn, cornmeal
Cornstarch, corn flour
Croscarmellose sodium
Crystalline dextrose
Crystalline fructose
Cyclodextrin
DATEM (a dough
  conditioner)
Decyl glucoside

Decyl polyglucose
Dextrin
Dextrose (also found in IV solutions)
Dextrose anything (such as monohydrate or anhydrous)
D-Gluconic acid
Distilled white vinegar
Drying agents
Erythorbic acid
Erythritol
Ethanol
Ethocel 20
Ethyl cellulose
Ethylene
Ethyl acetate
Ethyl alcohol
Ethyl lactate
Ethyl maltol
Fibersol-2
Flavorings
Food starch
Fructose
Fruit juice concentrate
Fumaric acid
Germ/germ meal
Gluconate/gluconic acid
Glucono delta-lactone (GDL)
Gluconolactone
Glucosamine
Glucose
Glucose syrup (also found in IV solutions)
Glutamate
Gluten
Gluten feed/meal
Glycerides
Glycerin
Glycerol

Golden syrup/treacle
Grits
High-fructose corn syrup
Hominy
Honey
Hydrolyzed corn
Hydrolyzed corn protein
Hydrolyzed vegetable protein
Hydroxypropyl methylcellulose
Hydroxypropyl methylcellulose phthalate (HPMCP)
Inositol
Invert syrup or sugar
Iodized salt
Lactate
Lactic acid
Lauryl glucoside
Lecithin
Linoleic acid
Lysine
Magnesium citrate
Magnesium fumarate
Magnesium stearate
Maize
Malic acid
Malonic acid
Malt syrup from corn
Malt, malt extract
Maltitol
Maltodextrin
Maltol
Maltose
Mannitol
Methyl cellulose
Methyl gluceth
Methyl glucose
Methylglucoside

- Microcrystalline cellulose
- Modified cellulose gum
- Modified corn starch
- Modified food starch
- Molasses (corn syrup may be present; know your product)
- Mono- diglycerides and diglycerides
- Monosodium glutamate (MSG)
- Natural flavorings
- Olestra/Olean
- Polenta
- Polydextrose
- Polylactic acid (PLA)
- Polysorbates (e.g., polysorbate 80)
- Polyvinyl acetate
- Potassium citrate
- Potassium fumarate
- Potassium gluconate
- Pregelatinized starch
- Propionic acid
- Propylene glycol
- Propylene glycol monostearate
- Semolina (unless from wheat)
- Simethicone
- Sodium carboxymethylcellulose
- Sodium citrate
- Sodium erythorbate
- Sodium fumarate
- Sodium lactate
- Sodium starch glycolate
- Sodium stearoyl fumarate
- Sorbate
- Sorbic acid
- Sorbitan (all forms)
- Sorbitol
- Sorghum (not all is bad, but the syrup and/or grain *can* be mixed with corn)
- Starch (any kind that's not specified)
- Stearic acid
- Sterols
- Sucrose
- Sugar (not identified as cane or beet)
- Threonine
- Tocopherol (vitamin E)
- Triethyl citrate
- Unmodified starch
- Vanilla, natural flavoring
- Vanilla, pure or extract
- Vanillin
- Vinegar, distilled white
- Vinyl acetate
- Vitamin C and vitamin E
- Vitamins
- Xanthan gum
- Xylitol
- Yeast
- Zein
- Zea mays

Here's a good rule of thumb: If it's processed, there's a good chance there's corn in it. We probably cannot avoid eating all processed foods, but we can avoid some and eat more real food. On a side note, if you're having a hard time killing ants with deadly chemicals, go for something with a little more kick. Throw popcorn seeds in a blender and grind them up. Take the powder (i.e., cornmeal) and set it down for the ants to eat. They will all die.

Of course this doesn't mean that corn is bad for you altogether. Corn is bad for you because it's a major migraine trigger, highly allergenic, responsible for a large portion of the obesity epidemic, and not recommended for gluten-sensitive people. Corn is inflammatory, and processed corn products are highly inflammatory. Corn is a major headache factor in the growing Western headache diet.

Chronic Trigger #10: Soy

If you're a vegetarian or vegan or hippie or some combination of those three, please don't read this. I know how much you all love soy, but it's a top headache trigger. I apologize for the bad news. Soy protein has 17,000 mg of glutamic acid per 100 g (that's more than a lot). To be fair, you're not going to straight-up consume 100 g of soy protein—unless you're bulking up with protein shakes.

On the other hand, you can easily consume 100 g of whole soybeans with a whopping 7,000 mg of glutamic acid. This is more than double the amount of a gluten product like French bread. That's the highest amount of naturally produced glutamic acid found in any food. And get this—soy was also once used to make MSG.

Now, this next sentence will really upset all of our veggie/hippie friends: Tofu from soybeans (kori-dofu) has 9,500 mg of glutamic acid! Some tofu and soy products contain very little glutamic acid, but they are processed, and that means they include "free glutamic acid." Let's put this in perspective. When monkeys are given a total of 20 g of free glutamic acid in one-gram MSG doses, they develop brain lesions within five days. Those little boxes of tofu are about 400 g. If you eat the whole box, you will have ingested almost 40 g of free glutamic acid in one sitting! This is scary. But you're no baby monkey; you shouldn't get brain lesions, right? How about headaches?[289]

The Asthma and Allergy Foundation of America estimates that soy is among the eight most common allergens.[290] Soy causes an overreaction to the immune system that may lead to severe physical symptoms for millions of people. Soy was first reported allergenic in

1934. A small number of fatal reactions to soy have been reported.[291] Any top allergen could also be a top headache trigger.

Studies show severe villous atrophy as a result of intolerance to as many as 28 soybean proteins. According to Medscape, "The degree of villous atrophy may be similar to that found in celiac disease."[292] All of this information is a disappointment because many people attempting a healthier diet go to soy products. But sadly, soy is a major headache trigger, it's outrageously high in glutamic acid, it's hard on your stomach, and it's highly allergenic.

Other Headache Triggers to Avoid

Though the headache triggers listed here are not necessarily heavy hitters or chronic triggers, they are still major sources of migraines for a lot of people. They don't fall into this "other" category because they're not important. The triggers detailed here are no joke. And this is where we start getting into more of the migraine triggers that are not related to food.

Headache Trigger #1: Biogenic Amines

> *My English might not be very good, because I am from Germany, but I have had migraines for 20 years and I have found the cause for my migraines…and* **haven't had a single migraine since***. When I told my doctor I no longer get migraines when I avoid histamines, she said it is well known that histamines cause migraines. But none of my doctors who I have visited in the last 20 years has ever told me, that is the reason for my posting. I want to let other people know that it's worth a try.*
>
> *Best wishes,*
>
> *Annette*[293]

Annette is one of thousands of documented migraine sufferers treated for the symptoms of migraines instead of the cause. And Annette's doctor was right, because histamines, and all of the other amines, are often responsible for triggering migraines. Let's go back to Parma, Italy with the highest prevalence of migraines in the world and where the citizens consume heavy amounts of Parma ham. Parma ham has four ingredients: meat from Italian pigs, salt, air, and time. It cures, hanging from the ceiling, for one to three years, and as it ages, its biogenic amines grow.[294]

Aged cheese also grows biogenic amines. We can rapidly digest these foods with biogenic amines because they are not bound to fiber and nutrients, which is the case with spinach. This means that even small amounts could trigger a migraine. In susceptible individuals, the 4 mg of histamine from a glass of sparkling wine has caused negative reactions.[295] These amines all add up, so a meal in

Other Headache Triggers to Avoid

Italy that includes Parma ham, cheese, pasta, bread, and wine truly tests the headache threshold!

Once again, it's processed food that's dangerous to the headache threshold. The top headache triggers in the biogenic amine category include anything canned, jarred, fermented, pickled, aged, or spoiled. There's also the problem of tyramines. You'll find tyramines in old cheeses, processed meats, leftovers from two days ago, wines, pickles, olives, overripe bananas and avocados, chocolate, and soybeans. Tyramines can trigger headaches. The foods that contain them are on hundreds of headache trigger lists.

Tyramine, histamine, phenylethylamine, and all of the other amines may raise the levels of glutamate and inflammation in the brain, but they're also critical in maintaining the natural levels of neurotransmitters, such as glutamate, serotonin, and dopamine. Your brain is not a mop bucket of chemicals. All of these chemicals act together in a symphony of crescendos and decrescendos in very specific areas of your brain—the specific areas that we do not have the technology to fully understand.[296]

So what does modern medicine do with this lack of understanding? It throws a bucket of chemicals at the brain and hopes for the best. Monoamine oxidase inhibitors (MAOIs) were the first drugs for treating depression. Pay attention now, because this may hold the secret to migraines. Scientists knew depressed people needed more serotonin and amines to raise their levels of the happy chemical dopamine. Eureka! MAOI drugs inhibit the breakdown of both serotonin and amines, all the while raising dopamine levels, which will make you happy or numb, depending on whom you ask.

During the 1960s, a British pharmacist noticed that his wife developed headaches every time she ate cheese while taking an

MAOI antidepressant. This became known as the "cheese effect," and, as it turned out, the headache was simply a trigger for the tyramine-induced hypertensive crises that often followed her consumption of either cheese or draft beer.[297]

Today, dietary restrictions while taking MAOIs include: aged cheeses and meats, banana peels, spoiled meats, soybean products, and draft beers. All migraine triggers, right? But what do tyramine-restrictive diets allow? Avocados, bananas, chocolate, fresh or mild cheese, meats, and properly stored and pickled foods when consumed in moderation. The ill effects of this drug gave us a headache of insight into overdosing on tyramine since the first symptoms of hypertensive (high blood pressure) crises include headaches.

Here comes the defining moment of stupidity: Some doctors prescribe MAOIs as a migraine treatment. In addition, some doctors don't acknowledge that foods may trigger migraines. Those doctors then often prescribe a drug that magnifies our top food triggers, because they don't believe food triggers exist. An average unmedicated person would need to eat two pounds of cheese in 30 minutes to induce a rise in blood pressure. No sane person would eat two pounds of cheese in 30 minutes.

Thus, for most individuals, tyramine is not an issue. A patient on certain MAOIs may only eat 50 g (two slices) of cheese before it induces hypertension and headaches. Those two slices of cheese are the threshold that migraine sufferers should look at, because we don't know how these amine-rich foods are triggering headaches.

It is true that there are no conclusive studies on why amine-rich foods trigger headaches.[298] Pulling amines out of food and testing them alone doesn't work. This is because a food could contain multiple amines and multiple amino acids. The breakdown of amino acids can produce more amines. For example, measuring the Parmesan sprinkles on a pizza isn't going to tell you anything about the high levels of glutamic acid in the pizza crust or in the other amine-rich ingredients that will all add up to break the headache threshold. Some processed foods contain a bundle of amines and amine-reactive substances, such as tyramine, phenylethylamine, histamine, nitrites, and sulfites. Add all of these amines together with processed wheat, soy, MSG, and corn, and you may have the headache trigger of a highly processed combination pizza.

We do know that "amines are involved in the mechanism of food intolerance"; we just don't know exactly why.[299] But when we start looking at the digestion of amines and how it relates to headaches, things get fascinating. This is extraordinarily exciting. Amines are processed in your gut and become detoxified as they enter the bloodstream. There are full amines in the gut, oxidation happens in the gut lining, and the proper amount of filtered amines enters the blood. The enzyme that prevents the toxic buildup of amines is called monoamine oxidase (MAO). Do you see how incredible this is for migraineurs?

MAOI antidepressant drugs are not the only way to screw up the detoxification of amines. The negative effects of amines (tachycardia, hypertension, increased blood sugar, headaches, migraines, etc.) depend on the amount ingested, individual susceptibility, and the health of your gut. These are three known factors in today's limited understanding of amines.[300]

Your individual susceptibility is your genetic ability to produce MAOs and DAOs—another amine enzyme. Yet another reason that migraineurs have a higher probability of passing headaches on to their children. You can do something about that gene, but you'll read about that later. For now, we'll worry about the health of your gut.

We know that a leaky gut may pose a number of problems for migraineurs—from the increased number of food allergies to more frequent and severe headaches. Now we can add the inability to detoxify amines to the migraineur's leaky list of problems. Alcohol is especially of concern to amine toxicity because it increases the permeability of the intestinal wall. This happens when we drink alcohol that contains amines and when we pair alcohol with amine-rich foods.

Alcohol opens the gut's door and says, "Come on in, amines, conditions are perfect." Getting extremely drunk may inhibit stomach digestion altogether, a term known as "gastroparesis," which is why some alcoholics vomit undigested food that they don't even remember eating the night before. This is an example of just how inflammatory alcohol can be on your gut.

Smoking is another risk factor as it enhances the probability of suffering amine-associated symptoms. Cigarette smokers show a 30% reduction in their MAO abilities.[301] As my friend Dr. Dani says, "If you smoke and have migraines, you should quit, and if you smoke and don't have migraines, you should quit." Maybe you can't stop smoking or drinking or change your unlucky genes; however, you may still have a fighting chance. Lucky for you, the largest factor is the number of amines you ingest.

The Amine Content of Foods

We want maximum food pleasure with minimum amines. There are some foods we don't need to sacrifice as long as we eat them from the right package. With other foods, we may say something like, "I know this may give me a headache, and I don't care, but I will not eat a second slice, and I will not wash it down with amine-rich beer," or "I will do whatever I want, and I will know exactly where my pleasure and pain came from."

Bear in mind that this is not an exact science, and the amine content in foods is directly influenced by which company makes the food as well as the type and freshness of the food. Here, I've broken down all of the amine-rich headache triggers, which is something you've never seen. Not only are these lists not found on the internet, but studies have yet to combine the limited amount of amine information we do have. Yeah. Everyone tells us to limit amines, but no one tells us where the highest concentrations are. Don't worry about the numbers at first. I'm going to throw a lot of information at you, but it's summarized for easy digestion. If you have read a number of articles in this area, you will soon question the integrity of the almighty internet and most of those giving migraine-related dietary advice.

Take a look at the histamine and tyramine levels of these fresh vegetables from a 2005 study:[302]

Food (100 g)	Histamine (mg)	Tyramine (mg)
Broad beans	0.2	1.0
Broccoli	0	0
Cucumbers	0	0.2
Lettuce	0	0.1
Parsley	0	0
Spinach	2.0	0.8
Tomatoes	0.7	0.2

Not really that impressive. They recorded 0 mg for vegetables with less than 0.05 mg of histamine or tyramine. There was a list of other vegetables not worthy of mentioning that had minimal amounts of amines. Let's see what happens when we leave a few veggies out to rot. These are three of those vegetables after three weeks of aging:

Food (100 g)	Histamine (mg)	Tyramine (mg)
Broccoli	0.2 mg	0.3 mg
Cucumbers	0 mg	0.1 mg
Parsley	0 mg	0.2 mg

What happened? Not much. The amines in parsley and broccoli went up a little, and the amines in cucumbers actually went down. So what about all those migraine articles that attack fruits and vegetables with amines?

I expected a heavy rise from amines in preserved vegetables. Tomato sauce had only a trace of histamine and 0.4 mg of tyramine—less than that of a fresh tomato. But don't think it's OK to eat all the tomato sauce you want; it's still heavy in free glutamic acid and whatever else is hidden in the can. Other preserved vegetables showed no real difference until they tested sauerkraut.

Food (100 g)	Histamine (mg)	Tyramine (mg)
Cabbage	0	0.3
Sauerkraut	1.3	4.9

So cabbage is just fine, but once you turn it into sauerkraut, its amines skyrocket. Sauerkraut has 16 times the tyramine of cabbage. The reason: Sauerkraut is fermented. Some commercial sauerkraut averages 5.1 mg of histamine per 100 g, although many brands average under 0.1 mg per 100 g. The low-histamine sauerkraut typically goes through a shorter fermentation process. You probably won't be able to find out how long your store-bought sauerkraut was fermented, so if you're going to eat it, you may be eating dangerous levels of amines.[303]

The 2005 study concluded that fresh and preserved vegetables do not pose a risk for healthy consumers, with the exception of fermented foods.

OJ

You already know orange juice is a wicked heavy hitter, but let's talk a little more about how the synephrine added to commercial orange juice can increase its biogenic amine levels.[304]

A 2007 study out of Brazil checked the amines in seven brands of orange juice. Histamine ranged from 0.03 mg to 0.26 mg per liter, and tyramine ranged from 0.02 mg to 0.67 mg per liter.[305] We're talking about liters now. A liter is a measure of volume, so you can have a liter of Coke, water, juice, or sand, and each item will be one liter. The tyramine before was taken from 100 g of food, and that is a measure of weight. A kilogram is 1,000 g and a liter of water happens to be 1,000 kilograms. But a liter of soda or sand will weigh more than 1,000 kilograms. So a liter is at least 10 times more than our 100-gram samples of food.

So 0.67 mg of tyramine per liter is not a huge concern, but because this is processed, your body may digest it much faster. You should consider even small amounts of amines in processed liquids a threat.

The OJs tested in this study also contained the amine synephrine. Synephrine ranged from 10.1 mg to 21.8 mg per liter. That means the most potent orange juice they tested had over 30 times more synephrine than tyramine. You already know synephrine is bad—and sure, its adrenaline-like substance is found in orange skin, but the way commercial orange juice is made isn't natural, and it's dangerous for migraineurs. Even with low histamine and tyramine, OJ's synephrine content poses a giant headache threat.

Raspberry Juice

Raspberry juice makes OJ look like baby stuff. A study done in the 1990s showed raspberry juice has 66.66 mg of tyramine per liter.[306] Take a look at how that stacks up against OJ:

Juice per Liter	Tyramine (mg)
Orange juice	0.02–0.67
Raspberry juice	66.66

Is it possible to have a raspberry juice with 100 times the amount of tyramine as orange juice? Yes. One study showed that whole raspberries range from 1.3 mg to 9.3 mg of tyramine per 100 g. We're back to 100 g again, which is basically 10% of a liter. A later study tested multiple samples and found that fresh and frozen raspberries range from zero to 2.1 mg of tyramine per 100 g, with frozen raspberries being slightly more potent. The raspberries that registered with zero tyramine were fresh, but they began to show minimal amounts of tyramine four days later.[307] Given that fresh and frozen raspberries have a tyramine range that high, you can imagine that the pounds of raspberries required for commercially squeezed juice will have a wider range of potency.

Other Headache Triggers to Avoid

Do we really need to add raspberries to the towering list of things we can't eat? Despite their tyramine content, raspberries were deemed safe for those who can't properly digest tyramine. While raspberries are on many migraine trigger lists, some resources list raspberries as a headache helper because they contain vitamin C and antioxidants.

Raspberries are higher on the allergenic scale than most fruits, which doesn't say much considering that all fruits are low on the allergy totem pole. Raspberries have the potential to contain 9.3 mg of tyramine per 100 g or no tyramine at all. Raspberries are a risk. If you take the risk, just make sure the raspberries are organic and fresh. And don't put a kilo of raspberries in the blender. You could also switch from raspberries to cranberries. Cranberry juice was found to have zero tyramine.

Bananas

What about bananas? Bananas are kind of like chocolate, a well-documented migraine trigger with little scientific data. Dr. Buchholz, author of *Heal Your Headache*, is adamant that bananas are a top trigger for many of his patients. And if you look at the reviews of his book, patients are also saying that bananas cause migraines, but no one knows exactly why.

The same fresh raspberry study I mentioned earlier found that fresh bananas contained zero tyramine, while the overripe banana jumped the tyramine up to 1.3 mg per 100 g.

Food (100 mg)	Tyramine (mg)
Fresh banana	0
Overripe banana	1.3

The fresh banana may not have contained tyramine in the pulp, but a single peel had 1.42 mg. Just the skin (30 g) of an overripe banana had 2.58 mg of tyramine. It appeared the tyramine had increased, but the study noted that this could easily have been from the variability of content in bananas. The study concluded that the pulp from an overripe banana is very safe for those who have a hard time processing tyramine.

This doesn't make sense. Most lists of headache triggers say not to eat overripe bananas (and avocados) because of the tyramine. What really happens to an overripe banana? This question was answered in 2005 when a study looked into the ripening effects of Prata bananas, a popular banana out of Brazil—one of the world's largest producers of bananas.

Green bananas have a pulp to peel ratio of 1.49, which is another way of saying 60% banana pulp and 40% peel. As green bananas ripen, the sugar in them continues to increase until the skin becomes yellow and the pulp is sweet. Two ripe bananas equal about the sugar of a can of Coke. As the sugar is made, osmotic pressure sucks in the water from the peel, creating a pulp to peel ratio of 2.36, which is another way of saying 70% banana pulp and 30% peel. Banana pulp went up, and the peel went down.[308]

Why do we care if the banana pulp becomes infused with the peel? For one, we don't want more tyramine. Keep that garbage inside the peel. We also don't want pesticides or any of the other vasoactive substances that are found in higher concentrations in the skin, including serotonin, dopamine, and noradrenaline.

I love all three of these. Serotonin and dopamine are happy brain chemicals mixed in with the upper of noradrenaline (fight or flight). Brain serotonin actually relieves migraines, but apparently the serotonin in bananas does not cross the blood-brain barrier.[309] The problem is that we don't know exactly how these substances affect headache sufferers when mixed with tyramine.

Now back to tyramine. Is tyramine from fresh fruits and vegetables a true headache threat? Check out these tyramine numbers referenced in a 2005 study, all from 100-gram samples:

Food (100 mg)	Tyramine (mg)
Avocados	2.3
Banana pulp	0.7
Orange pulp	1.0
Tomatoes	0.4
Spinach (multiple samples)	0.4–3.2

Spinach has the highest amine levels, and more headache resources list it as a headache preventative than as a headache trigger. Some of the foods listed above could be triggers for you, despite their low levels of tyramine, but that's probably because there's more in them that causes you headaches than the tyramine.[310] The amine levels in all fruits and vegetables are considered much safer than other types of food.

Fish

Let's take a look at the amine levels in a few types of fish:

Food (per 100 g)	Histamine (mg)	Tyramine (mg)
Fresh fish	2.34	6.18
Fish (two days old)	20.9	19.8

Tuna (canned)	2,000	0
Smoked mackerel	1,788	0
Anchovies (canned)	1,625	?
Sardines (canned)	850	?

Note: "?" indicates the food was not tested, whereas "0" indicates the food has zero mg of tyramine.

Canned tuna and smoked mackerel also have large amounts of the amines putrescine and cadaverine, which are pretty gross and may produce similar amine problems. Studies show that amines in fish will increase when stored at room temperature, raise slightly when cooled, and become stable at subzero temperatures. This makes canned fish especially dangerous.[311] Fish aged in salt will fare better than fish aged in oil. However, both brined fish and fish aged in oil will form histamines at room temperature.[312]

A biogenic amine study on salted Korean fish found that there were few changes in fish when stored at cool temperatures. However, one brand had a substantial increase in amines when stored for more than 10 days. This may relate to the quality of the packaging and storage process.[313]

High-quality canned tuna may produce low numbers of amines. The 2,000 mg of histamine per 100 g of tuna is ridiculous. In fact, far lower histamine numbers are documented in food poisoning cases of tuna, meaning not every brand and can are equal. This is a problem. The European Food Safety Authority out of Parma, Italy, found that the fish and fish products it tested had amine totals of 8 to 9 mg/100 g. That's not bad because "total amines" included histamine, tyramine, putrescine, and cadaverine—all of the amines combined. But when we look at the top 5% of the heaviest amine-producing fish and fish products from the same study, the amine totals jump to 55–57 mg/100 g.[314]

Food (100 mg)	Total Amines (mg)
Fish and fish products	8–9
Top 5% of fish and fish products	55–57

This kind of variance is the problem with *all* processed foods. A small percentage will contain dangerous risks, and we have no clue which brands are dangerous. You just need to ask yourself one question while eating processed foods: "Do I feel lucky?"

Alcohol

You've probably already read enough bad news about booze, but the amine levels in beer and wine are noteworthy. Here are the results from a few studies:[315,316,317]

Fermented Drinks per Liter	Histamine (mg)	Tyramine (mg)
Wine	25	19
Red wine	19.6	18.2
White wine	1.1	2.3
Beer	3.0–8.8	3.6–10.5
Beer (Becks)	?	1
Draft beer	?	27–113
Multiple white wine study	3–120	?
Multiple red wine study	60–3,800	?
Multiple beers study	21–52	?

The study with draft beer noted that "storage and contamination of the hose from the keg to the tap may provide conditions conducive to the production of tyramine." I only buy that tyramine explanation to an extent. Anyone who has seen wine or beer made knows that thousands of ingredients and combinations of those ingredients change everything about the final product. It is possible that once a keg is opened, the amine levels can rise just as they do with food, but we will never know until a study compares canned beers to their kegged versions.

I bet you could test 100 different beers and 100 different wines and you would have nearly 200 different levels of amines. Just as the sulfites in wine vary drastically (which you'll see when you get to the chapter on sulfites), amines vary with all types of alcohol. So don't drink beer, but when you do, drink Beck's. Amines belong in the list of congeners, so they may contribute to hangovers. Don't forget how acetaldehyde tears up the stomach and formaldehyde may leave you blind. Multiple factors in alcohol make consuming amines dangerous, but not quite as dangerous as what you'll read next.

Soy

Some interesting soy information from multiple samples:[318,319]

Soy Products per Liter	Histamine (mg)	Tyramine (mg)
Soy products (fermented)	4,620	35,680
Soy sauce (sample 1)	?	293
Soy sauce (sample 2)	?	878
Soy sauce (Kilman)	?	941
Soy milk	?	2
Tofu (100 g)	?	.80

Look at these numbers! They say not to eat an overripe banana because it has 1.3 mg of tyramine per 100 g. They say to watch out for red wine because it has 18.2 mg per liter. And if that's not bad enough, something as seemingly innocent as raspberries have 67 mg of tyramine per liter. But now, here are these fermented soy products with an unimaginable 35,680 mg of tyramine per liter. Even the soy sauce with the least amount of tyramine (293 mg) is way too much. Fish sauce, shrimp sauce, and the like reveal similarly high amine numbers.

The fermented soy (e.g., soy sauce and Asian pastes and seasonings) also has about six times as much putrescine as canned tuna, 14 times as much putrescine as raw blue cheese, 123 times as much putrescine as red wine, and 1,000 times as much putrescine as most vegetables.

We know amines may combine to break the headache threshold, and soy sauce has high numbers of multiple amines. Soy products are very dangerous, and many cause the "Chinese food headache." Even a splash of amines in concentrations this high will be dangerous. Soy milk and tofu may seem innocent, but they have unnaturally large amounts of free glutamic acid and a number of other amino acids that may impact an amine headache.

Meat

Moving on to meat. Take a look at these numbers:[320][321]

Meat (100 g)	Histamine (mg)	Tyramine (mg)
Dry fermented sausage	5.7	27.3
Italian sausage	0	21.4
Fresh meat	0	3.8

Pork	0.14	1.8
Chicken	?	0.83
Chicken liver	?	0.63
Chicken liver (aged nine days)	?	213
Pastrami (deli 1)	?	1
Pastrami (deli 2)	?	6.9
Cooked ham	?	0.43
Cured ham	11.4	10.4
Chorizo	1.8	28.2
Salami	?	3.9–18

Fresh meat is usually safe. Fermented or aged meats are usually not. Typical deli meats are either made with preservatives or cured with a fermentation process. Don't confuse deli meats with meats from an actual deli. Many delis have high-quality fresh meats that are not preserved or fermented, and if you want to stay away from tyramine, those are the meats to eat. Just take a look at what happens to chicken liver after nine days at room temperature:

Meat (100 mg)	**Tyramine (mg)**
Chicken liver	0.63
Chicken liver (aged nine days)	213

A previous study found that fresh chicken liver with zero tyramine went up to 0.51 mg per 100 g when stored in the fridge for five days. Clearly, leftovers are a bad idea. Something to think about the next time you're in a sandwich shop or picking at a party platter with cheese, crackers, and meats that have been left out in the sun. The thought of old meat is repulsing, but when we age meat, enzymes break it down, which brings out flavors that simply weren't there before. Many fine restaurants let beef sit from days to months to improve its taste.

In addition to the foregoing, studies note that air-dried sausage and salami should be avoided as they contain microorganisms that can convert amino acids (tyrosine) into tyramine during the drying process; however, all sausage seems to be on the same dangerous level. With unreal flavors come unnatural levels of unwanted byproducts. Don't eat aged and preserved meats. Just don't.

Remember that the biogenic amines in aged meats are growing unnatural biogenic amines with time. They are an unbound science project, unlike the amines in lettuce or even fresh tuna. And they typically are rich in the other amines that impact glutamate levels, such as putrescine and cadaverine. For example, the European Food Safety Authority found the total biogenic amines in sausage averages 28 mg per 100 g, yet the average goes above 89 mg per 100 g in a small percentage tested.[322]

Dairy

Here is some interesting dairy information:[323]

Dairy (100 g)	Histamine (mg)	Tyramine (mg)
Yogurt	1.3	0
Feta cheese	84.6	24.6
Goat cheese (pasteurized)	0.63	1.09
Goat cheese (raw)	4.31	32.46
Blue cheese (pasteurized)	12.7	52.66
Blue cheese (raw)	104.1	105.1

Milk cheese (raw)	11.08	23.33
Milk cheese (raw/ripe)	51.92	45.37
Milk cheese (pasteurized)	6.02	2.2
Milk cheese (pasteurized/ripe)	6.54	30.1
Mozzarella (pasteurized)	?	1
Mozzarella (five days old)	?	1

Cheese has high amounts of the amines putrescine and cadaverine. Amines seem to rise when cheese is unpasteurized and aged. The blue in blue cheese turned me off at a young age. My mother told me that the blue was a form of mold, and I immediately associated it with the time I accidently sipped from a jug of rotten milk. I couldn't even tell anyone, because you never want to let anyone know you sip straight from the milk jug.

Years later, I slowly grew to love blue cheese and all of the old stinky cheeses, which is why I don't like this list. Raw blue cheese has 105.1 mg of tyramine. Absolutely don't eat aged meat, like salami, they say. And with 4–18 mg of tyramine, they're right. Raw blue cheese has more than five times the tyramine of salami and 80 times the tyramine of an overripe banana. This clearly shows that ripened or unpasteurized cheeses are dangerous for headache sufferers.

Mozzarella that was part skim milk and pasteurized seemed to beat the odds. We usually find that over processing food makes it more of a headache trigger. But in the case of cheese, low-fat content and pasteurization seem to lower the tyramine levels. Because most people lack enough enzymes to properly digest milk and many are allergic to milk, migraine sufferers should avoid all cheese and dairy products.

Olives and Pickled Foods

Here's what a couple of food studies report about olives and pickled food:[324] [325]

Food (100 g)	Histamine (mg)	Tyramine (mg)
Spanish-style green olives	0	0–0.26
Uncured black olives	0	0.02–0.21
Ripe olives (can)	0	0
Capers (bottled)	0–3.7mg	0.02
Pickles (cucumber)	0	0.07

Ripe black olives are washed, creating an oxidation process that removes amines. Multiple olives and pickled food samples were used in these combined studies, and about half did not contain amines, with the exception of uncured olives. No one wants to eat bitter, uncured black olives. Besides, all of the amine levels here are of little concern.

But take a look at how these pickled foods fared in a Turkish study:[326]

Pickled Food (100 mg)	Histamine (mg)
Mixed vegetables	1.7–5.8
Hot peppers	2.0–7.5
Pickles (cucumbers)	2.7–4.5

These results are considerably lower than pickled foods like sauerkraut, which averages 5 mg per 100 g. One study reported sauerkraut histamine levels as high as 22.9 mg per 100 g. Both this

Turkish study and the study that measured the amine levels in Spanish olives noted that the quality of the fermentation process plays a large part in lowering overall amines. Quality standards involve factors such as temperature, brining (salting), and packaging.

Concerns about eating pickled food have recently been in the spotlight due to a rise in cancer in Asian populations that love pickled foods. One 2012 review examined over 30 studies that showed a positive association between stomach cancer and pickled foods, with the strongest association in Korea and China.[327] The study suggested a potential 50% higher risk of gastric cancer associated with the intake of pickled foods. Many people refute this fact in the United States, because we eat fewer pickled foods than they do in China or Korea.

Our pickled foods typically come from commercial distributors that use precise measurements and pasteurization processes. In some parts of rural China, they actually pickle foods in the ground. We have known since the days of Columbus that pickled foods need a certain amount of salt to stay preserved over a long period of time. This was vital for the long journey to America, because preserved pickles, rich in vitamin C, prevented sailors from dying of scurvy.

We can speculate that pickles in the United States are fine, but we don't know for sure because information on amines is extremely limited. I went to great lengths to find this information; it is not made public by the companies that profit from our consumption of their food. Pickle juice can definitely be harsh on the stomachs of some. I recently visited an old group of friends in New York. We all had picklebacks, a fairly popular drink in Brooklyn. A pickleback is a shot of whiskey with pickle juice to back it up. Sounds terrible, but it is disgustingly good. We all had a couple except for one Brooklynite by the name of Bob.

Bob said he couldn't do it. He physically could not drink it. Bob likes pickles and he loves whiskey, but every time he drinks a pickleback, he immediately becomes sick to his stomach. Not the next morning—immediately. It seems most people can only stomach a few of these gut bombs. In comparison to other amine-rich foods, pickled foods are considered safe and can be eaten in moderation. I would suggest not eating pickled foods as part of an elimination diet. Reintroduce them with caution and an awareness of how you feel. A pickleback is certainly a bad idea.

Beans

Here is what you need to know about black beans:[328][329]

Food (100 g)	Histamine (mg)	Tyramine (mg)
Black beans (fermented)	?	45
Black bean ("douchi")	29–81	?

"Douchi" black beans are actually black soybeans, and they too are fermented. Why would you want fermented beans? It's not as strange as you might think. Soaking beans overnight starts the fermentation process to make the beans softer and easier on the stomach. (At this point, we're going off the biogenic amine topic, because looking at foods as a whole gives you an understanding of how their amines could break the headache threshold in combination with other factors, such as antinutrients.)

Oligosaccharide is a sugar that we don't have the enzymes to break down. These sugars begin to rot in the stomach and give us terrible gas. Soaking beans and periodically discarding the water gets rid of oligosaccharides, lectins, and other antinutrients. Antinutrients are a natural defense mechanism that protects the seeds from predators like you and me until the seeds are ready to sprout. Not only does soaking beans break down the antinutrients, it makes the nutrients inside the bean accessible for digestion.

In 1988, a hospital launched "healthy eating day" in its cafeteria and served 31 portions of red kidney beans to staff.[330] At 3:00 p.m., one of the surgeons vomited in the operating theater. Over the next four hours, 10 more hospital workers suffered from profuse vomiting. It was found that the beans were high in lectins. Some lectins are toxic, inflammatory, and resistant to cooking and digestive enzymes. However, lectins are easily blocked from binding to the cells by oligosaccharide.[331] That should make your head spin.

So do we soak beans to remove lectins, or do we not soak beans to keep the oligosaccharides that block the lectins? We don't want the oligosaccharides in the first place because they can create gas and headache problems. It would seem that soaking beans would cancel out the lectins and the oligosaccharides, but many of the lectins will remain, and this is especially true of soybeans. And this takes us to the general theme of the Paleolithic diet: It may not be healthy for us to eat certain types of foods if we don't have the ability to produce the enzymes to digest them.

It certainly isn't what I want to hear about beans. Beans are double-edged swords. On one hand, beans are a staple food of low cost and steady energy, fiber, magnesium, protein, selenium, folate, and iron. They are also making a comeback with popular new diets like *The 4-Hour Body* diet plan. Known as part of a "slow-carb diet," beans give sustained energy without the "crash" that comes with many unhealthy carbohydrate-cutting diets.

Other Headache Triggers to Avoid

I've taken lectins out of context in this section. Many natural foods include lectins, and not all are going to kill you. Countless studies show that some lectins, especially in high quantities, have the ability to damage the gut.[332,333] Others, like okra lectins, have recently been found to kill breast cancer cells.[334] Many people do fine with the high levels of lectins in beans, while some even have trouble with the limited amount of lectins in spinach, tomatoes, potatoes, and rice.

When you put beans or natural foods next to food additives or processed foods, there is no comparison. Beans and natural foods pose a much lower risk, but there is still a risk you should be aware of. Many people on diets that contain lots of beans are going to have gas and stomach problems. That's expected. The possible high levels of tyramine pose an even larger bean risk for headache sufferers. If you take the bean risk, eat freshly made beans in moderation.

Canned beans may come with a number of unwanted added ingredients, from MSG to BPA—that stuff they took out of water bottles because of an increased risk of cancer. Make sure to get your beans hot, because undercooked lectin can lead to serious problems. Beans are a headache trigger because of allergic reactions, lectin, oligosaccharides, tyramine, histamine, and antinutrients.

Food Amine Summary

Now let's take a look at all of these foods and their amine levels together. This list was compiled from multiple studies.

Food (100 g)	Histamine (mg)	Tyramine (mg)
Fresh vegetables	0–2.0	0–1.0
Spinach	2.0	0.4–3.2
Orange juice	0.03–0.26	0.02–0.67

Raspberry juice	?	66.66
Raspberries	?	1.3–9.3
Bananas	?	0–0.7
Bananas (overripe)	?	1.3
Avocadoes	?	2.3
Blue cheese (raw)	104.1	105.1
Fresh fish	2.34	6.18
Fish (two days old)	20.9	19.8
Fish (canned)	850.0–2,000	0
Red wine (liter)	19.6–3,800	18.2
White wine (liter)	1.1–120	2.3
Beer (liter)	3.0–52.0	3.6–10.5
Draft beer (liter)	?	27–113
Soy product (liter)	4,620	35,680
Soy sauce (liter)	?	293–941

It's confusing, which may be why no one has properly addressed this known problem. The information is limited and it changes drastically by brand, so we have no way of knowing the specific amine levels of the actual foods we buy. However, the information is also blunt. Processed foods, poorly stored foods, and spoiled or aged foods have the greatest potential for biogenic amines.

But wait a minute. Aren't migraines related to a rise in inflammation and an increase in glutamate? What do amines have to do with it? Monoamine oxidase (MAO) is known to prevent the toxic buildup of glutamate. Amines can raise glutamate. Thus, the breakdown of amines stops glutamate toxicity and inflammation, which you already knew.[335]

What Does It All Mean?

You need a healthy gut to break down amine migraine triggers. This means severely reducing the foods that are most likely to cause inflammation in your stomach and immediately limiting your amine intake. That's it. You can't change your genes, but that doesn't mean you can't solve the problem.

Remember Annette from the beginning of the chapter? I bet you can't guess which enzyme told her how to "cure" her migraines. She said, "I had a blood test which showed that I haven't got enough enzyme (diamine oxidase) to catabolize histamine in the body, meaning I have a histamine intolerance." Annette had a low blood count of diamine oxidase (DAO). DAO will be a breakthrough area of migraine research in the years to come. Some pregnant women have a complete remission of allergies due to a 500-fold increase in DAO.[336]

An increased DAO production is used to protect a mother from the histamine created by the fetus. Add to that the interesting fact that many women report complete remission from migraines after the first trimester of pregnancy, despite the countless hormonal and biological changes going on,[337] and you can see a clear connection between migraines, histamines, and DAO.

After the first trimester, the increased DAO production lowers the amount of histamine in the blood throughout the remainder of the pregnancy. How cool is that? Both migraines and allergies are gone from the natural breakdown of histamine. On the other hand, low production of DAO during pregnancy is associated with a higher risk of pregnancy complications. This is a concern for migraineurs. Pregnant migraineurs need to do whatever it takes to heal their guts for the healthy production of DAO.[338]

A 2015 study found that a genetic defect in DAO production and its ability to break down biogenic amines may double a woman's risk for migraines.[339] It is becoming increasingly challenging to argue that migraines are never triggered by foods or that migraines have nothing to do with allergens. The gut is the center for breaking down amines, and amines are known to trigger migraines. Foods known to damage the gut are migraine triggers, so when will we begin to focus our medical energy on the problem instead of treating the symptoms of the problem?

And why can't we cheat and just take a DAO pill? You can. In fact, recent studies have shown that there is a high prevalence of DAO deficiency in migraine patients. DAO supplements, which you can buy on Amazon, have proven to reduce the frequency and duration of migraines.[340] The author of *The Daily Headache* blog wrote about her success with DAO in a blog post titled "The Post I Never Thought I'd Get to Write." Kerrie, the author, points out that there is no reliable way to check for low DAO production because blood tests don't show the DAO levels in your gut, where you need it.[341]

Kerrie notes that DAO helped relieve her migraines, but it did not completely cure them. DAO doesn't take care of other amines, such as tyramine. MAO supplements are not on the market. Even if they were, we would still be treating the symptoms instead of the problem. In order to fix the problem, you need to reduce your intake of amines and make sure you have a healthy gut.

Headache Trigger #2: Rice

The glycemic index of one serving (150 g) of white rice is 89. One serving of the soft drink Fanta has a glycemic index of 68. Sure, a Fanta serving is only 8 oz., but it's like drinking straight sugar. A carb-packed serving (180 g) of something like macaroni has a glycemic index of 47. A 150-gram serving of black-eyed peas has a glycemic index of just 33. None of this takes away from this heavy hitter: a 30-gram serving of bread with a ginormous glycemic index of 71.[342] No matter how you compare it, white rice spikes your blood sugar to unnatural levels. Why?

White rice was once brown rice. Brown rice has a glycemic index of only 50, as opposed to white rice with a glycemic index of 89. So how was this little sugar monster made? White rice is milled to remove the husk, bran, and most of the germ layer. Polishing further whitens the rice and takes away essential fatty acids that reduce the shelf life of rice. The end product is the more palatable white rice in which most of the vitamins, minerals, macronutrients (like fiber), and beneficial fats have been destroyed. What does that even mean for us?

The fiber in brown rice acts as a slow-releasing nutrient dispenser, meaning you can fully absorb nutrients over time without a sugar spike. White rice takes the antioxidant vitamin E from 1.4 mg down to 0.46 mg. More importantly, white rice no longer has the nutrients we need to absorb antioxidants in the first place. The lost fiber and broken amino acids will also create free glutamate from rice's moderate amount of glutamic acid. Also, the majority of a great source of magnesium is lost in processing white rice.[343] Magnesium is a natural calcium channel blocker that can help with high blood pressure, migraines, and seizures. Brown rice also contains a substantial amount of GABA (gamma-aminobutyric acid), an amino acid that helps with stress and may also play a role in seizure and migraine prevention.

Wait. You just read the nutrition label of your white rice and found that I'm completely full of it. White rice has a ton of nutrients, maybe even more than some brown rice. But look again, and you will also see "enriched" on the label. In the process of making brown rice white, its benefits are removed, and several nutrients are depleted: zinc; potassium; manganese; selenium; vitamins B6, B3, B1, and B2; omega-3 fatty acids; and about a dozen others. So, since white rice does not meet the FDA's minimum nutritional requirements, it's required to be "enriched" with the vitamins that were lost. Some extra nutrients may be added, and this is referred to as "fortified." Many doctors disagree on whether supplements are beneficial or even harmful for healthy people. The entire medical community does seem to agree that vitamins are best absorbed in their natural forms. White rice is not the same as brown rice. Sprinkling vitamin powder on an empty carbohydrate does not recreate a "healthy" food.

Brown rice has a lot of benefits. It contains nutrients that help fight disease and aging that also maintain balanced sugar levels that promote weight loss and energy. Eating brown rice will also help you make friends with hippies, because it is their preferred rice. But what if you want to make new Chinese friends? A billion Chinese people eat white rice every day. How could they all be wrong?

That's not the way to look at food. If you're starving, is rice bad for you? In some parts of the world, "to eat" literally means "to eat rice." If rice were to vanish from the earth today, millions of people would die of starvation. That doesn't mean I personally need (or want) the sugar spikes and extra cushion in my winter coat that eating white rice can cause. And really, what millions of Chinese and

American people *don't* need is more sugar pumping through their veins.[344] White rice is associated with an increased risk of type 2 diabetes. In some Asian populations, the risk of diabetes is doubled with heavy rice consumption. Doubled.[345] Sumo wrestlers eat five to 10 bowls of rice per day to stay fat and don't live long, despite being powerful athletes.[346]

Allergic reactions are also a concern for populations that eat more rice. Rice supplies half of the daily calories for 50% of the world's population. In Japan, a rice allergy is present in 10% of allergy sufferers.[347] It's all about moderation. Of course, the people who consume large amounts of rice are more likely to have rice allergies, the same way people who consume heavy amounts of low-nutrient white rice will increase their risk of diabetes. In contrast, consuming brown rice lowers your risk of diabetes. This could be attributed to the fact that people who eat brown rice are more health conscious in general. Or maybe brown rice in moderation is good for you.

During a 30-day wheat elimination diet, rice is not recommended because of its cross-reaction. Brown rice is recommended by many migraine diets for its nutritional content (especially magnesium), although some nutritionists advise against brown rice because it contains more toxins, such as arsenic and lectins—the defensive mechanism of plants, which can be hard on the stomach.

But let's go back to the glycemic index. It's important to remember that it's just one measurement of how the foods you eat become sugar in your blood. It's a great tool but not a complete health guide. You wouldn't live your life based on obtaining the lowest glycemic index number possible. In this case, you would pick a

211

Snickers bar with a glycemic index of 51 over a ripe banana with a glycemic index of 62. That's crazy.

A Snickers bar is high in calories and low in nutritional value. Fructose and high-fructose corn syrup may convert to fat faster than glucose, giving Snickers and bananas a less than accurate glycemic index. Brown rice has about the same glycemic index (50) but is packed with nutrients. White rice has a much higher glycemic index but a very low number of nutrients, so it will give you a sugar spike. Studies and common sense tell us that we need to look at all of the qualities of a food to understand if it's healthy.[348]

The Snickers commercial that shows a hungry guy turn into an angry Joe Pesci is a sound example of how we feel when we have a rock-bottom blood sugar level. Unfortunately, the fix of a Snickers bar is temporary—and volatile—relief. Fast rises come with fast falls. White rice, wheat, or a Snickers bar will give you the type of short-lived relief you easily become reliant on. Relying on a sugar spike is not a sustainable way to stay headache-free. But it is a great way to market junk food.

The story of rice is a sequel to American obesity, or perhaps it's a rerun. Brown rice is considered a whole grain, while white rice is a refined grain. The studies for brown rice parallel the weight loss observed in any large group that consumes more whole grains.[349] Across the board, studies show that eating brown rice improved people's overall health and overconsuming white rice negatively impacted it.

The Dark Side of Brown Rice

Lectins are considered antinutrients because they bind to areas that process nutrients in the stomach, and that means you can't fully absorb the nutrients. Small amounts of brown rice don't seem to be a problem for most, but an advocate of the Paleolithic diet would argue that all rice is just like beans and can cause various digestive problems. An allergic response, a special concern for those with gluten sensitivity, would definitely pose the risk of poor nutrient absorption.

I say that brown rice is very different from beans, because you won't have the same level of gaseous problems. People generally digest brown rice with ease, and rice does not have the same level of allergic reaction as beans.

The Paleo argument deepens when you look at the omega-6/omega-3 ratio of rice. A cup of white rice has a 5 to 1 ratio of omega-6 to omega-3. Not bad, but it's definitely not great. White rice polishes off those essential fatty acids. Brown rice has an omega-6 to omega-3 ratio of 22 to 1.[350] This is bad.

A 22 to 1 ratio is in the range of the Western diet that is responsible for big waists and everything else that comes with buying a bigger belt. You don't want to promote inflammatory and autoimmune diseases by eating something as boring as rice.[351] Other grains, breads, and pastas will also contain high omega-6 ratios. This is a hit for brown rice and a win for the Paleo argument.

The final Paleo argument is that rice is low in nutrients and will pull minerals out of the body in order to stabilize pH levels. Let's add rice to the simple equation of glutamate + inflammation = migraine. Rice = negative minerals, which may create inflammation. Try frying massive amounts of rice in omega-6-rich vegetable oil, soy sauce, MSG, processed meat, and who knows what else. Can you feel tightness in your chest, dizziness, fatigue, and a headache emerging? That's called "Chinese restaurant syndrome" and it's a common feeling for those walking away from their mall's Chinese-food restaurant.

Panda Express, a Chinese food restaurant chain, does not represent how a billion Chinese people eat. Most of Asia's rice equation will look something more like this: a moderate amount of rice, plus fresh vegetables, plus a tiny portion of organic meat, plus natural seasoning, plus a few dashes of soy from organic crops. The Western diet's large portions of unnatural food with low-nutrient content is what makes an American airport distinguishable from any other airport in the world—you can tell by the size of our people.

So what is the right rice? Both brown and white rice come with problems. Both should be eliminated during an elimination diet for possible reactions. However, brown rice and white rice in moderation, when eaten along with a nutritious diet, pose very little threat in comparison to top headache triggers.

Headache Trigger #3: Eggs

We know that eggs contain a large amount of glutamic acid, which is easily digested by you and soon-to-be baby chickens, and we know that eggs are one of the top eight most allergenic foods, which together account for 90% of all allergic reactions. Eggs cause major reactions in all of the large migraine-allergy studies.

We also know that corn-fed, store-bought eggs contain up to a 20 to 1 inflammatory to anti-inflammatory ratio. But truly free-range chickens may produce eggs with more anti-inflammatory benefits since their eggs have an omega-6 to omega-3 ratio closer to 1.5 to 1. But none of this fully explains why natural eggs disproportionately produce unnatural headaches.

We can look at diet soda for the answer. Eggs are heavy in aspartic acid and phenylalanine. I'll sum it up briefly: Aspartame is made primarily of aspartate (aspartic acid) and phenylalanine. Aspartate is considered an excitotoxin that may increase glutamate and inflammation in the brain. Large amounts of aspartate may trigger migraines in the same way that large amounts of the excitotoxin glutamate triggers migraines. This may be why both aspartame and MSG have thousands of complaints filed with the FDA.[352] According to WebMD, phenylalanine increases a mother's risk of birth defects.[353]

Eggs are different from aspartame in that the aspartic acid and phenylalanine are not held together by poisonous methanol. However, eggs contain exorbitant amounts of aspartic acid and phenylalanine. Milk has quite a bit of aspartic acid, but eggs have seven times more.[354] This may produce weight gain in a similar way to MSG or aspartame.

Here is where we really screw ourselves. Dried eggs (eggs from a box) have more than four times the aspartic acid as whole store-bought eggs and 26 times the aspartic acid of milk. Dried eggs also have one of the highest amounts of glutamic acid seen in any food product. Dried eggs contain more than 6,000 mg of glutamic acid, which is more than Popeye's fried chicken![355] That will be sure to cause significant weight gain, as will weight-gainer protein shakes with a comparable amount of glutamic acid. Eggs, even whole eggs, test the limits of the amino acids we can consume.

It hardly seems reasonable to say we can't eat a food that's been around since the beginning of time. Right? Eggs have been around as long as we have, and you know damn well that the cavemen were scavenging those eggs from any nest they could unearth. Cavemen slurped eggs that were not cooked and therefore contained fewer "unbound" amino acids (a good thing). These eggs were not from a box. In fact, they were even better than most of the organic eggs found at your local health food store. What you want are eggs from free-range chickens that eat what nature intended. Easier said than done.

The FDA's definition of food labeled "free-range" misleads the American public into thinking we're eating something healthy when we eat free-range eggs. Here's what the FDA requires: "The poultry has been allowed access to the outside."[356] Most of the time this means that the chicken can walk outside on a small patch of concrete while continuing to eat food with toxic pesticides, hormones, and antibiotics. If they are certified organic free-range chickens, their most common meal will be a mix of highly inflammatory corn and soy feed. We know that grass-fed cows produce meat that closely resembles the omega-3-rich Mediterranean diet. What would happen if chickens ate what they were supposed to?

Mother Earth News compared official USDA nutrient data with eggs produced from hens raised "on pasture." *Mother Earth News*? Yes. *Mother Earth News* has been a reputable magazine, supporter of family farms, and a pioneer of health since the 1970s. The hens *Mother Earth News* compared were truly free to range on pastures and eat "all kinds of seeds, green plants, insects and worms, usually along with some grain or laying mash."

Mother Earth News found that true free-range eggs contain:[357]

- One-third less cholesterol
- One-fourth less saturated fat
- Two-thirds more vitamin A
- Two times more omega-3 fatty acids
- Three times more vitamin E
- Seven times more beta carotene

A study published in the *Cambridge Journal* in 2010 echoed those results. It found that the amount of omega-3 in pasture hens was two and a half times greater than the amount of omega-3 in caged hens. This cut the omega-6 to omega-3 ratio in half.[358]

Real free-range eggs are healthier than "organic eggs." Organic eggs are healthier than boxed eggs. Boxed eggs are what most migraine studies use to test eggs as a headache trigger. So where does that leave eggs in terms of a headache trigger?

Aside from migraines, many people are allergic to several proteins in eggs. A high number of headache sufferers will have reactions to eggs regardless of their nutritional benefits. It's not clear which of the proteins or numerous amino acids are triggering migraines. However, eggs are not up for debate as a headache trigger and will be in nearly every headache elimination diet. Eggs were the number two trigger in the 1983 study and the number three trigger for the 1979 study. The 2010 migraine allergy study that tested 266 foods identified eggs as a problem for nearly half of all migraine patients. If you have migraines on a regular basis, it is critical that you eliminate eggs from your diet.

Gonna Eat Eggs Anyway?

The abundance of easily digestible amino acids in eggs makes them very dangerous. What do eggs go best with? Eggs and bacon with sourdough toast are a delicious headache conglomeration. How about a Sausage McMuffin with Egg? What about a three-cheese baked omelet with ham (processed of course) and mushrooms, topped off with a glass of milk? Eggs go great with other headache triggers. Very few foods that complement eggs will slow the progression of their quickly converted amino acids.

While a large physicians' health study shows no greater risk of death in healthy individuals who eat one egg per day, diabetics double their risk of death by consuming more than one egg per day.[359] A Greek study shows a fivefold increase in cardiovascular death for diabetics who consume one egg or more per day.[360] It's no secret that most diabetics get there by way of unhealthy processed foods. It is also likely that the diabetics consuming eggs (mostly boxed, store-bought eggs) are doing so in combination with cheeses, breads, and processed meats, and that combination can be deadly. With respect to headaches, no trigger should be devoured with a plethora of other headache triggers.

Other Headache Triggers to Avoid

It's not that hard to find a real free-range pasture farm. Ask your local health food store or checking out these websites:

- Local Harvest: www.localharvest.org
- USDA's farmers' market listing: www.search.ams.usda.gov/farmersmarkets/Default.aspx
- Eat Wild: www.eatwild.com

It may seem like hippie overboard to visit your local farm, but it could be fun. These are the people who live for good food and health, and they are very passionate about what they do. You may learn more from visiting just one farm than you ever could from reading a book, including this one. You will also bring home some delicious food and knowledge for your friends and family.

Headache Trigger #4: Chocolate

The craving for chocolate is a major headache trigger. This is not to say chocolate itself is a trigger. The myth that chocolate causes migraines is also dependent on what your definition of chocolate is in the first place. Let me explain.

If you were to say chocolate in its pure form is a well-known headache trigger, then you would be sadly mistaken. Cocoa is packed with antioxidants that are likely to benefit insulin resistance, cardiovascular disease, and protect nerves from injury and inflammation.[361] We don't know for sure, because conclusive studies have not been performed on pure cocoa. With that said, there is potential for pure chocolate to be beneficial for migraineurs.[362]

What about the 1983 study, the 1979 study, the 2007 Mexican migraine study, and numerous others that all label chocolate as a top headache trigger? It's not "chocolate"; it's a mixture of headache triggers processed with chocolate. The top headache triggers are also the top allergy triggers. While many people are allergic to processed milk chocolate, cocoa allergies are so rare that pure chocolate is not included on a number of large allergenic-food lists.

Instead of saying "chocolate can trigger migraines," we should say "processed candy bars that may or may not contain milk, nuts, wheat and gluten, soy, eggs, corn syrup, and caffeine can trigger migraines." And that's a powerful combination of triggers. The people who add "chocolate" to a headache trigger list without an explanation of what else is in the chocolate are about as helpful as the people who add the scientific term "pizza" to undefined food trigger lists.

One of the best articles on the internet for chocolate and migraines merely states that "phenylethylamine, tannin, and caffeine may be the culprits when chocolate is a migraine trigger." The problem is that, beyond stating popular thought, no one has evaluated the potential of these ingredients to trigger a migraine. So let's evaluate the phenylethylamine, tannins, and caffeine in chocolate.

Phenylethylamine

When you hear the suffix "amine," you should think "methamphetamine" before you think "antihistamine." Abnormally low concentrations of phenylethylamine are found in people suffering from ADHD, whereas abnormally high concentrations are found in people with schizophrenia. Too little phenethylamine is bad; too much phenethylamine is bad.

Phenylethylamine, not to be confused with the phenylalanine found in eggs and aspartame, is a stimulant, and in high doses it will have similar effects to cocaine or methamphetamine.[363] Will phenylethylamine in the extremely low dose found in chocolate affect a headache? To be answered shortly.

Tannins

Tannins produce the mouth-puckering bitter taste in wine, unripe fruit, chocolate, and teas. They were designed by nature as a defense mechanism to let us know that the fruit is not ready for the seeds to be carried off or that the plant doesn't want to be consumed in the first place. Along with an astringent taste, the tannins disrupt the digestion process in an effort to halt the body's ability to consume the entire plant.[364]

Tannins are a concern to migraineurs because they bind to nutritional components (like starches) and even to the digestive tract itself. These nutrients are needed for the body to produce serotonin. Low levels of serotonin are associated with migraines.[365] The theory that tannins cause headaches is likely incorrect since headache sufferers inconsistently react to foods with higher or lower tannins. If tannins were the cause of a red wine headache, the sufferer should find that consuming the greater amount of tannins found in soy, berries, tea, and chocolate would cause the same type of headache. Tannins have more recently been in the limelight for their antioxidant properties that protect us from cell damage, cancer, high-blood pressure, and the growth of many diseases and viruses.[366] Saying that tannins are unhealthy would be like saying all fruit is bad for us.[367] To their credit, research has revealed that tannins actually protect the brain from the oxidative stress associated with migraines.[368]

Caffeine

Chocolate also contains theobromine, which can be deadly for dogs. For humans, it has a similar effect as caffeine, although it isn't as strong. Caffeine is in chocolate, but it contains less than a serving of decaf coffee.[369] Tyramine is in chocolate, and most foods that contain tyramine are also headache triggers. Tyramine-rich spinach is not a major migraine trigger, and pure tyramine did not result in headaches in the 1983 study. All of these media-hyped theories are isolated triggers that do not in any way represent natural chocolate (or any food) as a whole.

Does pure chocolate trigger headaches? That is a relevant question. Thousands of migraineurs will tell you without a doubt that chocolate is a headache trigger. Thousands of people have documented in headache diaries that when they consume chocolate, the probability of getting a migraine goes through the roof. If only we could take the people who have experienced chocolate-induced headaches and put them in a controlled study.

In 1974, this was accomplished by taking 25 migraine patients and putting them on a double-blind chocolate test, which essentially meant that the migraineurs were given two types of perceived chocolate in multiple sessions and did not know that one was a placebo that didn't actually contain any chocolate. Only two patients responded consistently with chocolate as a headache trigger. The placebo effect alone should have produced more headaches, as these patients were sure that chocolate was a personal headache trigger.[370]

The study concluded that either all of the patients were incorrect about their prior chocolate-induced headaches or other factors were involved, such as stress, with the latter being more likely. A 1987 study involving 39 children confirmed this theory with a diet that was both heavy in vasoactive amines (like chocolate) and fiber. The patients actually experienced a significant decrease in their number of headaches, and it was not dependent on the consumption of amines.[371]

These studies lacked the subjects and control measures necessary to identify that chocolate was definitely *not* a headache trigger. That leads us to 1997, when a University of Pittsburg study aimed to add what the older studies lacked. This study involved 63 patients in a double-blind chocolate challenge. In addition, researchers closely monitored the patients' diets and restricted other vasoactive amine-rich foods. Contrary to the belief of patients and physicians, chocolate did not play a role in triggering migraines or tension headaches.[372]

Jump forward to 2015, the year that *Back to the Future* promised the release of flying cars and hover boards, and we still don't know if chocolate causes headaches. By "we" I mean the majority of doctors and patients and the mainstream media. But you just read that pure chocolate is not a confirmed headache trigger. So if chocolate doesn't trigger headaches, what's going on?

There are two possibilities. Either chocolate is desired as a symptom of a migraine that has already started, or the desire for chocolate is a symptom of the precursors to a migraine, such as fluctuating hormones, stress, and fatigue. Again, this is pure chocolate we're talking about. At this point, you already know eating a candy bar processed with a mixture of chocolate, sugar, caffeine, milk, soy, and wheat is a bad idea for migraineurs.

Headache Trigger #5: Sulfites

If you Google "sulfite migraine trigger list," you will find over two million articles that somehow relate sulfites to causing headaches. Then try to find a study that holds sulfites directly responsible for causing headaches. You won't, according to Dr. Waterhouse of UC Davis's Waterhouse Lab. So, are all of these articles completely wrong or just 50% wrong? I would like to say 50%, but who knows?

Dr. Waterhouse studies sulfites in wine (an area long in search of headache cures) and writes that "medical literature has virtually no reports on sulfites inducing headaches." Without any kind of medical research, there is no way to know if headaches are induced by sulfites or something else in wine. Sulfites are most often the blame of white wine headaches, although red wine may contain the same amount.

Here's where things get gray. Most people who get headaches from wine don't get headaches from dried fruit. They usually find that they don't even get headaches from certain kinds of wine that have the same amount of sulfites. Wine has an average of 80 mg of sulfites per liter. Orange-colored dried apricots typically have 2,000 mg of sulfites per kilogram.[373] As with most dried fruit, these sulfite levels are very high. In theory, if you had a sulfite headache from wine, you should definitely get a headache from dried fruit that is preserved with sulfites.

In 1986, the FDA banned the use of sulfites on fresh fruits and vegetables. Restaurants were notorious for dumping sulfites all over the salad bar to prevent the fruits and vegetables from browning or wilting. The ban was based on a government report of some 500 "allergic reactions" that included 13 deaths.[374] The FDA estimated that 1% of the population was sensitive to sulfites, but a more recent study that was published after the FDA ban took effect lowers that number to just 0.05% of the population.[375]

I put "allergic reactions" in quotations above because adverse reactions to sulfites are more like an overdose than a true allergic reaction that gives you an immune system response. The human body produces about 1,000 mg of sulfites per day, so it would seem that adding a glass of wine, or even a liter of wine with its 80 mg of sulfites, would not be a problem. People with severe sulfite sensitivity will argue this generalization to the grave, but those folks may be deficient in the enzyme that breaks sulfites down, which can cause a number of problems.

The people most likely to have a problem with sulfites are also the ones who may be inhaling sulfites on a regular basis. You can find several sulfite articles on the internet that label asthmatics as being most at risk for sulfite reactions, but there's more to it than that. Anywhere from 4–7% of severe asthmatics are susceptible to sulfite-induced asthma. Mild asthmatics don't appear to be susceptible. This gave the year 1986 a sulfite-sensitivity prevalence of 1–1.5% for the entire asthmatic population.

You and I may not feel good from too much sulfite; an asthmatic can be at risk of death in just a few minutes. The problem: Many inhalers and bronchodilators for asthma contain sulfites. These medications might not just be adding to the problem; they contain the sulfite problem. If you know a severe asthmatic, you might be curious to know what he or she is constantly puffing on and if that is adding to his or her sulfite problem.

The author of the original 1986 findings went on to clarify this issue 10 years later in another groundbreaking study titled

"Sulfite-induced asthmatics display thresholds for sulfites." Sulfite levels lower than 100 parts per million (ppm) present little risk, and sulfite levels below 10 ppm present no risk, although the reasoning behind this problem is still unclear.[376]

What would you expect the problem to be? When a food has a 10 ppm sulfite level, the FDA then requires that food manufacturers add sulfite to its label. Ten parts per million is also the highest sulfite concentration found in nature, with just a few exceptions. As long as you're not the guy or gal who thinks that anything natural can be consumed in gigantic amounts, you've found the problem. The sulfites from those dried apricots had 2,000 mg/kg, which is exactly the same as saying 2,000 ppm. Think about multiplying the strength of a natural substance like coffee or coca leaves by 200. What would multiplying the concentration of sulfites by 200 times do to your system?

We don't know. With sulfites, all we have is speculation. Dr. Waterhouse acknowledges a number of complaints from sulfite headache sufferers. Nothing can be done with these complaints on an academic level without funding. He even urges people to contact him if they are interested in supporting this exploration by funding a master student's research project. So if you have $50,000 lying around, we could get some answers.

How do we stay away from giant piles of sulfites? I read an article on sulfite headaches in the *Examiner* that stated the following: "If you don't get a headache after snacking on dried mango slices from Trader Joe's, then your body is probably okay with handling sulfites."[377] This is where the headache help goes from 50% full of shish kebab to *completely* full of shish kebab. Traders Joe's sells dried mangos that contain no added sulfites. Even the chili mangos that are a personal headache trigger of mine contain no added sulfites. On the other hand, Trader Joe's sells a number of dried fruits that are loaded with sulfites.

I don't blame the author of this *Examiner* article, because there are numerous legitimate resources that label all dried fruit as the highest source of sulfites. This assumption is found in a number of headache food trigger lists that generically label all "dried fruit" as headache triggers. Saying a dried fruit that contains less than 10 ppm of sulfites is in the same boat as dried fruit that's smothered with 2,000 ppm of sulfites does not make any sense.

Consuming something we don't understand 200 times over is a bad idea. So where do we find them so we can avoid them? The list of products that don't contain sulfites is shorter than the list of products that do. Sulfites can be found in anything processed, such as fruit juice, alcohol, condiments, teas, snacks, and baked goods. Medications are not only a concern for asthmatics; they are a concern for anyone who has to take them. A large number of medications, including migraine meds, contain sulfites.

Fortunately, all you need to do is look on the FDA-regulated label to see if the food or medication contains sulfites.

Here are the sulfite names to look for:[378]

- Sulfur dioxide (SO2)
- Sodium bisulfite (NaHSO3)
- Potassium bisulfite (KHSO3)
- Sodium metabisulfite (Na2S2O5)
- Potassium metabisulfite (K2S2O5)
- Sodium sulfite (Na2SO3)

If you see any of these names on a food label, it means the product contains over 10 ppm of sulfites. You are not going to find the specific amounts of sulfites on the package. You probably won't even be able to find the sulfite levels for specific foods on the internet. The food could contain 2,000 ppm or 11 ppm of sulfites. This is where the FDA has failed us. The FDA allows a substance in our food that it claims is dangerous for 1% of the United States population, and the food manufacturers are not required to list the ballpark number of this potentially deadly product.

The only thing we can do is avoid sulfites altogether. If you're in a restaurant, you can't. The FDA found there is no way that fruit and vegetables should be allowed to have sulfites, but anything else prepared behind the closed doors of a kitchen can contain sulfites. The restaurant is not required to notify you if the cooks dumped sulfites all over your visually pleasing food, which happened to be sitting in the kitchen for over a week. But that shouldn't worry you more than any of the other additives and preservatives they're not telling you about.[379]

Back to dried fruits. Are they healthy? There are two stances in the medical and fitness communities.

The bad: Dried fruit has had most of the water content removed, while concentrating all of the sugar. This tricks your stomach into thinking there is only a small amount of nutrients, and you will remain hungry. Dried fruit often contains preservatives and extra sugar. This is fructose and sucrose, which is a bad combination in excess. Overeating any dried fruit could spike your blood sugar and put you at risk for diabetes and obesity.

The good: Naturally dried fruit contains the same amount of nutrients and antioxidants as the whole fruit. This could be beneficial if you're lacking those nutrients, especially for headaches.

Because dried fruit is a concentration of nutrients, it is also a concentration of proteins. This is how I found out that I have a problem with mangos. Dried mangos may contain some of the unwanted oils from the skin that are similar to poison oak. I don't know if I'm allergic to the oil in mangos, the concentration of its protein, or both. I'm fine when I eat fresh mangos, but this is in smaller amounts with more water to dilute the problem. The point is that dried fruit is considered processed, and that comes with more headache problems.

I would personally lean toward eating fresh fruit as a safer alternative. However, in moderation, there doesn't appear to be a large risk with dried fruit. Fruit is a much smaller migraine trigger than headache triggers from highly processed foods, preservatives, and additives. If the choice is between MSG bacon and organic dried fruit, eat the dried fruit. If the choice is between no fruit for the entire day and organic dried fruit, eat the dried fruit. Be cognizant of what you're eating and the amount you're eating.

Headache Trigger #6: Nitrites

One late afternoon, my engine company responded to a 911 call for chest pain. We walked into the gentleman's house—let's call him "Frank"—anticipating the fast-paced race to add drugs to his blood flow before his heart became incapable of circulating those drugs. Frank stopped us at the door in a cold sweat and said, "Sorry, guys, I just had some anxiety. I'm fine now. You don't need to be here." The funny thing about a heart attack is that no one wants to admit that the unfamiliar feeling could be the end of the road.

Frank spent about five minutes convincing us he was fine, but before we left, our medic firmly said, "Just let me put you on the monitor, take a quick picture of your heart, and we'll leave."

Frank said "Fine," in a tone that signaled he would do anything to get rid of us.

I was under the impression that this was just a precaution since the 4-lead monitor showed a normal heartbeat. The medic asked me for the 12-lead monitor.

This was a normal extra precaution for a patient having heart-related signs and symptoms. However, this man no longer presented any symptoms and made it clear that he was against our medical help.

But the 12-lead, which takes a slightly better picture of your heart, showed that the man was having a full-blown heart attack.

We immediately gave him four baby aspirin followed by a spray of nitroglycerin. The nitro immediately opens up the arteries in the heart and increases blood flow before the heart is depleted of oxygen and dies. The nitro turns your little pipes into giant mains of blood flow. Frank went from lying down to jerking himself up into a sitting position.

Imagine filling every bathtub in an old 50-story apartment building at the same time. What would happen? The guy living on the fiftieth story would have a bathtub spout that's dribbling as the bottom bathrooms overflow with water. The tub on the 50th story was Frank's brain, and the nitro opened up every pipe in his body. As soon as Frank made it to his sitting position, his face lost all pigment, and he collapsed. His blood pressure took a dive and he stopped breathing.

Nitrites, nitrates, and nitroglycerin all turn into the powerful vasodilator nitric oxide (NO). Nitrites and nitrates, terms used interchangeably, are found in a number of fruits and vegetables and are well-known food preservatives. And this is where things get stupid in migraine treatment. We think of nitrates as stuff that's in processed meats, such as hot dogs, sausages, bacon, and lunchmeats. But there are migraine articles out there that specifically state you should not eat beets, celery, lettuce, radishes, and spinach because they contain high levels of nitrates.

A 2008 report by the European Food Safety Authority sided with common sense after evaluating the dangers of vegetable nitrates. Vegetables contain vitamins and nutrients that inhibit the formation of nitrogen oxide and outweigh the nitrate risk.[380] Nitrate preservatives are isolated, concentrated, and stripped of fiber. While studies show that vegetables do a number of great things, preserved meats have been linked to heart disease, cancer, and diabetes. The toxic effects of preserved meats worsen with the buildup of biogenic amines and nitrites, and there's a lot of unsubstantiated evidence around all of this.[381] One thing is certain: What we should be concerned with is preserved meat, not vegetables.

Other Headache Triggers to Avoid

Nitrites and nitrates are currently up for debate as some critics argue that lettuce, at 3,500 mg per kilo, can have more nitrites than hundreds of hot dogs—and your saliva contains more than both. This means your body produces your largest nitrite threat, so don't get spit on your food when you eat! Most samples of fresh meat do not contain nitrites. Preserved and packaged meats are regulated to contain less than 200 mg per kilo. Hands down, vegetables have more nitrites than processed meats.[382]

Look, there's conflicting information out there. Just as nitric oxide was used to improve the blood flow in Frank's heart, it was responsible for a lack of flow to his brain and a devastating drop in blood pressure. Your body uses nitric oxide for the vital regulation of your pipes.

What happened to Frank after he stopped breathing? His body quickly adjusted to the nitroglycerin, and he was able to breathe on his own. Of course, he probably ended up with the most common side effect of an unnatural rise in NO: a headache.

The greatest threat of nitrites in meat is type 3 diabetes, a term coined by the brilliant doctor Suzanne De La Monte. Her breakthrough research in Alzheimer's disease revealed that the drug nitrosamine can induce insulin resistance in the brain and causes dementia in lab rats.[383]

Nitrosamines—the same nitrosamines associated with cancer from cigarettes—can be formed in the human body from nitrites and nitrates. Cured meats such as bacon or Parma ham may form nitrosamines before ingestion because of the amine and nitrite chemical reaction during curing.[384]

Nitrosamines kill the good bacteria that help process migraine triggers—biogenic amines—and impair the function of the migraine gene, MTHFR.[385] [386] We will discuss the MTHFR gene in the section on vitamins. Dr. De La Monte believes that the low levels of nitrites and nitrates in our food supply could be to blame for all major diseases related to insulin resistance.[387]

Women are most at risk because the amyloid plaque responsible for Alzheimer's disease is found in the white matter of the brain—women have 10 times more white matter than men.[388] Research shows that similar white matter brain lesions found in migraine sufferers also may be caused by amyloid plaque.[389] Women are twice as likely to have Alzheimer's disease and nearly three times as likely to have migraines.

NO Headache Triggers

At the age of 19, I questioned not who I was, but what I wanted to become. I wanted to be a meathead. I thought that having huge muscles would somehow increase the size of my ego. I bought the strongest supplement on the market, N.O.-Xplode. In two months, I went from benching 145 pounds to benching over 275 pounds.

N.O.-Xplode works by increasing your nitric oxide levels for vasodilatation in your muscles. Your muscles expand, allowing for heavier reps and the intake of more nutrients. Unfortunately, many people experience the side effect of headaches from the unnatural increase in nitric oxide. At the beginning, I only had headaches directly after a workout.

After about three weeks of taking the supplement, I began to have a sustained headache that did not go away until I stopped taking it. I was 19 years old and unconcerned and unmoved by headaches. I could stay up all night drinking and go to class in the morning, yet the headaches were the reason I stopped taking this supplement. So the next time you see a meathead angry, be nice. He probably has a tremendous headache!

"I've finally found out what has been the primary cause of my daily migraines for the last five years! Hair loss cream." This was the enthusiastic reaction of a man who found out his migraine trigger was nitric oxide. NO has vasodilatation properties that are believed to improve perfusion to the cells of hair follicles and stimulate regrowth. This man's powerful headache trigger shows that triggers can take a lot of different forms, from your shampoo to the air you breathe. Which means there are even more things to consider eliminating when you start looking for the sources of your own headaches.

The most famous use of NO is in the penis. Viagra stimulates the production of nitric oxide in the penis. Using drugs to target a specific area is often not effective. The most common side effect of Viagra, according to Viagra, is headaches. When Googling "Viagra headaches," you will find a number of questions from people who may have migraine symptoms.

A study out of the University of Copenhagen found that Viagra induced migraines in 10 out of 12 migraine patients.[390] So why is nitric oxide causing such headaches?

My answer lies in a University of Cambridge study titled "Inflammatory neurodegeneration mediated by nitric oxide, glutamate, and mitochondria."[391] Neurodegeneration is the umbrella term for progressive loss or death of neurons. You're probably thinking about Alzheimer's, Parkinson's, or how our thoughts slow down with old age. This study details how NO causes a rapid glutamate release from both astrocytes and neurons, which leads to excitotoxic death! It all goes back to glutamate exciting cells to death in the brain.

I am still excited when I see studies that clearly display the glutamate/inflammation theory. All of them relate to a rise in inflammation or glutamate, but it seems they don't acknowledge it. The NO migraine study shows that NO triggers migraines. Studies on NO show that nitric oxide, nitrites, and nitrosamines each cause an increase in glutamate and inflammation.[392,393] The studies on MSG show that free glutamic acid triggers migraines. The largest study on the genome sequence of people with migraines shows that migraineurs have a gene in the area of the brain that regulates glutamate, so it's time we start looking for a cure instead of continuing to treat migraine pain.

What Can You Do?

The same drugs used to lower toxic levels of glutamate in Alzheimer's disease are also successful in migraine treatment,[394] and measures to lower glutamate have been successful in both Alzheimer's disease and migraine prevention—you'll learn more about this in the chapter on ketogenic diets.[395,396] This information suggests that we need to both lower our intake of nitrites and fight insulin resistance with diets that control both glutamate and insulin resistance.

In general, avoid high levels of nitrites, nitrates, nitrosamines, and NO.

Headache Trigger #7: Weather, Mold, Allergies, and Other Airborne Triggers

There are a vast number of airborne migraine triggers—some of which you can't control. You may not be able to pick up and move simply because of the airborne triggers around you, but it's important to know how they may affect you and your headache health.

Barometric Pressure

It's now commonplace for something like barometric pressure to influence where a migraine sufferer chooses to live. Accuweather.com now features migraine, sinus, headache, and allergy forecasts. Migraines have finally hit the weather map.[397]

Although the internet is full of raw barometric pressure data, no one has compiled the data to find safe habitats for migraine sufferers. Nobody until Jonathan Taylor, that is. Taylor, a tech executive, wanted to find migraine-safe cities for a client as well as himself. Taylor noticed that a minute change in barometric pressure (0.2 inHg) triggered a migraine for him nearly every time. He then created a list of major US cities with the least barometric variation based on the number of days per year with less than a 0.2 change. Here's that list:

- Honolulu (0 days per year)
- Miami (4)
- San Diego (7)
- Los Angeles (7)
- Tampa (11)

- San Jose (14)
- Sacramento (18)
- San Francisco (18)
- Phoenix (22)
- New Orleans (22)
- Jacksonville (22)
- Birmingham (29)
- Houston (29)
- Atlanta (37)
- San Antonio (37)
- Austin (37)
- Memphis (44)
- Las Vegas (47)
- Little Rock (48)
- Charleston, SC (48)

This list has helped headache sufferers remove the trigger, as opposed to treating the symptoms of that trigger. If you're questioning your environment, check out the other cities in his article titled "Avoiding Migraines Resulting from Changes in Barometric Pressure."[398]

Pressure Changes on Airplanes

Aircrafts are pressurized, so we're told that pressure changes are not to blame for the numerous migraines that occur during flight. However, my popping ears flying over the Pacific say that's not true.

Sea level atmospheric pressure is around 29.92 inHg, 1013 hPa, 14.7 psi, or 760 mmHg—these are just units of pressure that you might see on a barometer. A new Boeing 747 during flight will have a pressure that ranges from 23.45 to 24.98 inHg. In plain English, that's like instantly jumping from a 5,000 ft. summit to a 7,000 ft. mountaintop.[399]

In Honolulu terms, this would be a greater change in pressure than its record high (30.32 in 1919) and record low (29.34 in 1936).[400] Jonathan Taylor needs a 0.2 change in pressure for a guaranteed migraine. A flight is a 1.53 change in pressure, almost seven times greater than Taylor's trigger. Older planes are even worse. Yes, flying is a major migraine trigger. Taylor's law of 0.2 is actually quite high. Some migraineurs claim a 0.1 reduction in pressure will trigger a migraine, while one study found that a 0.15 pressure drop bumped up the likelihood of migraines in 64% of patients.[401]

Why Pressure Drops Trigger Migraines

A quick drop in barometric pressure over a short period of time indicates a storm is likely in the next five to six hours. Fluid and air expand when the barometric pressure begins to drop, which most people can't feel. However, people with inflammatory conditions, such as arthritis, migraines, or sinus infections, may feel pain from the pressure that is expanding and is trapped within areas of inflammation. According to new research, people with inflammatory conditions might be able to accurately predict a storm coming.[402] In theory, the pain is a defense mechanism that would warn a sick person to find shelter before a storm arrives.

Some migraineurs find that taking antihistamines, such as Benadryl, or decongestants, such as pseudoephedrine, will prevent migraines that occur during pressure changes.

High Altitudes

The Rocky Mountain range is also known as the "suicide belt" because these mountains fall in states that consistently have the highest suicide rate per capita, aside from Alaska where locals endure subzero temperatures and months of darkness. A 2010 study found that suicide rates begin to rise at 2,000 and 3,000 feet of elevation in all US regions.[403]

Perry Renshaw, a leading Utah neuroscientist of high-altitude suicide, thinks he knows why. Low oxygen levels are associated with decreased serotonin, the happy brain chemical.[404] This is particularly important for women, because they synthesize a fraction of the serotonin that men do.[405] Accordingly, Utah women lead the nation in antidepressant use.[406] The concern of headaches is only growing under Renshaw's theory, although he does have opposition—probably most of Utah—as many people thrive in mountain towns. And that's where genes come into play.[407]

Guess which gene? Low MTHFR function is associated with pulmonary hypertension, which basically squeezes down on the little pipes in your lungs that are attempting to gain oxygen.[408] This is a genetic predisposition that you don't want at high altitudes. According to the European Respiratory Society, the homozygous MTHFR C677T mutation you get when you have two migraineur parents was threefold higher in patients with high-altitude pulmonary hypertension.[409] This means that high altitudes are going to suck the life out of many migraineurs.

Winter Darkness

You are not going to get much sunlight during the winter, especially if you live in Barrow, Alaska. Living there can be devastating for your vitamin D levels and the production of serotonin, although you won't be using too much serotonin without light. Your body has an internal light sensor that starts the production of melatonin when it becomes dark. This increases sleepiness. It also inhibits the production of serotonin—which turns you into Sleepy and Grumpy.

The loss of vitamin D and serotonin can be calamitous, and migraines are only one way calamity may strike. But we can't presume that weather triggers for migraines are independent of nutrient deficiencies and other rises of inflammation that flow within the canals of one human system.

Other Airborne Migraine Triggers

My worst headache trigger is mold. I would get a headache after about three days of living in a beach house. These houses sit in a wet atmosphere and many have stale water under the floors from poor drainage, creating the wretched fungus we all know and hate: black mold.

My headaches are on one side of my head and accompanied by heavy sinus pressure between my eyes. My eyesight becomes blurred. At times my headaches are so bad that I can't formulate thoughts without confusion. Driving is also out of the question.

Mold allergies can create numerous conditions that are far worse than my headaches. Luckily, I had a second home at the firehouse while living in a moldy environment, and I would stay away from the house for days. My symptoms disappeared almost immediately—within hours. Many people aren't as lucky and continue to live in environments that are killing them, often without realizing it.

Pet hair, pollen, and dust can have the same effect as mold. Air purifiers with UV (a life saver for me), ozone generators, humidifiers, and dehumidifiers often help with air conditions that contain allergens or irritants.

The Worst Airborne Trigger of All

There is also one that isn't discussed as a migraine trigger. It is negativity. Misery breeds misery. Living or working in a place with constant negativity and little inspiration can make you miserable. Some firefighters spend more time on duty than they do at home, and the people they're spending time with might be great, or they might be miserable.

I was lucky to have a very happy crew, and it made it that much harder to leave the fire service. Being around people who do not share your values will have a large impact on your positive outlook and stress levels. But, new research shows that people rate even extraordinary experiences as poor when they don't experience those events with others, so if you need to change your environment, make sure you don't change it to one of solitude.[410] Surround yourself with happy, positive people who have values and interests similar to yours. Look for a job that inspires you. Get involved in a new activity where you can meet new people. Sure, misery feeds on itself, but so does positivity.

Headache Trigger #8: Smells

Is it possible to smell a migraine? Yes. In fact, there are two ways. The first is to smell an unpleasant odor that bursts your already volatile headache threshold—often an easy task to accomplish for female migraineurs, many of whom have heightened sensitivity to smells. If you don't get migraines and are wearing a strong cologne or perfume, there may be a migraineur across the room who wants to kill you.

The second way to smell a migraine is to experience a change in your sense of smell during an attack, which is common for about half of migraine sufferers. It's been proven that auras bring smells to mind that are not real. Garlic is one of them. This is the phenomenon in which senses become jumbled from the electrical thunderstorm in the brain. Whether it's real or not, the smell is often confused as a trigger because it can happen before the pain stage of a migraine.

The top smelly triggers (real ones) are as follows:[411]

- Perfume and colognes
- Foods
- Cigarette smoke

A Brazilian study found that odors could both trigger and worsen migraine symptoms. The top triggers were similar to the above: perfume, cigarette smoke, and cleaning products. The questionnaire responses from 98 male migraineurs shows odors to be a top migraine trigger, second only to stress.[412]

Most people can't fathom that a cleaning product could cause migraines. But I bet you can. After you read about the migraine gene and how it is negatively impacted by the detoxification of chemicals, it will be easy to see how bleach fumes can be a headache trigger. But it will not be until you read about hypothyroidism and migraines that you will realize how significant products like bleach are. Understanding these teeny triggers may help someone remove the toxic items that are actually causing their headaches.

Sure, cigarette smoke and cleaning products can kill us, but what about sweet perfume? In a report by the Environmental Working Group titled "Not So Sexy: Hidden Chemicals in Perfume and Cologne," researchers detail how 3,100 chemical ingredients are used in secret blends to hide the scent of you dying. "The average fragrance product tested contained 14 secret chemicals not listed on the label. Among them are chemicals associated with hormone disruption and allergic reaction, and many substances that have not been assessed for safety in personal care products."[413]

We can lump perfume into the larger category of endocrine disruptors, which are also referred to as hormone disruptors. Those include everyday products, such as metal cans, detergents, food, toys, cosmetics, and pesticides. Your doctor is not going to suggest that perfume or metal cans are causing a hormone disruption, because how could anyone pinpoint an individual exposure from the millions of daily exposures? Yet according to one 2015 study published in the *Journal of Clinical Endocrinology and Metabolism*, perfumes and other endocrine disruptors are estimated to take a $170 billion per year chunk out of Europe's healthcare costs.[414]

The fact that this is an "estimate" means that we actually have no idea how endocrine disruptors are affecting peoples' health or if the exposure to hormone disruptors is the cause of your headaches. Hormone disruption and allergic reactions are going to hit the MTHFR gene like a freight train, but you knew that.

What to Do About It

You can start by avoiding smell triggers and chemical exposure by any means possible. You also might find that, once you learn about and start avoiding the largest headache triggers, a trigger like a smell won't take you over your migraine threshold. As we saw with the 1983 elimination diet, other factors such as smells and light no longer triggered migraines. This theory also aligns with the understanding of the migraine gene and the headache threshold.

Neuro-Linguistic Programming

You can also use neuro-linguistic programming to create positive scent associations that could help you heal a migraine. Neuro-linguistic programming is the hard science of how thoughts are programmed. Have you ever taken a memory course? I did and went from barely remembering a name to being able to easily remember 50 words in order, in just a few minutes, and in any language. The program worked by having people visualize objects in places they knew very well. For example, I would visualize a cat in the doorway of my house, a silver fork in the mirror next to the door, a red car on top of the desk next to the mirror, and so on. The program would then add in more visuals if you needed to remember complex words or numbers, and it made memorizing anything easy. Why? Memory has nothing to do with intelligence. Even a dog can remember its way home through thousands of visualizations (and smells). Thoughts and emotions are categorized in the brain through chains of firing neurons. It's about making connections.

Let's say that currently, the smell of toilet bowl cleaner gives you a migraine—every time. That, too, is a connection your brain has made with those firing neurons. You can overwrite those connections easily by reprogramming the thoughts that were previously connected with them. And this is how Tony Robbins cured a man's 30-year stutter in a few minutes—by getting him to associate his childhood memory of a stuttering Bullwinkle with the man he is today, a man that does not stutter.[415]

Creating a healing association from a smell is easy. You may not be able to stay away from toilet bowl cleaner your whole life, but you can create positive smell associations to help you heal your headaches.

Here's how: You can take a natural smell, such as peppermint oil or menthol, and smell it when you feel great. You can also smell it when you finish a job, achieve a goal, or feel healthy, or after a great workout. Now take that peppermint oil and smell it when you have a developing headache. The mental association will increase your dopamine, serotonin, and endorphin levels, and that has been proven to reduce inflammation, glutamate, and migraines. Your brain creates new memories and associations in the same way it retrieves old ones. While it sounds like BS, it's science, and it is how memory develops and associates. Smell can be as much of a migraine reliever as it is a migraine trigger. I say, "John F.," and you think, "Kennedy." You smell peppermint oil and…

Headache Trigger #9: Smoking

If I can't get behind something as seemingly innocuous as whole wheat bread, you know I'm not going to get behind smoking, but did you know that smoking might actually be good for a headache? Nicotine relaxes the body and may prevent the onset of a migraine. Studies show that nicotine helps patients with Alzheimer's fire off neurons.[416] It also lowers depression and is even beneficial for the growth of new blood vessels.[417] So according to a number of articles on the internet, we should consider smoking.

According to Stanford, "Nicotine promotes the growth of new blood vessels and can also stimulate tumor growth and the buildup of plaque inside arteries."[418] The potential benefits of nicotine do not outweigh the more than 7,000 chemicals that tobacco smoke is made up of, including cyanide, formaldehyde, methanol, and ammonia.[419] Hoping for tobacco to fix your problem is kind of like using crack to relieve depression, headaches, and weariness. I don't think crack cocaine has 7,000 chemicals in it, but you get the idea.

Formaldehyde is the nasty byproduct in cheap liquor that causes headaches, death, irritability, and all that not-so-fun stuff. Methanol is in aspartame and quickly turns into formaldehyde. Excess ammonia in the brain causes inflammation, seizures, and a buildup of glutamate—which may trigger a migraine. Most of us increase ammonia by tearing up our stomachs with inflammatory foods—which lowers the glutamine production used to break down toxic ammonia. And cyanide? That's what the WWII "kill pills" were made of—little pea-sized pills of cyanide they carried in case they needed to avoid being tortured or killed some other way. The Nazi's "extermination efforts" also made cyanide gas infamous. None of this sounds like good stuff, right?

Well, here's the thing: We consume these products on a daily basis. Cyanide is found in a number of foods, such as almonds, lima beans, apricots, and apples. The concentration of cyanide in natural food is so low that it's not harmful, which is why we like whole foods. Whole foods don't kill us—most of the time.

Look up "healthy cigarette ads," and you will find some good old doctor-approved smoking ads. Tobacco is natural and must be good for you, right? One day we will look back at our food preservatives in the same way we look at our classic tobacco ads.

Are you still wondering about smoking? It's bad. It destroys the pipes that bring oxygen and water to your brain. This is common knowledge. The 1983 food elimination diet basically made all other triggers (e.g., exercise, stress, bright lights) irrelevant except for one category: "perfumes and/or cigarette smoke."

There are very few studies on migraines and smoking. In 2009, a Spanish study found that smoking more than five cigarettes per day might provoke migraine attacks.[420] The study looked at 361 medical students and found that the prevalence of migraines in active smokers was 29% higher than in nonsmokers, and migraine risk increased for those that smoked the most. The study cautioned that this is particularly dangerous because 90% of migraineurs self-medicate, often with cigarettes.

If you smoke, quit. You'll feel better all over.

Headache Trigger #10: Sweet Lies

The calorie myth is the largest catastrophe in American health. What gives you more calories: 100 calories of broccoli or 100 calories of a candy bar? What generates more fat: 100 calories of broccoli or 100 calories of a candy bar? The latter question is easy; candy bars make us fatter. But why?

The answer is in the thermic effect, which is the process of burning calories as you digest food. The thermic energy burned to digest fat is 2–3% of the fat calorie intake, for carbohydrates it is 6–8%, and for proteins it is 25–30%. So when you take in 100 calories of protein, you burn 25 to 30 calories as you digest the food, and you're left with around 70 calories of energy. Carbohydrates leave you with about 92 calories after digestion, and fats leave us with around 97 calories. A simple carbohydrate that's highly processed, such as sugar, will use very little thermic energy, and you may end up burning just a couple of calories.[421]

Broccoli is a low-calorie food with a lot of fiber and protein, making it a great example of how a calorie becomes less than a calorie. Broccoli is very controversial right now in the war between carnivores and herbivores. Made famous by Dr. Joel Fuhrman, 100 calories of broccoli has more protein than 100 calories of beef. One hundred calories of broccoli is 10 ounces, or more than three cups. The carnivores argue, "Who eats three cups of broccoli? One hundred calories of beef is only around two ounces. That's not even an appetizer, and beef has more protein, according to the USDA."

I agree with both sides. There are thousands of beef products, and some will have more protein and some will have less protein than broccoli. It's not a pissing match. Measuring food in calories doesn't work well. I don't believe that a small amount of organic grass-fed beef is bad for you. "Who eats three cups of broccoli?" Not many people—you got me there. That's a problem that is increasing our national medical expenses. I say take the best of both worlds: Make beef and broccoli.

What do you think is going to keep you fuller, a big bowl of beef and broccoli or a Snickers bar? The Snickers bar has far more calories but a fraction of the protein. Studies show that diets high in protein cause a significant weight loss from the increase in metabolism, but the other reason they're so successful is because they satisfy the appetite.[422][423] One study out of Seattle found that people unintentionally ate 441 fewer calories per day on a high-protein diet, resulting in the loss of 11 pounds in two weeks.[424] That's a lot of weight.

We also have celery's negative calorie theory. Digesting the high fiber in a six-calorie stick of celery may require more than six calories of energy, resulting in negative calorie intake. Fiber requires a lot of energy to digest. Let's take that celery and shove it through a juicer. Most of the fiber is stripped away and spit into the little bucket next to the machine. The end result is a juice that requires very little energy to digest.

Dumping the discarded fiber back into the juice will not create a celery stick. The fiber will certainly require calories to break down, but the final calorie absorption will be significantly different from eating a whole celery stick. When you eat vegetables whole, your body absorbs the bound nutrients slowly. You also have fewer sugar spikes, and your body doesn't need to store fat. The same calorie intake from whole foods will produce fewer calories in your body. Your brain will also be happy about the consistent flow of nutrients.

Brown rice has a glycemic index of 50. Removing nutrients and fiber turns it into white rice and spikes the glycemic index to 89, as we learned. Brown and white rice have roughly the same calories, plus or minus 20% depending on their variety, yet white rice creates 78% more blood sugar.

The greatest lie that breakfast ever told is that highly processed cereal makes a healthy meal. A bowl of Corn Flakes has got to be healthier than a candy bar. Wrong. The glycemic index of Corn Flakes is 93 for only a 30-gram serving. That's a higher glycemic index score than a cup of Coca-Cola at 63.[425] Let's look at the nutritional value. Corn Flakes are highly processed, so all of the added vitamins are about as good as a sprinkle of a multivitamins.

The ingredients include corn, sugar, salt, and butylated hydroxytoluene (BHT). Corn is a top genetically modified food used to make fructose, it's highly inflammatory, and it comes with little nutritional value. The National Toxicology Program said that BHT was "reasonably anticipated to be a human carcinogen" on the basis of experimental findings in animals.[426] So what is healthy about this breakfast?

I'll tell you what's sad about breakfast. Corn Flakes are the low-calorie breakfast recommended for obese children. The 2014 documentary *Fed Up* shows a number of kids who are struggling to fight diabetes and insulin resistance. You'll watch these kids crying, but it's not from the torturous remarks of classmates; it's because they're told they will die if exercise and low-calorie diets don't dramatically change their weight. The film slams Michelle Obama's "Let's Move!" campaign for promoting low-calorie diets and shows exactly how the low-calorie lunch line is the biggest threat to young people in America.

The terrible rise in childhood type 2 diabetes is causing a movement for change.[427] Bill Clinton was in the film to say that the current administration is not doing enough for this epidemic and his administration "missed it." I highly recommend watching *Fed Up* as it exhibits why a calorie is not a calorie.

So what does this all mean for your headaches?

Judging food in calories alone may lead to eating foods that spike glucose, glutamate, and inflammation and leave you feeling hungry, irritable, dehydrated, and nutrient deficient. Headaches and migraines will be extremely difficult to eliminate if we don't understand the sweet lies that large corporations sell us every time we walk into the grocery store.

Soda is the best example of the calorie lie. Soda has calories from fructose. The calories from excessive fructose have the potential to make more belly fat than glucose and create an insulin resistance that will lead to uncontrollable weight gain. Diet soda has "zero" calories, yet studies show that lab animals gain weight while on artificial sweeteners, and large population studies have found that people don't lose weight when switching to diet soda. The leading theory is that this is caused by the increase in insulin production caused by anything that tastes extremely sweet.

When you drink diet soda, your body produces insulin to say, "Energy is on the way. Don't burn fat. I got this." However, the energy never comes. The insulin burns all your glucose, you keep your fat as stored energy, and your brain is left without the beloved glucose it was anticipating. Meanwhile you keep drinking your diet Big Gulp because you're craving sugar for your glucose-depleted brain, and the insulin continues to spike. Insulin comes knocking on the cells' doors with nothing to offer. The cells don't want to tell insulin to go away, but insulin is on drugs and acting crazy.

Insulin starts stealing all the glucose it can to get its "fix." The cells get together and say, "We've got to stop enabling insulin."

A few cells say, "No, we can't do that. Insulin is family, he needs us, and we need him."

Another cell speaks up, "Insulin is causing a rise in inflammation! At this rate he's going to kill all of the cells in the brain. Best-case scenario, we will have more headaches. Worst-case scenario, tumors, cancer, and maybe death."

Insulin has gone too far, so the cells become insulin resistant. Insulin completely goes off the deep end and is unable to function as the manager of glucose and fat. The weight gain and deterioration of your headache health will be exponential.[428] That is why a calorie is not a calorie.

Companies add ingredients that will make you eat more of their products. They will add anything from MSG to processed corn in order to stimulate your appetite. Calories don't measure insulin and sugar spikes. The calories in food tell us nothing about the calories you will keep. Why would we allow calories to measure our health?

MSG rats are not safe, and neither are you. The same companies that produce chemicals in food produce drugs in your local pharmacy, and the FDA has almost no ability to uncover the dangers of chemicals once they are approved.[429] At least that's what top FDA officials claimed after the makers of the drug Vioxx hid high death rates from the FDA and killed more than 55,000 people from 1999 to 2004.[430][431]

Not to change the subject, but what kind of peanut butter do you buy? Do you buy real peanut butter? Have you looked at the ingredients? Most people buy peanut butter that is premixed and contains roasted peanuts, corn syrup, sugar, soy protein, hydrogenated vegetable oils, palm oil, and about five other ingredients that you can't pronounce. People pay slightly less money for fewer peanuts and more products that may eventually kill them. What you want is peanut butter that includes peanuts, period. Don't buy poison when other options that make both nutritional and financial sense are available.

Natural peanut butter tastes much better anyway, and fresh peanut butter machines produce something phenomenal. It's not like people are buying peanut butter that's mixed with vegetable oil for the taste. The sweet lie is that companies market this inflammatory concoction as healthy, when it is loaded with migraine triggers that will raise inflammation.

You only truly realize the cost benefit once you understand the negative impact products such as hydrogenated vegetable oils and corn syrup have on your body. I refuse to believe that a parent would say that it's in their best interest to purchase a product with substances that promote obesity, insulin resistance, headaches, and poor health. This is not a conscious decision. People make the assumption that peanut butter is healthy before they read or understand the impact of the ingredients.

The overall confusion stems from products that claim to be natural, healthy, free-range, nutritional, low in fat, low sugar, organic, or low calorie. Is a fish organic when it swims in its own filth and eats processed corn and soy? How about the products that claim to be low in fat and end up having more sugar? Is a chicken "free range" when it is exposed to only a small patch of concrete with outside air? These "healthy" and subtle taglines are disastrous.

My father is prediabetic and trying his best to eat foods that are healthy. I convinced him that diet soda is a bad idea, but buying "healthy" foods is another story. The ingredients of "healthy" foods often mirror the ingredients of junk food. You will find processed corn, soy, high-fructose corn syrup, whey, glutamate, and a million other insulin producers in candy bars and health bars alike. Don't even get me started with the hundreds of ingredients in "healthy" TV dinners.

How is my father going to fight diabetes when his recommended diet allows the very foods that are causing diabetes? He made the healthy choice to switch to agave sugar instead of artificial or refined sugar. Unfortunately, agave is primarily fructose and will cause faster weight gain. Natural stevia may be the best bet for his sweetener.

It's important to remember that we should use anything that's extremely sweet in moderation, especially those with insulin problems. And don't confuse actual stevia sweeteners with Truvia. Truvia only uses 0.5% percent of an extract of stevia. The rest of Truvia is a mixture of a sugar alcohol from genetically modified corn and "natural flavors." The slogan "Born from the leaves of a stevia plant" leads the less suspicious consumer to believe that the product has more than 0.5% of stevia. If you don't know what you're consuming, how will you know what is causing your headaches? Companies market single teensy-weensy ingredients as healthiness. It's easy when most consumers do not read the labels.

A diabetic will be prescribed a drug long before he or she understands the ingredients that cause insulin resistance. My greatest fear is that my father's "healthy" diet will cause type 3 diabetes. The loss of one's own thoughts may be the same threat that causes diabetes and migraines. I believe the answer to this encompassing insulin resistance problem is education. The only way to change the problem is to understand that the back of a package is more important than the front. The back of the package is one internet search away from finding out what causes insulin resistance, diabetes, and headaches.

How do companies get away with producing lies? In the TED Talk, "What doctors don't know about the drugs they prescribe," Ben Goldacre describes how he and other doctors are misled by research that only shows the positive effects of drugs.

Industry-funded trials are four times more likely to get positive results than independently sponsored trials. Individual trials are allowed to remove 50% of the data and still publish the study. This is the equivalent of tossing a coin one hundred times and only using the fifty results that showed heads, leading you to believe that all coins are two headed.

Thousands of studies are completed on drugs, yet very few of the negative findings are published to benefit the doctors prescribing these dangerous drugs. Dr. Goldacre references a very negative study on a drug for abnormal heart rhythms, a study that was never published. A high percentage of patients died from the drug. It presented a risk so high that researchers completely abandoned the development of the drug. In the years following the unpublished study, other researchers and doctors replicated this mistake until over 100,000 people died.

The Séralini study mentioned in the GMO chapter was criticized for only having 10 rats per sex group in order to be consistent with a study published by Monsanto. The Monsanto study did, in fact, publish the results of 10 rats' blood and urine chemistry, but the actual number of rats in the study was 20. Why didn't they publish the results of the other 10 rats? So remember, don't believe everything you read.

The sweet lies we are told could be the worst headache trigger. Reducing processed food and eating more truly natural foods may eliminate this headache trigger.

Want to Learn More?

- *Fed Up*, the film – Exhibits why a calorie is not a calorie
- *Sweet Deception* by Dr. Joseph Mercola
- "Battling bad science," Ben Goldacre, TED Talk – An entertaining and disturbingly hilarious discussion of how the publication of one-sided research in our medical system is killing humans
- "What doctors don't know about the drugs they prescribe," Ben Goldacre, TED Talk – A discussion on how doctors can be misled by medical studies
- "Atul Gawande: How do we heal medicine," YouTube – A compelling argument that inspired this book

Headache Trigger #11: Ice Cream

It's a warm, sunny day, and you are enjoying homemade ice cream. Then, suddenly, something is wrong. Everything between your forehead and mouth has the sensation of a cryogenic freeze. Your brain's blood vessels begin to dilate in an effort to rush in warm blood, but it's too late. You're having a brain freeze. There's nothing you can do. The next 20 seconds are debilitating. Finally, your brain vessels constrict and the pain subsides.

What's this got to do with migraines? "Apart from a few for whom an ice cream headache may trigger a migraine, the ice cream headache seems not to have any special significance for migraine patients," according to a study from 1992.[432] A more recent study found that the ice cream headache is more prevalent in kids with migraines. Many children reduced their consumption of ice cream or abstained from it in fear of headaches.[433]

The epic failure in ice cream and migraine research mirrors any type of study that attempts to recreate a migraine. An ice cream headache will not induce a migraine if the current headache threshold is not at risk of overflowing. It's essentially the same as the chocolate-induced migraine. Many people document the immediate migraine, but researchers are not able to repeat this exact scenario in a lab setting.

Anything cold may play with the size of your pipes and may break your headache threshold. This is the acute portion of the ice cream headache. Let's look at the chronic attributes from some of ice cream's common ingredients. Propylene glycol, ethyl acetate, yellow dye #5, diethylene glycol, and aldehyde C-17 make the top headache triggers found in ice cream look harmless—you know, the soy, dairy, eggs, and sugar. What else is in the 31,000 flavors of ice cream? Chocolate, coffee, MSG, aspartame, nuts, sulfites, wheat flour, and hundreds of other ingredients.

Chemicals such as diethylene glycol are meant for antifreeze and paint thinner. Do you remember those commercials with the youngest and cutest kids attempting to read chemical ingredients from typical ice cream, followed by the child clearly reading Breyers' ingredients: milk, cream, sugar, and vanilla?

Ice creams don't have so few ingredients today, including Breyers. Some people say, "How dare you, Breyers! You're feeding us bad stuff!" This is not Breyers' fault. Breyers wants to market that pure ice cream to us. The problem is that we don't give a flying fudge about what's in our ice cream. People stopped purchasing the pure ice cream for significantly cheaper products. So Breyers made smaller containers to offset the cost. We, the public, choose the larger bucket of ingredients meant for under the hoods of cars instead of delicious natural ice cream.

This is the case with any food. People vote every time they make a purchase. We pick up the cheaper box. We choose the products that are more likely to cause headaches. A company cannot compete when the public is willing to choose dangerously cheap ingredients.

What Can We Do?

- We can vote by purchasing ice cream made from whole ingredients.
- We can make our own ice cream.
- We can limit our intake of sugar and dairy.

- We can keep ice cream away from the roofs of our mouths.
- We can decide not to eat ice cream, since it's loaded with headache triggers.

Headache Trigger #12: Caffeine

Time is critical in migraine treatment. Taking 1000 mg of aspirin is still one of the most effective ways to stop a migraine—even when compared to triptans—but only if they're taken within 30 minutes of the first symptoms.[434] Caffeine will accelerate anti-inflammatory drugs to meet the migraine deadline.

The makers of effective headache medications that contain caffeine (Excedrin, Midol, Migranal, Anacin, Fioricet, and Darvon Compound) understand this very well. Many are confused when they hear that migraine meds use caffeine when caffeine is also a headache trigger. The drugs are using caffeine in an acute manner to fix the problem now. There's no guarantee that the headache won't come back. The drugs may even cause a worse headache, as some people have negative results from caffeine.

This is where the theories begin to spin out of control and fingers point in every direction. In reality, a 90-pound female may be able to down five cups of coffee and feel great, while a heavyset man may have the jitters as he becomes anxious, stressed, and clammy from just one single little espresso.

One study suggests that two cups of coffee per day is great, while another claims that one cup of coffee per day will increase the risk of chronic daily headaches by nearly threefold.[435] My personal tolerance is dramatically changed by how many cups of coffee I drink per day. Consistently drinking two mugs (four cups) of coffee per day will guarantee me a withdrawal headache after I miss my morning cup; four mugs of coffee and the headache will rise before the day is over. This is consistent with the advice of the Mayo Clinic, which suggests that having over 500 mg of caffeine in a day—two tall

Starbucks coffees—is likely to produce unwanted side effects. Why does this happen?

With every action, there is a reaction. Regularly using caffeine to constrict your blood vessels may act as a crutch for your pipes. After your pipes are done constricting, they open up. Whether it's from too much caffeine too quickly or from a slow buildup of the tolerance effect, the more you tighten, the more the pipes eventually loosen. You don't want wide pipes.

It represents the "rebound effect," a major problem with all acute or fast-acting migraine medications. This bounce comes back with a kick. Caffeine lowers adenosine in the brain, which then raises glutamate.[436] With something like MSG, this would be the easy equation of more + more = inflammation. However, caffeine may temporarily constrict inflammation.

So what happens to the glutamate? It's still there, building. Adenosine regulates glutamate and dopamine, so without it, you will continue to rapidly fire those glutamate thoughts.[437] The inflammation that would come with too much glutamate is squeezed as your mind runs wild with the dopamine feeling of success; you know, it's that morning-cup-of-coffee feeling. I wish that feeling could last forever, but apparently it can't even make a 15 km run.

A 2013 study of athletes, by the Research Institute on Health Science, found that those who consume caffeine before a 15 km run show significantly higher levels of IL-6 cytokines and oxidative stress.[438] I don't really care about this because I'm not running 15 km unless a lion is chasing me. But what happens when I just sit at a desk for eight hours and have a few cups of coffee?

Caffeine boosts cortisol secretion, which is great if a lion really is chasing you. But how long is a lion realistically going to chase

Other Headache Triggers to Avoid

you in our theoretical world? Fifteen seconds? An hour? You will either become a meal or survive, and your cortisol levels (stress hormones) will quickly return to normal.

A 2006 study by researchers from the Veterans Affairs Medical Center in Oklahoma found that including coffee with mental exercise will magnify cortisol secretion.[439] Just you, coffee, and some desk work could equal a little lion running through your mind. The elevation also happened when caffeine was taken prior to exercise, even though exercise alone did not increase cortisol. Researchers tested these levels eight times per day and found a steady rise in cortisol with caffeine consumption, no matter the stress inducer.

What happens when your body thinks a lion is attacking you every day for 18 hours straight?

Your body makes you feel terrible to encourage you to stay away from lions. But do you? No, you go back to your place of work, drink more coffee, and continue to stress out with more cortisol. The bump in cortisol causes increased insulin production, which causes inflammation and makes you feel icky.

Increased insulin or caffeine may decrease insulin sensitivity by 15%, which will help destroy your brain and belly.[440] That's one big reason to quit coffee. There are about 50 other common symptoms that stress itself will embrace, including insomnia, stomachaches, forgetfulness, pain, heartburn, depression, and frequent crying spells.

Coffee may cause a number of headache problems without the caffeine. The acidity of coffee may imbalance gut flora, leaving many stomachs turning. Coffee's diuretic properties may excrete magnesium and potassium, causing electrolyte imbalances. See the cycle? Coffee may impact the gut and hydration, which may impact the gut, which leads to dehydration, and on and on and on.

Is Coffee an Allergy Trigger?

You may recall that coffee triggered headaches in 40% of the participants in the 1979 study and showed an 83% reaction to gluten antibodies on the cross-reaction study. Past studies may have falsely accused coffee of allergic reactions from the gluten that contaminates most instant coffees. Gluten is not found in pure coffee.

This brings us to our next false judgment: Many people have headaches not from coffee but from what they add to coffee. Milk, sugar, soy, and artificial sweeteners cause more of a headache threat than coffee itself. I don't always drink coffee, but when I do, it's as black as a panther—unless it's Bulletproof.

So is coffee terrible?

For every negative study mentioned, there is a positive coffee study. Caffeine is in nearly every weight-loss supplement and can boost your metabolism. Studies actually show that coffee lowers your risk of diabetes for unknown reasons.[441] The bump in dopamine means you are less likely to jump off a bridge after a cup of joe. Coffee's additional benefits include antioxidants, nutrients, improved liver function, and an improved fight-or-flight response to battle lions.

What *Not* to Buy

Don't buy decaf coffee or cheap coffee, which are essentially the same thing. The beans used by bargain coffees are often the beans that didn't make the cut, possibly loaded with pesticides and mold. This is particularly bad for decaf, because caffeine kills some of that mold. The worst coffee beans are used to produce decaf, because decaffeination strips the flavor anyway.[442]

The molds (mycotoxins) will not be a problem for the majority of those who drink quality coffee because the drying and roasting process eliminates nearly all molds.[443] [444] Low toxin levels are necessary for the premium coffee to receive a decent rating when graded. In reality, the levels of mold toxins from even average coffee beans make little difference to your health. A European study found that 28 cups of coffee per week (four cups per day) result in only 2% of the mold exposure considered to be harmful.[445] This is great news for most people, but if you are like me and feel like you're going to die when you're exposed to certain types of mold, you may want to stick with good, quality coffee.[446]

What to Buy

Any premium coffee will do, and there is, of course, the self-certified, low-mycotoxin Bulletproof coffee. Most people think that Dave Asprey is out of his mind because he suggests people consume his Bulletproof coffee in the strangest way. I thought he was crazy until I tried the Bulletproof method and was blown away by results that included increased mental stamina and a healthy loss of appetite. Asprey was a migraine sufferer who spent over $300,000 to cure himself of disease.

Although I am impressed with the new way to drink coffee, overall I feel remarkably better when I don't drink any coffee. Coffee is a big headache trigger. Many headache sufferers, including migraineurs, lose the headaches when they lose the caffeine. Try cutting caffeine for a few of days and see how you feel. Remember to gradually decrease your coffee consumption, since withdrawal symptoms for heavy coffee drinkers will peak in one to three days.[447] Slowly lowering your caffeine intake should make the 3-day transition a breeze.

Other Headache Triggers to Avoid

Headache Trigger #13: Blue Light

Everyone knows migraine sufferers stay out of the light like vampires, but everyone may not know the new science behind this headache aggravator. A study conducted at Harvard Medical School on blind migraine sufferers found that light was not a trigger for those with eyes that had zero function—no surprise there. However, the sufferers who were blind but still had melanopsin receptors experienced pain from light during a migraine.[448]

Melanopsin receptors don't help you see shapes, but they do react to *blue light*—this is a big deal. Melanopsin receptors play a role in synchronizing circadian rhythms and producing melatonin for sleep. Circadian rhythms are your internal clock that can go haywire with jet lag, the nightshift, booze, or artificial light. An out-of-whack circadian rhythm can alter your insulin sensitivity and cause hypertension and inflammation. While we're dazed and confused, our bodies asks for something sweet to treat the bitter feel of a broken internal clock.[449] To make it even worse, blue light is also known as high-energy visible (HEV) radiation and can cause macular degeneration, the leading cause of vision loss in Americans 60 and older.[450]

Researchers found that when blue light triggers the melanopsin receptors, calcium levels increase and signals are sent to the pupil of the eye. The question the researchers had was, how do we stop this influx of calcium? In 2013 they found their answer in a drug called an opsinamide, which blocked the calcium, ending the entire process of light sensitivity without affecting vision.[451] Opsinamides are currently being tested and give hope to migraine sufferers who have light-sensitivity triggers and may be at risk of irreversible eye damage.

What to Do About It

So how do we block the blue light now? By bringing back 1986, a time when BluBlockers were not only functional but also stylish. These retro shades have made a small cameo in hipster fashion but may be ready for a full comeback in our battle against new technology that blares blue light. You see, people like to sleep and are having a hard time doing so with too much blue light—it's like someone pulled the plug on your body's internal clock. You can simply avoid computers, TVs, fluorescent lights, and all light, for that matter. But you won't. That's a recommendation people never follow. (Vampires, yes. People, no.) But that's OK because there are other products you can use as well.

BluBlocker Shades

The concept of BluBlocker sunglasses is simple: Orange and yellow (amber) block blue light, so let's block blue light in style. NASA invented the technology to protect astronauts from strong UV rays and specifically to block blue rays so that the retina could focus, allowing objects to appear sharper and clearer.

Where to Get Them

BluBlocker sunglasses are still available at www.blublocker.com, but they might not suit your style.

You can try some other knockoff brand if you want a different style, and most quality sunglasses will block a good amount of blue light. The problem with cheaper shades is that they dilate your pupils but continue to let in all of the UV and HEV rays. You would do better to go out and stare into the sun, because then at least your eyes would be able to constrict some of the harmful light. Most

Other Headache Triggers to Avoid

people only use dark shades during daylight—with the exception of maybe a few cool cats and some Vegas high rollers—leaving no protection from the powerful blue light of car headlights, LEDs, fluorescent lights, and computer screens. Migraineurs sensitive to blue light may want to consider wearing sunglasses all the time.

Search for a variety of quality shades that have UV and HEV protection. It's also critical that the shades block some of the light that sneaks past the sides of the frame. It's not clear how blocking blue light during the day will affect your sleep, but it's certain that blue light during the night has a large impact on our sleep patterns, making orange or yellow lenses a great solution for blocking blue lights in less than sunny conditions.

Other Ways to Eliminate Blue Light

Stopping use of your TV and computers probably isn't reasonable, but even shutting down the laptop, iPad, and TV near bedtime is an achievement—an achievement that will show immediate results.

While you're looking at your screens, however, you can block that blue light with any number of products. I'm currently using a product called f.lux, which turns down the blue light on my laptop so I can work longer hours without eyestrain. You can also get "blue light screen covers" for just about any electronic device you own.

Light bulbs, fluorescent lights, and LEDs can easily be swapped out for blue-blocking bulbs. You can buy lenses, contact lenses, and shades that have varying levels of blue-light protection. Many new products are being developed for the newly found threat of blue light.[452][453]

Headache Trigger #14: Poor Sleep Patterns

Samantha Hall has just finished a stressful week using every bit of her master's degree in English. Tonight, she is waiting tables at a high-end restaurant that is understaffed. She's almost done with her double shift as she takes mental notes of the order for the last member of a party of 10—this is the type of establishment where notepads are forbidden.

Samantha makes it home, her head hits the pillow, and everything goes blank. Ten peaceful hours later, Samantha is reminded that life is painful by awakening to a Saturday morning migraine.

How did this happen?

The first theory is that oversleeping causes a fluctuation of serotonin, which will cause ups and downs in glutamate levels. A second theory is that stress constricts and inflames the blood vessels all week long until complete relaxation is found. Tighter constriction ends with a wider relaxation—especially if you also miss your morning coffee. As we know, wide pipes can trigger a headache.

Sleep patterns have long been associated with migraines, as too much or too little sleep is a well-known trigger. Because sleep produces dopamine and serotonin, depression also goes hand in hand with sleep disturbances.[454] Why do you think your body hates the sound of an alarm clock?

Sleep Loss: Cause or Symptom of Migraines?

Sleep loss is both a trigger of migraines and a symptom of migraines. Those with chronic migraines (15 or more migraines per month) report that they have trouble sleeping, which can reduce productivity by as much as 50%.[455] And what about sleep loss as the cause of migraines? Sleep deprivation can lead to an increase in inflammation and glutamate, which keeps your thoughts chaotically running as triggers reach the top of the headache threshold.[456] [457]

In an interview of 147 women with chronic migraines, not a single one reported feeling refreshed upon awakening. It seems that sleep loss can cause or be caused by migraines. What a nasty cycle.[458]

The Midnight Migraine

Want to know why you sometimes wake up in the middle of the night with a migraine? As you dream inside a fully developed make-believe world, your primary neurotransmitter, glutamate, is firing rapidly to create that dream world. According to Los Angeles neurologist Vincent Fortanasce, the dream stage of sleep (REM) often causes the powerful migraines that occur 5 to 6 hours after sleep begins.[459]

Interestingly, late night meals may raise your glutamate levels long after your last bite. Although most food is digested within three and a half hours, the release of glutamate in your brain can take much longer. This is especially true if that food triggers inflammation. The glutamate rise during REM sleep may break the glutamate threshold that has been building for hours, days, or even months.[460]

Many other factors are involved with sleep. Dreams can bring on stress, muscle repair at night can raise inflammation, and the billion other neurological functions we don't yet understand may play an immeasurable role in the nighttime migraine.

Getting Better Sleep with Fewer Migraines

Sleep is so important for every part of your life, so it should be your goal to get better sleep. In one study, these things helped chronic migraine patients sleep better at night:[461]

- Going to bed at a scheduled time
- Not watching TV, reading, or listening to music in bed
- Having dinner more than four hours before sleeping at night
- Discontinuing naps*

*Some recent studies show that naps are beneficial.

The results of these patients getting a better night of sleep might blow your mind. Fifty-eight percent reverted from chronic migraines to episodic migraines. The study listed the success of episodic migraines as fewer than 13 headaches per month with at least four headache-free days. While that may sound like a terrible definition of success, every extra day that a sufferer is headache-free matters. These women went from an average pain scale of 46.7 for the month to 28.3. The calculation was based on a three-point headache-ranking scale: The number of days they had severe headaches were multiplied by three; the days with moderate headaches were multiplied by two; each day with mild headaches counted as one; and then they took the sum of those numbers.

Here's the crazy part of the study: 74.4% of the patients were overusing various acute medications, and all of the subjects that reverted back to episodic migraines were the ones who lowered or eliminated their medications.[462]

Other Headache Triggers to Avoid

Why was medication hurting these patients? Acute-migraine medications have a rebound effect, but there's something you should know about medication and sleep. Certain medications will reduce or eliminate REM sleep, which should scare you because many of these sleep-altering medications are prescribed for patients with migraines.

How to Get Great Sleep

Start off by eliminating caffeinated beverages and medications that are made to stop sleep. Eliminate bright lights in the evening. Nature has our sleep cycle planned according to the sun, so stick with that. This means don't shine a floodlight while brushing your teeth or reading a nighttime story.

Stop crazy thoughts from exciting your brain. TVs, laptops, or other visually and mentally stimulating devices should get the boot from your bedroom. Get some exercise, but not too late, because exercise promotes immediate energy and happiness.

Lower your daily intake of glutamate and foods and drinks that cause inflammation. Reduce alcohol, sugar, MSG, and any other bad stuff before bed.

Sleep Apnea and Migraines

Sleep apnea is a huge problem for many migraine sufferers. NFL player Percy Harvin has had debilitating migraines that have claimed numerous practices and games, and one nearly claimed his life. In 2010 he collapsed during practice and was rushed away in an ambulance.[463]

He was diagnosed with sleep apnea and now uses a CPAP breathing machine—we call them Darth Vader machines at the firehouse. We prefer these machines for firefighters with breathing problems to the roar of snoring. Percy is migraine-free—for now. It's unknown whether his near-death experience was the result of sleep apnea or migraine medication. It is clear that sleep loss severely affects migraines. Sleep apnea is also responsible for doubling your risk of developing dementia, according to a study of 1,300 adults over the age of 75.[464]

Talk to your doctor about seeing a sleep specialist if you suffer from sleep apnea. New CPAP machines are extremely quiet, and they even have mouth guards that work well for mild sleep apnea and snoring. It's also critical that you see a TMJ specialist for jaw alignment, as this could be the trigger of sleep apnea and migraines. There's a mouth guard for that, too.

Why Is Sleep So Important?

The average person sleeps 36% of his or her life. If you live to be 100, that's 36 years of sleep. Not Donald Trump though; he credits his success to only three hours of sleep per night. But according to sleep researcher Robert Stickgold of Harvard Medical School, sleep is undeniably important for forming memories. A tired brain has a hard time concentrating.

What most people don't know is that your brain is far from finished with the memories that have passed through your thoughts. The breakfast you had this morning is stored in a different place than the memory you will use to decide what you want for breakfast tomorrow.

Crazy fact: The brain shifts memories around and strengthens the neural connections as if it were recording memories on a computer's hard drive.

Other Headache Triggers to Avoid

This shuffling of information allows your brain to take the memory of yesterday's breakfast to form the memory and decision-making thoughts that will help you pick what you want for breakfast today. Dr. Stickgold believes this process happens most often while you sleep, although modern science has yet to prove how or when this actually happens—just that it does happen.[465]

Many scientists side with Dr. Stickgold, as people and rats increase their REM sleep after intensive language learning or successful maze completions, while other researchers state this is due to the stress response and not to learning itself.

As a firefighter who has worked near a giant Halloween maze, I also confirm that people will freak out when they get lost in a maze. When the fire department comes to rescue these people, the employees of the giant maze will also freak out. This is because the fire department will eliminate the stress of a giant maze by breaking through every wall.

We do this for two reasons. One, the stress may actually cause (and has caused) life-threatening medical emergencies that shouldn't rely on a firefighter's ability to solve a maze. Two, firefighters like to break things. The point is that learning a maze could be enough stress to induce the need for more REM sleep.

So is sleep for memory consolidation or stress reduction? Does the answer matter?

The physiology behind memory consolidation or stress relief doesn't change the end result of sleep. Sleep improves memory and lowers stress—this we know for sure. Trust that your body knows more about sleep than the internet does.

Sleep-Deprivation Headaches

The light bulb of Thomas Edison—who regarded sleep as a waste of time—has led to a growing number of walking zombies. Aside from cognitive decline, sleep deprivation is associated with increased stress, high blood pressure, impaired control of glucose, inflammation, diabetes, obesity, stroke, mood disorders, damaged immune systems, alcoholism, and heart disease.[466]

Many busy fire departments have permanently jet-lagged firefighters. Thirty-seven percent of firefighters have one or more sleep disorders.[467] Accidents happen when we are deliriously sleepy. It destroys the brain. There is a reason why sleep deprivation is used for torture and mind manipulation.

The real importance of sleep has yet to be discovered. The first evidence at the molecular level of the basic purpose of sleep was just discovered in 2013. The brain clears waste products during sleep with cerebrospinal fluid. Waste products cause inflammation and can trigger headaches.

What's spectacular is that the study found that amyloid proteins were cleared from the brains of sleeping mice as if by a "dishwasher" or "brainwasher."[468] You read previously about amyloid plaque as the link between Alzheimer's, migraines, and brain damage. Sleep is more important for headache health than we know.

First Sleep and Second Sleep

In the fifteenth and sixteenth centuries, people slept a full eight hours, but not the doctor-prescribed eight hours that you're thinking of. Writings from these two centuries reveal a "first sleep" and a "second sleep." People would go to sleep soon after dark for four hours and then wake up. The in-between hours were reserved for reading, relaxing, recalling dreams, and sex. The "second sleep" would then last another four hours.[469]

How would I feel with a first and second sleep?

A famous study in the 1990s had students experience a 14-hour dark schedule every night for a month. After a week, subjects fell into a natural rhythm of two hours of quiet wakefulness followed by four hours of sleep, another two hours of quiet wakefulness, a "second sleep" of four hours, and another two hours of quiet wakefulness before light.[470]

The students said that they "never felt so awake." Tests showed they were unnaturally alert for modern-day humans. Maybe it's like the movie *Limitless* where the brain can access 100% of its intelligence so you can do things like stop time and learn Italian in a day. How would you know if you've never slept a natural day in your life?

WTF Can I Eat?

The Elimination Diet Process

Seriously, what the fork can you eat now that you've read enough to start thinking about Safeway as mine field? If you're frustrated and not sure how you're going to manage eliminating even a few of the headache triggers I mentioned, just remember: The key is in moderation and balance. It's about finding what triggers your headaches and limiting your intake of those things. If you find that not eating gluten (or anything else, really) makes you feel so fantastic you're ready to go gluten-free forever, that's great. And if you only avoid eating gluten when you know you have other triggers on board just waiting to hit you with a migraine, that's great, too. But there's no quick answer to the question—WTF you can eat is what we are here to find out.

During your elimination diet, you will find your own 3-day "cure" for your headaches. For many people, it only takes three days of eliminating the top headache triggers from their diets before they start to feel infinitely better. For others, it may take a little longer to start feeling the benefits of the cleanse. Don't get discouraged during this process. Elimination diets are hard, and you may find yourself screaming, "WTF can I eat?!" over and over again.

And listen—all the information out there can be very confusing. Don't let a healthcare professional steer you in the wrong direction. There is simply too much information and there are too many variables to create the perfect diet. As such, *there is no perfect diet*, and there doesn't need to be. Instead, this book shows you how to eliminate the major migraine triggers, lists the foods least likely to cause reactions, and displays the steps you can follow to evaluate your personal triggers. Don't worry; you will not be required to eat like a pigeon.

Once you've determined what your triggers are, peruse the guidebook for a list of excellent, free websites with top-rated, delicious, healthy, natural recipes you can use. I'll also recommend some outstanding recipe books, but any natural food recipes will do. The Headache Help Checklist was designed to help you navigate your elimination diet and includes a list of foods that are dangerous or questionable so you can choose from thousands of other tasty foods.

This massive amount of information all points to eating more real food and limiting your intake of the other stuff. It's simple. Just pay attention, look for the healthier, whole-food options when they're available, and, if you can't swing a full elimination, balance what you know produces migraines for you with healthy foods that aren't triggers, foods that are healing for you, so you don't break your headache threshold.

Sadly, there are no headache-safe foods! You may have an individual reaction to any kind of food. The large migraine-safe food lists online are typically useless and sometimes even harmful. They may be well-meaning and based on solid research, but if you see anything that lists something like diet soda (or anything else with Splenda or artificial sweeteners), cheese, milk, bread, or Frosted Flakes, beware of what you're reading.[471,472,473,474,475]

How in the world are you going to pull this off? It's actually pretty easy, willpower notwithstanding, and you have options. The first thing you should know about starting on either option is this: It is not a true elimination diet if you are eating processed foods. Our FDA-regulated foods allow food companies to add many hidden ingredients in small amounts to their foods. There's also cross contamination from large manufacturers using the same machines for multiple foods. Cross contamination makes it very difficult for people on elimination diets, especially for people with gluten sensitivity. So eliminating processed foods and replacing them with whole foods is your first step in this process.

Dear Diary

You know who your best friend through this process is? Your headache diary. You're going to tell that diary everything—and in return, it's going to tell you what your headache patterns are so you can find the path to prevention.

What if the culprit were something as simple as diet soda? You could instantly eliminate extraordinary amounts of pain. A headache diary is where many people find their problem triggers. Keeping a headache diary can keep you accountable for your headache triggers, and you can use that information to help guide your medical care. A headache diary allows you to quickly share information about your headaches and triggers with healthcare professionals, and that lets them know you're not messing around.

You can simply search online for a migraine diary, and you'll find a number of free and printable diaries. Warning: Most are very limited and only look at moments before the migraine. I like Migraine Diary by The Migraine Trust[476] because it has an extensive daily record of possible triggers, a monthly diary of migraines—easily viewable by doctors—and it comes with a medication list.

There are also a number of headache diary apps for the iPhone and Android. The two best apps I've found thus far are

Migraine Buddy and My Pain Diary: Chronic Pain and Symptom Tracker. Both apps make it easy to add in multiple headache factors and generate graphs to send to your doctor.

A regular calendar and notebook would also work great, because your knowledge base of headache triggers is more extensive than any headache diary currently available. The more information you include, the more steps you can take to eliminate the problem.

Headache diaries should include:

- Sleep – Record your bedtime, wake up time, and hours of sleep.

- Foods – The more details you can include, the better. Try to include every food, ingredient, preservative, and additive you consume, along with anything else that might be relevant, such as whether something you've eaten is processed. A single food dye could be more powerful than any other triggers combined. Equally important are the vegetables and foods that may reduce the risk of a headache. Portion size and timing are also huge factors.

- Drinks – You should record everything: alcohol; soda, juice, caffeinated beverages, sugary processed drinks, water, mineral water, coconut water—all of it. How much do you drink and how often?

- Activities – Record your activities, such as work, driving, traffic, meditation, rock climbing, exercise, smoking, fun in the sun, etc.

- Headaches – Here, you should record the time of the headache, whether you had an aura or warning, the locations of the pain and how you rate it on the 1–10 pain scale, the types of relief and medications you used and their side effects, the symptoms of your pain, and whether the headache caused you to miss activities or work.

- Happiness – Were you happy? Stressed? Crying? Indifferent? What caused the feeling? Stress is a major headache trigger.

Identifying even the small roots of a stressor can open up much larger solutions. Are you unhappy at work? Problems at home? Is it the dog? Are you worried about public speaking? Are you just not that happy? Use your diary to look for patterns and try to discover the reasons behind your feelings.

- Menstrual cycle – Tracking this pattern can help you learn when your most common migraine days are so you can spend the days prior ensuring you don't break your headache threshold.

- Other conditions – If you have other medical conditions, you can record those symptoms as well.

- Medications – You'll list the names of your meds, your dose, how long you've been using it, side effects, and anything else. Many people continue to use drugs that gradually become toxic. Even migraine experts will find themselves back in a state of chronic migraine from the slow addition of rebound headaches from their once-lovely medications.

- Environment – Track the weather, barometric changes, allergens, mold, dust, etc.

- Anything you come in contact with – Record the soaps, solvents, deodorants, perfumes, smoke, etc. Anything that may have triggered a migraine for you is worth tracking.

Set Your Own Limits

Does all of this seem like a lot? Well, the same way you can with the elimination diet, you can set your own limits. If you're not willing to record the entire day, don't. You may find that it's easier to record the bare minimum, and that is far more helpful than nothing.

Just know that even the greatest thinkers may start by writing a problem down. As Charles Kettering put it, "A problem well stated is a problem half solved." Charles Kettering was an American inventor with 186 patents, including the electric ignition in your car and the lacquers used to shine your favorite color of paint on that car. If tearing apart a problem helped Kettering advance civilization, maybe it can help you solve the complex problem of a single headache.

Step 1: Choose Your Elimination Diet Option

Both of these elimination diet options consider the foods that may be individual headache triggers, and both have their benefits and drawbacks. No matter which one you choose, make sure you use the Headache Help Checklist along with your elimination diet, and if you don't already use a headache diary, this is a great time to start.

Before You Begin

If you have a health condition other than migraines, or if you're vegetarian or vegan and concerned about finding the right foods for a balanced elimination diet, you should consult with your doctor and do some research on your own. You may even consider consulting a nutritionist. Remember, what you eat can have a profound impact on your body—that's why you're doing this. So talk to your health professionals about your plan to try an elimination diet, and get some support for this process.

Plan #1: A Typical Elimination Diet

With this elimination diet option, you will eliminate all possible headache triggers on the Headache Help Checklist—all possible triggers, processed foods, and all questionable allergens—for three to 30 days and then slowly reintroduce each possible trigger, one at a time. During your elimination, you will choose only a few foods to eat. This option is a little more extreme, but it is also more successful overall, and it will help you figure out what your headache triggers are more quickly than option #2.

The preferred method in research is to follow this type of elimination and to choose two hypoallergenic foods to eat for the three to 30 day period you're on the diet. While it is true that eating fewer foods makes it easier to find one that is a problem, I think limiting yourself to only two foods for three days is challenging enough without thinking of stretching it to 30! And I believe that eating only two foods for an extended period of time can be dangerous and create mineral deficiencies. Keep in mind that you'll need a nutritional balance that includes vegetables and protein. In general, any natural foods that are not triggers, questionable allergens, processed, or hypoallergenic are OK as part of the diet. You'll read more on this after you choose your elimination plan.

When you eat fewer foods, it's easier to identify your problem foods, so definitely come up with the smallest number of foods you can limit yourself to without going crazy. Then go for it, keeping track of it all with your headache diary and the Headache Help Checklist.

Option #2: A Kinder, Gentler, Less Effective Elimination Diet

If you choose option #2, you will only eliminate the chronic triggers, heavy hitters, and the big eight allergens that are listed at the beginning of the **Main Eliminations** section below, and you'll take your chances with all of the less common triggers. Cutting out all of those main eliminations will significantly raise your threshold in three to 30 days. Because you aren't eliminating all of the less common triggers, make sure you're aware of them when you eat them. If you get a headache within three days of consuming one of those triggers, record it and add it to your list of eliminations. So, the same as you would with option #1, use your headache diary and the Headache Help Checklist to keep track of what you eat and your reactions to the common triggers as you reintroduce them.

Many people have found this route works just fine, although there are a couple of drawbacks. For one, it's not as effective as a true elimination diet is. The other drawback is sort of a good news/bad news thing. The good news is that this option, like option #1, will help you become more conscious about the foods you eat. The bad news is that some who have tried this option started to feel paranoid about ingesting the less common headache triggers—those that are harder to pinpoint. If you start your elimination diet with this option and you find it's too messy or simply doesn't work for you, stop it and try option #1.

Main Eliminations

Whether you choose elimination option #1 or option #2, you want to make sure you avoid the biggest culprits for triggering headaches. These are all listed on the Headache Help Checklist, and here, you'll learn which are the most important to eliminate along with some other foods you can consider eliminating as well.

Definitely eliminate all of the chronic headache triggers:
- Cooking oils
- Trans fats
- Sugar
- Refined grains

- Milk
- Artificial sweeteners
- Inflammatory meats
- Alcohol
- Corn

Also eliminate these two very important heavy hitters:
- Food additives
- Free glutamic acid (MSG)

Be sure to avoid the big eight allergens:[477]
- Milk
- Eggs
- Fish
- Shellfish (e.g., crab, lobster, shrimp)
- Tree nuts (e.g., almonds, walnuts, pecans)
- Peanuts
- Wheat
- Soybeans

There are four major headache triggers that will prevent you from reaching your goal if you do not include them on your elimination list: milk products, wheat, eggs, and soy products. Those four are the chronic triggers that will keep your headache cup consistently full. Fish, shellfish, tree nuts, and peanuts are tricky because they're packed with omega-3 anti-inflammatory fat and nutrients. Switching from corn-fed pork and beef to fish might be enough to cure your headaches. However, all of the big eight foods have the highest possibility to give you an allergic reaction.

Other Eliminations to Think About

I know cutting the triggers listed above narrows us down to only the foods that nature intended for us to eat. But there are a few of nature's delicious foods we should be careful of. The 100% successful 1979 migraine diet eliminated the foods listed below. (They are in order according to the most adverse reactions.) So, according to this list, you may also want to consider eliminating tea, yeast, mushrooms, and peas:

- Wheat (78% patients reacting)
- Oranges (65%)
- Eggs (45%)
- Coffee (40%)
- Tea (40%)
- Milk and chocolate (37%)
- Beef (35%)
- Corn, sugar, and yeast (33%)
- Mushrooms (30%)
- Peas (30%)

Citrus is always a top headache trigger. Remember, it's easy to overdose on one little glass of processed orange juice. There are hundreds of teas, so you are bound to find one that doesn't sit well in your stomach. Corn and mushrooms are on many headache trigger lists and should be a concern, even in their natural forms. Many of these foods were tested in powdered form, which makes them highly processed and may account for why peas are a trigger here but show no reaction in other studies.

And if we look again at the 1983 study, we see where some of the top IgE allergens match foods on the 1979 study's eliminations. Clearly, these are worthy of including in your list of eliminations: milk products, eggs, chocolate, oranges, wheat, and food additives.

A migraine study conducted in 2010 involving 266 antigens and 30 patients had a 30% success rate overall, but some patients had over a 50% reduction in migraines.[478] These numbers are statistically significant in comparison with all of the other headache studies. This study is extremely successful in the category of eliminating only personal headache triggers for each individual. The 1979 and 1983 diets had extremely low success rates for eliminating individual triggers. Following a diet that eliminated the groups' top triggers proved to be superior to following individualized diets. However, the success of the 2010 study shows promise for a diet that combines individual triggers with chronic headache triggers. Here are the results of that study:

- Spices (27 patients reacting)
- Seeds and nuts (24)
- Seafood (24)
- Starch (22)
- Food additives (21)
- Vegetables (21)
- Cheese (20)
- Fruit (20)
- Sugar products (20)

- Eggs (14)
- Milk (14)
- Mushrooms (9)
- Yeast (5)
- Meat (5)

At a glance, that list makes fruits and vegetables look like something we should stay away from, but this is out of context. The 20-some food reactions come from over 60 fruits and vegetables. These fruits and vegetables come with fibers and nutrients that we need for survival and a healthy headache threshold. It's possible that these fruits and vegetables won't actually trigger a headache on their own.

Compare all of the previous results with these from the 2007 Mexico study involving 108 foods and 56 patients:

- Eggs (26 patients responding)
- Cheese (24)
- Milk (24)
- Yeast (21)
- Casein (15)
- Pork (14)
- Tomatoes (17)
- Kidney beans (14)
- Pork (14)
- Chili peppers (13)
- Oranges (12)

- Corn (11)
- Lemons (11)
- Peanuts (11)
- Shrimp (10)
- Mushrooms (9)
- Bananas (8)
- Chocolate (8)
- Mustard (6)

These were not headache reactions but positive immune system responses. The more people affected by each trigger, the more likely the food may be a problem for you. Mind you, this is one study and doesn't demonstrate how critical an allergen is. For example, milk chocolate may only be a reaction for eight out of 56 migraineurs, but it may be a powerful reaction that triggers a migraine every time for those eight. In contrast, some of the vegetables that have an adverse reaction for only a select few may never actually trigger a headache in those individuals. So don't freak out and stop eating.

The most notable fact from the 2007 study has completely changed the way I think about headache triggers. As you read the study, you can see the number of positive food reactions for a migraineur was between six and 30, while it was between zero and four for nonmigraineur patients! The reactions are poles apart. Tomatoes had 17 migraineur reactions and only two nonmigraineur reactions. The 56 migraineurs had a total of 524 food reactions, and the control group of 56 nonmigraineurs had only 68 reactions. Is the pathophysiology of a person with migraines really so different from a "normal" person's?

Sure there is a migraine gene, and migraineurs are predisposed to headaches if their parents are also migraineurs. But does that account for the whopping 524 reactions? If you've read this far, you know the answer. An equally important question: If your migraines go away, do they take some of your food allergies with them? I would bet my life the answer is yes.

Step 2: Figure Out WTF You Can Eat During Your Elimination Diet

OK, you've chosen your elimination diet option and what you're going to eliminate. Now you have to figure out what you can eat. Option #2 leaves you with a lot more possibilities for mealtimes, but if you're going with option #1, you're probably really wondering what the fork you can eat, especially during this elimination diet. Take a look at the lists in this section and see which ones might be possible for you to include as staples during your elimination. These lists aren't perfect, and yes, you will see foods here that conflict with elimination diets based on low-allergenic foods. I go back to the fact that this is not an exact science. These are nothing more than guidelines for you to consider.

Foods that caused the least reactions in the Mexico study involving 56 patients were:

- Apples (0 patients reacting)
- Asparagus (2)
- Broccoli (2)
- Cabbage (2)
- Carrots (2)
- Cherries (2)
- Cranberries (2)
- Eggplant (2)
- Onions (2)
- Papayas (2)
- Parsley (1)

- Peas (1)
- Peaches (1)
- Pineapples (1)
- Potatoes (3)
- Pumpkins (2)
- Zucchini (2)
- Beef (2)
- Brazil nuts (2)
- Cinnamon (1)
- Ginger (2)
- Herring (2)
- Lentils (1)
- Lobster (2)
- Oregano (4)
- Salmon (1)
- Snapper (2)
- Sunflowers (1)
- Tuna (2)

Compare these to milk with 24 patient reactions. It's good to see the options that are less likely to harm you, but you already know shellfish, like lobster, is not recommended on an elimination diet, yet this study shows lobster as one of the safest foods to eat. What I take from this study is that natural whole foods are a safer bet than processed foods or meat from animals that are fed or injected with unnatural substances.

The foods that caused the least reactions in the 1983 study were:

- Cauliflower (1 patient reacting)
- Lettuce (1)
- Avocadoes (1)
- Dates (1)
- Rabbit (1)
- Peas (2)
- Lentils (2)
- Honey (2)
- Lamb (2)

The 1983 study shows rabbit and lamb as the least likely meats to actually trigger a migraine. Many hypoallergenic diets list wild game as low-allergenic food. This is on the basis that grass-fed and wild animals contain higher levels of omega-3, conjugated linoleic acid (CLA—another good fat), and vitamin E. This combination is found even though the meat is overall leaner with less omega-6 fat. You will see that deer, elk, bison, lamb, grass-fed beef, pasture-raised hens, and other organic animals are listed in hypoallergenic diets that are aimed at lowering food additives and inflammation.

Migraine diets usually contain green vegetables, such as spinach, Swiss chard, and collards. You already know spinach is relatively high in histamine and tyramine for a natural food, but this has yet to be identified as a problem. Orange vegetables are the most common recommendation, such as carrots or sweet potatoes. Cooked yellow vegetables, like summer squash, are also on some lists. Other migraine diets include all fresh fruits and vegetables that are not top migraine triggers. "Fresh" will be on nearly all recommended diets because the histamine levels go up due to additional mold toxins in food that's aged or spoiled.

Although these diets are "safer," they are not foolproof. The Physicians Committee for Responsible Medicine lists migraine-safe foods that "virtually never contribute to headaches or painful conditions."[479] The list includes cherries, cranberries, pears, prunes, rice, yellow vegetables, orange vegetables, and green vegetables. These may even be good recommendations in general, however, any person can have a reaction to any of these foods.

Ultimately, you know your body better than anyone else. You know that some foods upset your stomach, and you can look at others and think, "That seems like a soothing food to eat," or "that seems like a stomachache/headache/allergy attack waiting to happen." With other foods you feel less sure about, try eliminating them along with the other foods on the list, and then reintroduce them to find out if you have any reaction. How you do your elimination diet is up to you.

Want to Learn More?

- www.eatwild.com/healthbenefits.htm – For a list of health benefits for organic meat with studies to back them up

Step 3: Reintroduce Possible Headache Triggers

Make sure you have your headache diary handy, because you need to make sure you record what you eat during step 2 of your elimination diet. At the end of your three- to 30-day elimination period, begin to introduce one possible trigger at a time—and only that trigger—on an empty stomach and see how you feel.

While researchers typically monitor patients for a few hours after consumption, we know that it can take two to three days for some foods to trigger headaches. This presents a major problem because you're bound to eat more than one food trigger in three days, and some foods might not be triggers for you until you consume them with others.

This leaves us with the very basic concept of elimination diets. If a food gives you symptoms within hours of digestion, it's a trigger for you, and you should eliminate it from your diet or moderate your intake of it. And since symptoms can take up to three days to appear, make sure you look at your headache diary's list of foods for the three days before you recorded a symptom. That will give you a better idea of what's causing it.

Symptoms That Tell You a Food Is a Trigger

Your body will tell you in more than one way that it doesn't like something you've eaten—a headache is only one way. To figure out if a particular food is a trigger after you've reintroduced it to your diet, answer the following questions:

- Do you have any kind of digestive problems, even bloating?
- Do you have diarrhea?

- Do you have sinus symptoms?
- Do you have any allergic response?
- Do you have a headache or migraine?
- Does your heart rate go up?
- Are you tired, lethargic, or just don't feel great?

If you answer yes to any of these, mark this food on your Headache Help Checklist. It's that simple. Combinations of foods may seem impossible to pinpoint, but using a headache diary along with the Headache Help Checklist makes this much easier. For example, if I see someone's headache diary with a migraine every Saturday morning with whiskey, Diet Coke, cheese, bread, and a change in stress and sleep pattern within the three days prior, I can recognize the headache pattern and know there are six possible triggers this person can work to eliminate.

Eliminate whiskey, Diet Coke, cheese, and bread, and take the steps to improve your sleep schedule and stress levels for those several days prior. Try reintroducing triggers one at a time after the headaches are gone. This is a simple and easy way to pinpoint your triggers.

Actually eliminating *all* of the triggers may be practically impossible. For example, if you told me to eliminate stress and sleep disturbances as a firefighter, I would have laughed at you. But that doesn't change the fact that we can identify triggers and work on multiple ways to reduce the impact of those triggers with other eliminations and prevention efforts.

The fact that it takes multiple triggers to break a headache threshold can be an advantage. Lowering your intake of food triggers can make other triggers irrelevant, because reducing damage to the stomach will allow it to self-heal and more effectively process food triggers and nutrients.

The Dangers of Food Reintroduction

Reintroducing a food and discovering you have a reaction to it can be no joke. It can make you sick. Let's say you've been on your elimination diet for three days and you're feeling pretty great. Next, you start by reintroducing wheat. And maybe you go a little overboard with it. Or maybe you eat something exceedingly processed, like pancakes from a box mix or restaurant and put a little syrup on them, combining headache triggers (a bad idea for a food reintroduction, by the way). Or maybe you just eat something small and simple with wheat in it. Depending on your sensitivity to the trigger you reintroduced, you may have a lot of symptoms—any or all of the symptoms listed above, plus any others your body may decide to throw back at you. And they could be fairly severe.

To keep yourself healthy during your food reintroductions:

- Begin each reintroduction by ensuring that you reintroduce the food alone and on an empty stomach.
- After you log your reaction to the food, continue eating the safe foods you've been eating for your elimination diet so you can reintroduce another one once your reaction to the food has passed.
- Don't go overboard when you reintroduce a food.
- Choose unprocessed, whole foods whenever possible. You may not be able to accomplish this with wheat since finding truly whole, modern wheat is all but impossible—but since that's not the wheat you'll be eating later anyway, it doesn't make sense to try. You can, however, reintroduce wheat in two

phases: Before you reintroduce modern wheat, try something made with ancient sprouted wheat first. One person who has tried this two-phase wheat reintroduction found that she can eat ancient sprouted grains, but modern wheat gives her allergy symptoms that often lead to migraines.

- Take a break from reintroducing foods for a while if you need to. Go back to eating the foods you chose for your elimination diet for a little while. Maybe add the foods you found safe during the reintroductions you've already completed as well to make your restricted diet less painful. Then start again.

I understand elimination diets can be arduous, especially once you start reintroducing foods. It can feel as though you're continuously giving yourself a migraine on purpose. That's because you are, if you're finding several headache triggers. But knowing that doesn't make doing it any more comfortable—or any less confounding. Just remember that elimination diets are designed to help you create a new way of eating and a pain-free way of living going forward—something that works for you, specifically.

The Headache Help Checklist

On the next pages, you will see the largest list of well-documented migraine triggers and many successful treatments from numerous migraine studies. You can find a printable version of this checklist and the free guide that accompanies it at www.3dayheadachecure.com. Take the list with you when you visit your doctor, along with your headache diary, to discuss all of your treatment options.

Please keep in mind that this list compiles the top *possible* eliminations and additions to your diet and lifestyle. Simply because they are all in one place does not mean that I'm suggesting you eliminate or add *all* things listed. You should pick and choose what makes sense for you and consult your doctor when necessary.

Before You Begin

Don't start your elimination diet without starting a headache diary. You'll use it to record your reactions to each trigger you eliminate and then reintroduce, and it's a very important part of this process of figuring out what's causing your headaches. On this checklist, you'll record whether or not you had a reaction after you reintroduced the food, and then you'll mark on the checklist whether you plan to eliminate or moderate your intake of that food going forward. There is a legend for the **Food Eliminations** section that explains what the symbols next to each food mean. Other elimination sections include clear instructions.

My Headaches in a Nutshell

Before you begin, start by spending a little time thinking about your headaches, and then add your answers to these questions to your Headache Help Checklist. Here are the questions you'll answer there:

- How many headaches or migraines do you usually get in a month?
- What is the average level of your pain on a 1–10 scale?
- Write down all of the things you already know trigger migraines for you, such as mold, MSG, stress, certain foods, etc.

The Headache Help Checklist

Eliminations

Legend:

Top eliminations ★ Chronic triggers ◎ Big eight allergen ❽
Possible allergen ✿ Food additive ⊕

Food Eliminations	Date Eliminated	Date Reintroduced	Reaction?	Eliminate?	Moderate?
Aged, canned, jarred, pickled, fermented, or spoiled food ★					
Artificial sweeteners ◎					
Alcohol ◎					
Avocados ✿					
Bananas ✿					
Beans ✿					
Citrus ✿					
Coffee ★					
Chili peppers ✿					
Chocolate ★					
Cooking oils ◎					
Corn ◎					
Eggs ★ ✿ ❽					
Fish ❽					
Food additives ◎					
Free glutamic acid ◎					
GMO foods ✿					
Inflammatory meats ◎					
Milk products ★ ◎ ✿ ❽					
MSG, free glutamic acid ⊕ ◎					
Mushrooms ✿					
Nitrites ⊕ ◎					

The Headache Help Checklist

Orange juice ★						
Peanuts ○ ⑧						
Pesticides ⊕ ◎						
Processed foods ★						
Refined grains ◎						
Rice ○						
Seafood ○						
Shellfish ○ ⑧						
Soy ◎ ○ ⑧						
Spices ○						
Starch ○						
Sugar ◎						
Sulfites ⊕ ◎						
Tomatoes ○						
Trans fats ◎						
Tree nuts ○ ⑧						
Wheat ★ ○ ⑧						
Yeast ⊕ ◎						
Other Food Eliminations						

Lifestyle Eliminations	Date Eliminated	Write down the changes you can make in your life to help you eliminate these headache triggers.
Extra pounds		
Smoke		
Perfume		
Stress		
Cleaning products		
Barometric drops		
High altitudes		
Negative environments		
Molds and allergens		
Blue light		
Other Lifestyle Eliminations		

Additions

Note: Keep in mind that the food additions here are foods you could possibly eat on your elimination diet.

Food Additions	Date Added	Judging from your headache diary, has this addition helped reduce the number or severity of your headaches?
Hypoallergenic/anti-inflammatory foods		
Wild game		
Grass-fed, hormone-free, organic, and pasture-raised meats		
Fresh, organic vegetables		
Green vegetables (spinach, Swiss chard, collard greens, etc.)		
Orange vegetables (carrots, sweet potatoes)		
Cooked yellow vegetables (summer squash)		
Ketones (MCT and coconut oils, grass-fed butter)		
Natural fats and oils (fish, sunflower and pumpkin seeds, olive oil, etc.)		
Other Food Additions		

Hydration Additions	Date Added	Judging from your headache diary, has this addition helped reduce the number or severity of your headaches?
Mineral water		
Juicing (consult doctor)		
Salt (consult doctor)		
Epsom salt baths		
Hydration minerals		

The Headache Help Checklist

Other Hydration Additions		

Happy Chemicals	
Dopamine	Write down the ways you can discover, learn, and work toward your goals.
Endorphins	Write down several things you can do to boost your endorphins: your workout schedule, a list of things that make you happy, etc.
Oxytocin	Write out your plans to see friends and family, get intimate, and give some love.
Serotonin	Write down the ways you can make yourself feel and be important, a plan for giving, and the ways you can be thankful, get more sleep, get some sunshine, and eat some healthy fat.

Lifestyle Additions	
Exercise	What's your new workout routine? Set some reasonable goals here with regard to your time and energy levels.
Sleep	How can you improve your sleep schedule? Half an hour of gentle yoga and a brief meditation before bed? Going to bed earlier? Sleeping later?
Relaxation	List several ways you can make more time to relax and unwind.

Meditation	What meditation method are you willing to try? How often will you practice it?	
Binaural beats	Write down your plan for incorporating binaural beats into your routine. Will you use them for sleep, relaxation, migraine relief?	
Air purifiers	Try a **HEPA** filter with **UV** rays, humidifier, dehumidifier, or an ozone generator.	
Blue-blocking products	If you're light sensitive, give the blue-blocking products a try: sunglasses, light bulbs, computer products, etc.	
Hara hachi bu	Eat slower, and stop eating when you're 80% full.	
Ketogenic diet	If you plan to try a ketogenic diet, make a few notes here about how you plan to research the diet before you get started. Then set a date to begin and go for it!	
Natural foods diet	Your elimination diet will start this process for you, but if you don't do an elimination diet, simply following a natural foods diet will help you. Write down your plans here.	

Vitamins and Supplements	Date Added	Judging from your headache diary, has this addition helped reduce the number or severity of your headaches?
Magnesium		
Butterbur		
Coenzyme Q10		
Vitamin B2		
Vitamin B12		
Vitamin B6		

The Headache Help Checklist

Vitamin B9		
Active B12 lozenges with L-5-MTHF with B2 and B6 (to bypass the migraine gene, MTHFR)		
Vitamin D3		
Feverfew		
Omega-3s		
5-HTP		
Ginger		
Saltstick Caps		

Hippie Treatments	Date Added	Judging from your headache diary, has this addition helped reduce the number or severity of your headaches?
Acupuncture		
Massage		
Chiropractic care		
Medical marijuana		

The Doctor's Appointment

Take this list and your headache diary with you when you visit your doctor so you can provide all of the information possible to start solving your headache problem.

Medical Tests	Notes from your discussion with your doctor:
Blood test	
Urine test	
CT scan	
MRI	
EEG	
Eye exam	

Sinus X-ray	
Spinal tap	
Comprehensive metabolic panel	
Complete blood count	
Thyroid function test	
Micronutrient test	
Stool test	
Inflammatory marker test	
MTHFR test	
TMJ/TMD	
Sleep test	
IgG and IgE allergy tests	

Migraine and Anti-Nausea Drugs

Do not take any drug without first educating yourself and consulting with your doctor. Some of these popular drugs have dangerous side effects. Understanding how medications work and how they affect you personally can help improve your headache treatment and help you find natural alternatives.

Anti-Nausea	Using currently?	Used in past?	Helpful?	Side effects?
Chlorpromazine (Thorazine)				
Metoclopramide (Reglan)				

The Headache Help Checklist

Prochlorperazine (Compazine)				
Ondansetron (Zofran)				
Promethazine (Phenergan)				
Trimethobenzamide (Tigan)				
Benadryl				
Dramamine				
Pepto Bismol				
Pepcid				
Tums				
Acute Pain Relief				
Demerol				
Naproxen (Aleve)				
Ibuprofen (Advil)				
Acetaminophen (Tylenol)				
Aspirin (Bayer)				
Aspirin and caffeine (Anacin)				
Excedrin Migraine				
Others				
Diphenhydramine (Benadryl)				
Pseudoephedrine (Sudafed)				
Progesterone cream				
DAO histamine block				
Corticosteroids				
Dexamethasone				
Solu-Medrol				
Ergotamines				
Dihydroergotamine (DHE)				
Migranal				
Cafergot				
Migergot				
DHE 45				
Cafatine				
Cafetrate				
Ercaf				

Ergo-Caff				
Wigraine				
Triptans				
Sumatriptan (Imitrex, Sumavel, DosePro, and Treximet)				
Rizatriptan (Maxalt)				
Naratriptan (Amerge)				
Zolmitriptan (Zomig)				
Eletriptan (Relpax)				
Almotriptan (Axert)				
Frovatriptan (Frova)				

Rescue Medications

Opiates	Using currently?	Used in past?	Helpful?	Side effects?
Codeine				
Hydrocodone				
Morphine				
OxyContin				
Percocet				
Vicodin				
Opiate Mixes				
Tylenol with Codeine #3				
Percocet				
Empirin				
Nuerofen Plus				
Darvon				
Other: _____				
Muscle Relaxers				
Soma				
Skelaxin				

Zanaflex				
Butalbitals				
Fioricet				
Fiorinal				
Dr. Krusz's ER Protocol				
Magnesium sulfate				
Dexamethasone (Decadron)				
Valproate sodium (Depacon)				
Droperidol (Inapsine)				
Metoclopramide (Reglan)				
Dihydroergotamine (DHE 45)				
Promethazine (Phenergan)				
Lidocaine				
Propofol				
Tramadol (Ultram)				
Levetiracetam (Keppra)				
Ketamine				
Other Rescue Remedies				
IV saline				
IV saline/magnesium sulfate				
Oxygen				

Preventative Drugs

Anti-Seizure Medications	Using currently?	Used in past?	Helpful?	Side effects?
Topiramate (Topamax)				
Valproic acid (Depakote)				

Antidepressants				
Amitriptyline (Elavil)				
Beta Blockers				
Propranolol				
Metoprolol				
Timolol				
Atenolol				
Nadolol				
Other Medications				

Preventive Medicine

Hydrate

It's time to start talking about other preventative medicine—a few things that have less to do with radically altering your diet. These are things you can do regularly that may help reduce the severity and frequency of your migraines. We'll start with one of the simplest things you can do: Drink more water. An interesting but slightly vague study in 2005 found that an increase in daily water intake by 1.5 liters resulted in a headache reduction of 21 hours in a two-week period.[480]

"How much water should we tell them to drink?" one researcher must have asked.

Another probably replied, "I don't know. Maybe 1.5 liters more than they usually drink."

"For everyone? The fat people, the little people, the chronically stressed, everyone?"

"Yes."

And so the famous study determined that an additional 1.5 liters of water per day may reduce migraine hours per week.

A 2011 study published in *Oxford Journals* discovered that migraineurs enjoy a significant increase in quality of life when they increase their water consumption; however, no studies have identified a reduction in the number of headaches.[481] Yes, this is another murky headache "cure." If you ran the same study on people who are already hydrated, which doesn't apply for too many Americans, the results would be less significant. The facts are that water deprivation can cause headaches, and increased water intake can make life with headaches significantly better.[482]

One obvious headache trigger is from a reduced blood flow, resulting in a lack of oxygen and glucose to the brain. Around 65% of the human body is comprised of water. It is essential to every organ in the human body. The worst headaches occur from the toxic accumulation of something: It could be biogenic amines, glutamate, acetaldehyde, ammonia, or hundreds of other compounds.

Water-deprivation headaches are widely recognized by the public, but not in medical literature. A small water-deprivation study in 2004 found that water-deprivation headaches in most people could be cured within 30 minutes of drinking less than 16 ounces of water. The study speculated that water deprivation might play a role in migraines, particularly in prolonging attacks.[483]

The filtration process in your liver, gut, pancreas, and brain requires lots of water. If you choose not to drink copious amounts of water, you're saying, "I have zero interest in filtering my top headache triggers." Dehydration can cause poor digestion, but it can also be the result of an inflamed gut, meaning your dehydrated, leaky gut could cause a downward spiral of further dehydration, gut inflammation, and the destruction of enzymes meant to break down biogenic amines and amino acids.

Water may even allow you to eat all the foods you shouldn't, like glutamate-rich pizza. Glutamate in the brain is found to increase during a state of dehydration.[484,485] Histamine is also released to stimulate thirst and water retention, but that comes with the negative impact of stress and inflammation. This is how your body tells you to drink water in order to prevent imminent death.[486]

One 2009 study plotted a nearly 8% jump in headache-related emergency room visits for every nine-degree rise in temperature.[487] Headache calls often and quickly turn into much more serious emergencies. When a person is "circling the drain" with low blood pressure (BP), we push an intravenous solution of salt water to raise that BP to normal levels—salt water saves that person's life.

Fun fact: Antihistamines and painkillers can block the histamine thirst signal, leaving headache patients happy as they draw toward a state of severe dehydration. When the painkillers wear off, so will the happiness, and their bodies will feel like the dry creek beds of the Mojave Desert. Remember to drink water when blocking the histamine thirst signal.

Water and Weight Loss

Hunger is often mistaken for dehydration, according to the internet. I don't call this a mistake at all, because many foods, real foods, contain a significant amount of water. Hunger is a logical response to dehydration. Correspondingly, water can suppress appetite and improve weight loss. A recent 12-week study found a 44% greater loss in weight for those who consumed 16 ounces of water before meals.[488] Wow.

A Humboldt University of Berlin study—not to be confused with California's Humboldt—showed that 16 ounces of water increases a person's metabolic rate by 30%.[489] With so many fad diets and gimmicks, we forget that a healthy consumption of water can be a powerful diet on its own.

Next Stop: Hydration Station

So what is the best way to hydrate? The common advertisement-driven response is that a sports drink is the absolute best way to hydrate because of its sugar and electrolytes. But loads of sugar can actually dehydrate you. Those advertisements may not be correct on another point as well: We don't know how hydrating sports drinks are since most sports drink studies use urine tests that only measure a volume of fluid rather than an actual state of hydration. It's not their fault. Maybe hydration can't be measured.

Everyone has heard that we're supposed to drink eight glasses of water a day, but according to research from the University of North Carolina, "There are no adequate biomarkers to measure hydration status."[490] Hydration is not concisely measured, nor is there a consensus on what hydration is in the medical community. Dehydration is another story. A quick hydration test, such as the color of your pee, can generally tell you if you are dehydrated, assuming you haven't taken a vitamin or eaten nutrient-rich, yellow-pee-producing foods. It's possible to quickly drink water in excess and pee clear without hydration. This is the drawback of any hydration test that measures volume.

The Importance of Electrolytes

I was on a wildland fire a few years back, and the temperatures were well above 115 degrees. In California, we have inmate firefighters—low-risk inmates incarcerated for nonviolent crimes who are responsible for cutting through miles of brush to eliminate fire spread. It is one of the most physically demanding jobs you could possibly do. We had a crew of inmate firefighters helping us on that wildland fire. I was fully hydrated that day, or so I thought, after drinking plenty of water and Gatorade for several consecutive days before. An inmate firefighter went down from heat exhaustion, and we had to carry him on a backboard about half a mile up a steep canyon to a place where a helicopter could safely land.

This man was huge, and his fellow inmates did not think highly of him. This inmate firefighter was in serious need of medical attention, and only a couple of inmates were willing to help carry him.

"He look bad. I hope he die," muttered one inmate who decided he was too fatigued to help. I forgot about how my own body was feeling because I had become consumed by the thought that one man was so angry with another that he actually wished death on him, that making someone *that* angry was possible.

After the arduous task of making it up the mountain and sliding him into the back of the copter, I was tired. For the next couple of hours, I felt my muscles begin to weaken until I had to take a break. Then my muscles stopped working. They would not move. It felt like I was wearing concrete shoes. I continued to drink water and Gatorade, but neither was helping.

So I sat under the hot shade of the fire engine and ate a small bag of trail mix. It was the strangest feeling. My mind was still somewhat alert, but my muscles were paralyzed. The sensation that started in my legs had now spread throughout my body. About 30 minutes after eating the trail mix, incredibly, I was cured. I was back to feeling 100% and returned to the fire line. To understand what cured me, we need to understand what electrolytes are and how water and sports drinks may not contain all the electrolytes we need.

How did we survive in nature before there was Gatorade? When you think of electrolytes, you should think mineral water. Natural mineral water is a great source of electrolytes from magnesium, calcium, chloride, potassium, and sodium. You can learn more about these minerals that at www.3dayheadachecure.com by watching my video: *Hydrate with Migraine Minerals to Cure Migraines*. You'll find a number of other beneficial minerals for your muscles and headaches in the natural water that the earth provides. These essential minerals become electrically charged when dissolved in water and turn into electrolytes.

Distilled, filtered, and treated water may take some nutritional benefits away. Sports drinks provide high amounts of sugar and sodium. The average American ingests a large surplus of sugar from our typical and nearly unavoidable processed food diet. Do we really think that a sugary sports drink is healthy with all of the added sugar, fructose, high-fructose corn syrup, dyes, and additives?

High amounts of fructose and glucose can actually lead to a condition called hypokalemia. "Hypo" means low, "kal" is neo-Latin for potassium, and "emia" means it's a condition occurring in the blood. Low levels of the electrolyte potassium can paralyze you, which may be an explanation for why my muscles stopped working.

Large amounts of sodium and potassium are lost during profuse sweating. In this case, I may have benefited from Gatorade, but for some reason it was not working. The large amounts of sugar are not a problem during firefighting because firefighters burn all of the calories they ingest. This is a valid argument for Gatorade consumption because it contains heavy amounts of salt and potassium. The large amounts of filtered water I was consuming may not have contained any potassium.

A fraternity pledge in Chico, California died from the ritual of drinking gallons of filtered water during intense exercise. The electrolytes in your blood work as a balancing act to properly hydrate cells. Normally, your body will just pee out excess water and continue to search for essential electrolytes. However, large amounts of filtered water can become acidic and draw minerals out of your blood. Burning all of those electrolytes without replacing them can cause numerous cellular hydration problems, including death.

Drinking gallons of water during an exercise meant for torture, profusely sweating during a 24-hour shift on a wildland fire, and running a marathon are all unnatural conditions. The distance of a marathon can kill a horse. But we can do it. You know how humans hunted before inventing tools? We ran, and then kept running, until our prey was pretty much dead from exhaustion—a term called "persistence hunting."[491] Humans are able to do this because of our ability to regulate the body's temperature through sweat. Under normal and even heavy workouts, the pancreas effectively regulates the body's stored electrolytes. We just need to make sure we don't run out.

The human cells use electrolytes to send messages back and forth amongst themselves in order for you to be able to think, see, move, speak, and do any other basic functions. How did the trail mix fix my electrolyte imbalance? Under exercise-induced dehydration, tap water and natural foods provide enough electrolytes to restore the human body to a normal fluid balance.[492]

Some tap water and bottled water contain enough minerals on their own, but this varies widely depending on the location and filtration of the water source. Most Americans do not get the proper levels of electrolytes from water alone.[493]

In my case, it was a mix of nuts and dried fruit that balanced my electrolytes from the natural levels of potassium, sodium, calcium, and magnesium. Fruits and vegetables will carry a wide range of minerals. This is also dependent on the plant's water source, just like humans. We are what we eat.

This leaves us with several options. We can inquire about the mineral levels of our filtered tap and bottled water, but most are not sufficient. But don't stop using water filters, because they remove some toxins we don't want to ingest more of. We can eat mineral-rich fruits and vegetables grown with our local water source, which is proven to work under even extreme conditions. We can purchase mineral water that contains all the vital electrolytes, as well as about a hundred other beneficial minerals.

People living in the Stone Age must have relied heavily on mineral water for survival. Fruits and vegetables may not have been available year-round. Hydration is dependent on electrolytes that help cells absorb water. It is no surprise that mineral springs that were once referred to as "fountains of youth" are now showing medical benefits from increased hydration to preventing memory loss.[494][495]

Minerals are vital to a human's survival and may benefit your headaches. If you are really dehydrated, try coconut water. The fact that you can put coconut water directly into your blood means that it will have the exact nutrients you need for cellular hydration. One cup of coconut water has about 6 g of sugar, which is a fraction of a sports drink and contains very little fructose.

But Really, How Much Is Enough?

How much water, mineral water, or coconut water should you drink every day? There are too many factors for anyone to give even a ballpark number. We know that the thirst mechanism used for millions of years is now outdated with the consumption of filtered water and highly processed foods that contain very little water and nutrients. The answer to this question is to consume more water and minerals in sequence with those factors that dehydrate you. You can also use an app to remind you: Waterlogged for iPhone or Water Your Body for Android are apps I like.

There are huge health markets that bank on our trust. We regularly see words and terms like "vitamin water," "hydration," "sports water," "healthy," and "smart food" used for marketing purposes, but they're often misleading or inaccurate. If you compare these "healthy" ingredients to what's in soda or candy bars, your perception will change.

After I wrote this book, my uncle said to me, "I used to get migraines. They were bad, just awful. Turns out I wasn't drinking enough water. It took me a long time to figure that out, and I haven't had a migraine since. That was many years ago." This really made me think of the impact a migraine can have. My uncle was a captain in the United States Navy during times of war. The inability to function could have been deadly not only for him but also for the hundreds of soldiers who trusted in his judgment.

Just plain old water could make all the difference in the world—provided you have enough minerals.

Sodium, the Other Part of Hydration

People associate salt with high blood pressure, because excessive amounts of salt cause high blood pressure. However, this is temporary, and a healthy person will excrete this extra sodium within a few days. If you have high blood pressure, don't try this at home without consulting your doctor.[496] The culturally accepted salt myth began in the 1970s when a researcher induced high blood pressure by

326

feeding rats the human equivalent of 500 g of sodium per day, or 50 times more than the average human intake in the Western world.

That myth was disproven in 2005 and has since received a heavy opposition of studies that say restricting salt *does not* lower the risk of heart attack, strokes, or death in people with normal or high blood pressure.[497] That's one step forward for humankind and two steps backward in the trust of science.[498]

How did salt end up getting such a bad name? The word "salary" comes from the Latin root of salt, when the road from the salt pans to Rome was called Via Salaria, the "salt route." In the sixth century, an ounce of salt could be traded for an ounce of gold.[499] When cereals allowed for the expansion of civilization, people lowered their intake of salt-rich game, fruits, and vegetables. Sure, cereals have a longer shelf life, but the transition away from eating natural food left many people without enough salt. Gold was precious, but salt became vital because without salt, you die. Today, we have an entire industry of nutrient-depleting processed foods with low sodium that forget the history of salt. Salt could buy a life—and a lack of salt was the end of life.

If you want to learn more about salt, check out Chris Kresser's article, "Shaking up the Salt Myth."[500] He is an influential health professional whose work is regularly cited. This particular article on salt suggests that consuming between 1.5 to 3.5 teaspoons per day is healthy. Check with your doctor before taking in extra salt, as it could kill you if you have certain medical conditions. The salt myth is becoming well known with a ton of recent studies and buzz to back it up.

But what's this got to do with hydration? Or headaches? A lot, if you ask Dr. Angela Stanton. She has been migraine-free for over four years now and says it's "a result of proper and regular hydration assisted by apps on my smartphone."[501] She has a great blog post that explains how cells require salt to create the proper voltage for sodium-potassium pumps, which allow nutrients inside the cell. Nutrients like magnesium are required to open the pumps and allow water to enter. So without sodium, you don't have hydration.

Sodium is also required for calcium—that migraine bullet—to function properly with high voltage. We'll get to just how important magnesium, calcium, and, subsequently, sodium are in the vitamins and medication chapters. The topic of proper hydration is so large that you could write an entire book on it. In fact, Dr. Stanton recently has. It's called *Fighting the Migraine Epidemic*, and she has found many other migraine sufferers to have the same remarkable results that she herself has had. I see numerous Facebook fans thanking her for "curing" their migraines by way of hydration.

Sodium's effect on migraines is still a new area of research, but we already know that salt water can save a person's life. Without salt and without hydration, our neurotransmitters do not fire. This will raise inflammation and glutamate. This affects your ability to hold thoughts and become headache-free. Next time you get blood work done, ask your doctor for your sodium levels and compare them to the optimum levels. You might be low.

What to Buy

When you buy salt, go for the good stuff: sea salt. If you want sea salt from an ancient time before pollutants and three-eyed fish, try pink Himalayan sea salt or pink sea salt from Utah. Table salt tastes bland and often comes with anticaking agents that may contain aluminum or sodium ferrocyanide, which could produce cyanide.

Regular sea salt and pink sea salt come with magnesium and numerous other minerals required for headache health. Some argue that Himalayan salt is not as good as table salt because, in addition to all those minerals, Himalayan salt comes with plutonium, lead, mercury, and aluminum. It's not a valid argument, because the plutonium content is under 0.001 ppm, the mercury content is 0.03 ppm, the lead content is 0.1 ppm, and the aluminum content is 0.66 ppm. It's nothing. It becomes less than nothing when you add it to water or food. You should be more concerned with the EMFs radiating out of your cell phone.[502]

Yes, I did say plutonium. But with less than 0.001 ppm of plutonium that's millions of years old, you won't be generating a nuclear reaction. Even radioactive plutonium mixtures of up to 2 to 4 ppm are OSHA approved for human exposure.[503] Guess who cleans up radioactive plutonium off the highway after super-secret government trucks crash? Firefighters.

If you can't picture how small 0.001 ppm is, remember that one ppm is one part per million, so to get one part per million of a grain of salt, you'd divide that grain into one million pieces. So 0.001 ppm is the same thing as saying one part per billion. It's nothing, yet it is important to understand that all of these fractions are microscopic, since people advise not eating Himalayan salt because it has 0.66 ppm of aluminum. Vegetable garden soil that is considered "uncontaminated" of any metal may contain lead concentrations of 50 ppm.[504] Our vegetables and water sources and any food we eat will have some contamination at low levels. And the nutritional benefits of those things will detoxify the body.

As much as 2% of table salt can be anticaking additives, which include ingredients such as aluminum. To put this in perspective, 2% is 20,000 parts per million of poison that you don't need.[505]

Despite the anticaking additives, the nutritional benefit of salt far outweighs the risk. You can't detoxify the body without salt, and you can't live without salt. That being said, why not avoid the extra bad stuff? Buy premium coarse salt in those nice little salt grinders that don't need anticaking additives. Premium salt from today's oceans will have today's toxins—we dump eight million metric tons of plastic into oceans each year, not to mention oil and radioactive stuff. The salt that's millions of years old will have plutonium. But again, the toxins in natural salt will show up in tiny, nontoxic doses. If you're really worried about toxins, try Hawaiian black lava sea salt. It has activated charcoal that will detoxify any toxins that come from the ocean, and it also tastes great.

I prefer these natural salts that include numerous minerals strictly because of their taste. I'm not that concerned with the small amounts of toxins in any salt, including table salt.

Salt Water and Mineral Water

When I drink water with a pinch of salt in it, I feel more awake, my mind feels sharper, and I have more energy throughout the day. I wrote a portion of this book in Spain while drinking Vichy Catalan—a great-tasting, naturally carbonated spring water that is also naturally high in sodium. It has 1.1 g of sodium per liter.

People have been drinking from the springs of Vichy Catalan since well before Roman times, and guess what? They consider it healthy. Natural water, meats, fruits, and vegetables have salt, and it is nothing new. The more natural food you consume, the fewer pinches of salt you will need.

Stress, dehydration, or a salt deficiency can lead to adrenal fatigue or low adrenal function. The adrenal gland produces cortisol and DHEA, which then produces estrogen and progesterone. The result of adrenal fatigue can be low serotonin levels, loss of sodium, poor blood pressure regulation, low blood pressure, higher glucose levels, weight gain, general fatigue, waking up tired, depression, unstable blood pH, and frequent urination.[506] Consuming too little salt will impair the regulation of the adrenal glands, stress, blood pressure, and the migraine gene.[507] [508]

Epsom Salts

Hundreds of migraineurs take Epsom salt baths. They believe it detoxifies their bodies while replenishing the sodium and magnesium in their blood. Although spas rich in magnesium sulfate have been therapeutic for who knows how long, I've only found one study that suggests that a nice, long bath with magnesium sulfate has the power to raise magnesium and sodium.[509] Some migraine sufferers will also add in sodium bicarbonate (baking soda), and natural oils, such as lavender—depending on personal preference. Remember to drink plenty of fluids before this soothing detox. If it makes you feel great, why not? It's said to be very relaxing.

How Much Salt Do I Need Every Day?

You tell me. A meta-study of 23 observational studies found that 2.5 to 6 g of salt per day is associated with the lowest risk of cardiovascular disease.[510] (Six grams is about one teaspoon.) Chris Kresser recommends 1.5 to 3.5 teaspoons (8.5 to 20 g) of salt per day based on the amounts that have been associated with the lowest risk of disease over the last 200 years, suggesting salt is part of a diet that will keep you healthy when it's consumed with natural foods. However, he explains that our bodies have a natural sodium appetite that will allow us to salt foods to taste. Migraine sufferers are at risk of salt depletion from stress and may have a heavier taste for salt.

I've found the Bulletproof diet recommendation of mixing a half teaspoon of natural salt into a glass of water in the morning is almost the equivalent of a cup of coffee—almost. I squeeze some lime in it for flavor, which may be a problem for some. But it wakes me up, and I feel energized.

Juicing

I need to make something very clear before we make it to one of the largest misconceptions and debates about health: The fructose studies that suggest insulin resistance, obesity, diabetes, abdominal fat, and rapid fat storage have focused on massive amounts of isolated liquid fructose.[511] At this point, none of the studies have been performed on actual fruit. This is a massive critical error committed by our most trusted health experts.

Fruits and vegetables are associated with a reduced risk of cancer, heart attack, stroke, Alzheimer's disease, and the list goes on and on. Uncountable headache benefits are homegrown from fruits and vegetables. A large portion of the medical community believes that the proper levels of vitamins can only be reached by consuming them in their natural forms.[512][513]

Can't a vitamin supplement real food? Well, probably not, but we don't know. Science has yet to fully equate how a single piece of fruit affects the human body. Fruits and vegetables provide nutrients and phytochemicals that serve as antioxidants to reduce oxidative stress. Many of these nutrients are proven to boost happy brain chemicals, such as serotonin and oxytocin. They can also give your body some great anti-inflammatory benefits by boosting your omega-3 levels, which is a lot like taking a natural aspirin. A glass of vegetable juice will increase your energy level and clear your mind. The effects forge an incredible feeling of sustained happiness. That's right, vegetable juice equals happiness.

Search the internet for "juicing cured my migraines," and you will find hundreds of people writing about just that. Some say it was from a juice a day, others find the cure from the first day of a juice cleanse, and a few take weeks to fully resolve their problem. The film *Fat, Sick & Nearly Dead* awakened me to juicing with the inspiration of numerous health benefits, including a woman "cured" of migraines.

If a nutrition deficiency is causing you headaches, depression, fatigue, or any health problems, juicing is definitely for you. Many people claim that the common cold is never common for those who juice. I have to agree. I haven't had a cold since I started juicing. Many nutrition experts, however, will strongly advise us to only use vegetables, because there is too much fructose in fruit.

Juicing Drawbacks

There are a couple of drawbacks to juicing. If you have any allergies to a fruit, juicing will magnify those allergies into a potent little glass. Most people find that the nutritional benefits outweigh any of the possible negative effects. Fruit is seasonal, and it happens to provide your body with more fat-producing fructose, which has helped mankind's belly survive the winter for millions of years. Survival, though, does not have anything to do with having a big belly.

Nauru is a remote island in the Pacific, and it is the fattest country in the world, with 94.5% of the adult population overweight.[514] Many attribute this to their consumption of high-fructose corn syrup and sugar. A favorite drink on the island is a bucket-sized beaker of Coke. High-fructose corn syrup is around 55% fructose and 42% glucose. Table sugar is not so different and usually contains 50% fructose and 50% glucose.

Overconsumption of pure fructose by obese individuals has been found to cause excessive amounts of abdominal fat and insulin problems when compared to glucose consumption.[515] However, a large meta-study from 2008 shows that weight gain and insulin problems don't happen until a person consumes over 100 g of fructose per day—the study even suggests fructose consumption under 100 g per day may improve metabolic function.[516]

To consume 100 g of fructose in one day, you would either have to eat eight medium apples or eight whole pounds of strawberries.[517] This is why juicing fruit is considered dangerous. You would only need to drink about three cups of apple juice per day to consume over 100 g of fructose (in addition to a considerable amount of glucose, which is also found in apple juice). But let's not forget—these studies on fructose and weight gain are only from excessive consumption of isolated fructose (as found in high-fructose corn syrup) and not from actual fruit that contains fiber and nutrients.[518]

The myth that fructose, all fruit, and all fruit juice is toxic was nearly disproven in 2014 when researchers from Berkley, California found that mice that consumed grapefruit juice weighed 18.4% less than mice that consumed a similar high-calorie diet that included pure glucose. The grapefruit group also had lower blood sugar and triglyceride levels and achieved greater insulin sensitivity.[519]

While fruit juice may have some benefits, research is not conclusive, so I recommend limiting your consumption due to the risk of headaches from large quantities of fructose and glucose. The numerous people who have eliminated migraines from juicing fruit are often eliminating all other processed foods and their success does not imply that any quantity of fructose and glucose is safe.

Other risks from fruit juice apply to anyone on medications, because juicing may produce concentrated vitamins that can conflict with a drug prescription. For example, the potassium of a banana could kill you while on certain heart medications. Thus, five bananas in a blender could present a concentrated problem at high speed.

There is no argument that eating whole foods is a safer choice. However, you're probably not going to consume such massive amounts of nutrients in their whole form because of the sheer quantity of produce required for one small cup of juice. But try making homemade vegetable juice once, and your body awakens, making you feel wonderful. This is your body's way of saying, "Thank you for giving me all these nutrients."

Juicer or Blender?

The benefits of blending (using a blender, instead of a juicer) come from the fiber that stays within the juice to aid a longer digestion period that results in sustained energy and weight loss. The downside is that it creates juice with a heavy (but healthy) pulp. Some don't like that pulp, but I actually prefer it when juicing fruits and making smoothie concoctions.

Vegetable juice with husky pulp is not for the novice juicer, but it will leave you feeling full and healthy. It's a quick way to make a full meal in a cup with a superfast cleanup. I try to blend as much as possible for its health factor.

Juicing with a regular juicer nearly removes all of the pulp and creates a fast sugar spike. It's easy to overdo your daily allowance of fructose with a glass of juice and still have room for an entire meal. The upside: The juice is energizing, delicious, and nutritious. I usually blend fruits (in moderation) and juice vegetables to get the best of both worlds.

The smaller and faster the cut, the more nutrients will be exposed to the elements. This gives a blender an advantage over a juicer; however, a third option takes the cake on nutrient preservation. Cold press juicers (aka, masticating juicers) slowly crush nutrients, providing a maximum yield juice that has not been exposed to the oxidation of heat, and they produce the most pulp, juice, nutrients, appetite satisfaction, and health benefits of all the juicers. People who want the most bang for their juicing buck will end up saving money with the minimal food and nutrient loss of a cold press juicer.

Heating or cooking destroys nutrients, a common rant among raw-food dieters. This gives juice from a cold press the closest resemblance to raw foods that contain intact enzymes. If you can't handle heavy pulp, or if you're attempting to introduce juice to a skeptic, don't start with this type of juicer.

What to Buy

Juicing can go two ways: It can be delicious or leave you feeling "meh." Using fresh, organic ingredients gives you delicious juice with intense flavors that could leave you thinking it's the best drink you've ever washed down. On the other hand, juicing with mediocre, nonorganic, or slightly older ingredients may cause you to pour the magnified mediocrity down the drain. For this reason, and many others, go organic.

Genetically modified fruits and vegetables have a level of toxins that are tested as "safe" when they're consumed in their whole forms. Juicing concentrates those toxins, and those toxins are meant to kill insects by destroying their stomachs. In large concentrations and removed from nutrients, they may become toxic to humans.

I often drop my jaw when I compare the price of organic produce sitting next to all of that affordable produce that was mass-produced with the help of science. But you know what else is expensive? Missing a day of work for a headache is expensive. Cancer is extravagant. When we don't buy organic produce, we're paying less for more water content and fewer nutrients. We're buying produce modified with poison so more poison can be sprayed on the exterior.

I appreciate all of these health concerns, yet I still look at the prices and weigh my options. Farmers' markets can be the merger of the lowest price and the highest quality. You support local businesses; why not directly support your local farmers? Buying vegetables fresh means you are consuming them with their highest nutritional content and their lowest health risk. If the food is old, its probability of mold goes up, and food that can grow old without mold is flavorless. Remember, mold and migraines often go hand in hand.

Freshness is one of the largest benefits of juicing. If you cut an apple and leave it exposed to the air and sun, you will watch oxidation punch the clock as its crisp texture begins to brown. Juicing will disintegrate the apple and expose all of its nutrients and enzymes to a rapid oxidation process. Because of this, you should always consume your homemade juice within 20 minutes of making it.

Juicing Recipe Sources

I have two books that are excellent and have phenomenal reviews on Amazon: *Juicing Recipes for Vitality and Health* by Drew Canole and *The Healthy Green Drink Diet* by Jason Manheim. The newest and most popular juice book is *The Reboot with Joe Juice Diet* by Joe Cross. I like to keep the books on the coffee table so I can take a quick photo of a recipe and head to the grocery store for fresh ingredients.

Do you want more energy? They have a drink for that. Do want to instantly feel smarter? There are a few of those juices. How do you want to feel? There is probably a juice for that feeling too. I like the book form of recipes because the pictures propel my mind to actually want to get up and make a delicious drink that I've already associated with energy.

There are also numerous websites with great juice recipes. I use allrepices.com and juicerecipes.com. I often search online for the name of a fresh fruit or vegetable at the grocery store followed by "juice recipe" to find something new (e.g., "kale juice recipe").

Fruits and vegetables have numerous minerals that help hydrate you and reduce headaches and migraines. There is no formula to follow. You can do a quick internet search on "minerals of fruits and vegetables," and you'll find the exact numbers for potassium, calcium, magnesium, sodium, and other minerals. You will also learn that no food is complete.

This complex science comes down to simply eating a variety of produce. Each piece of produce will come with numerous nutrients that will all add up to hydration, filtration, and possibly a headache-free life.

Ketogenic Diets

Ketogenic diets, like the Bulletproof Diet, involve fasting and consuming a diet high in fat and low in carbohydrates. Ketogenic diets are often used in epilepsy treatment because they have the ability to reduce seizures, so we can assume that following a ketogenic diet will improve migraines as well. There is also emerging data that suggests the ketogenic diet can benefit a variety of neurological diseases.[520] In 1928, shortly after its success as an epilepsy treatment was realized, the ketogenic diet was given to migraine sufferers. Nine of 28 patients reported "some improvement." However, some patients admitted to cheating while following the diet, which definitely affected the success rate. In 2010, it was found that ketones might retard CSD—the start of a migraine and the link between migraines and seizures.[521]

You already tried the ketogenic diet long ago. Human babies are in ketosis shortly after birth and continue to burn ketones while breastfeeding.[522] The most insane development of the human brain is done on the ketogenic diet, yet many health professionals still believe that this is the same thing as diabetic ketoacidosis (DKA). The body can't store much more than 24 hours' worth of glucose and should starve in just a few days of fasting, but it doesn't because we're able to burn ketones from fat. It is our secondary source of energy and a damn important one at that.[523]

In fact, ketogenic diets have been used to rapidly change insulin sensitivity and reverse the "carbohydrate intolerance" that diabetes can manifest. Without an insulin problem, there is no ketone problem. Hyperglycemia, having too much sugar, is also a large part of the superacid levels of a ketone overdose.[524] When ketone production goes up, glucose production goes down. The result of a ketogenic diet is weight loss and improved energy production instead of that constant, desperately hungry feeling you get from traditional diets.[525] In fact, burning ketones reduces hunger, glucose levels, and insulin problems.[526]

One study in particular has made the ketogenic diet very relevant in the migraine world. In 2013, researchers did something amazing. They prescribed a low-calorie diet and a ketogenic diet for a group of 108 migraine patients.[527] The diet lasted for one month. The 56 migraineurs in the low-calorie group experienced no change. But more than 90% of the 52 migraineurs on the ketogenic diet experienced a reduction in headache frequency and drug consumption.

That gives the ketogenic diet a higher success rate than any migraine drug, yet in 2015, a doctor is more likely to prescribe opiates for migraines than suggest a ketogenic diet. Headaches are a sign that the body is not metabolizing energy, so why not try a diet that will help it do just that? Removing the top headache triggers from your diet while following a ketogenic diet just might be the most successful migraine treatment in history.

The Easiest Way to Burn Ketones

You can ingest either grass-fed butter or coconut oil to immediately burn ketones. Both contain medium-chain triglycerides (MCT oil).[528] Grass-fed butter will contain healthy omega-3 fats and butyrate—a strong anti-inflammatory that supports the digestion of headache triggers.[529,530,531,532,533] Using MCT oil along with a standard diet has been found to cause fat loss[534] and is so powerful that it has been used to increase the memory retention of patients with Alzheimer's.[535]

Risks

The high cholesterol levels that come with a diet high in saturated fat were once considered deadly. However, recent research shows that saturated fats help lower dense LDL ("bad cholesterol") and raise HDL ("good cholesterol").[536] And in 2010, research from the University of North Carolina at Chapel Hill found that there is no proof that saturated fat, cholesterol, or salt consumption cause heart disease.[537] [538] Another study published in the American Journal of Clinical Nutrition, looked at 21 studies with a total of 347,747 people and found that there is no significant evidence for concluding that dietary saturated fat is associated with stroke or heart disease.[539]

While cholesterol levels no longer increase your risk of heart attacks, seek a doctor's advice before trying any diet that could affect your health condition.[540] Cholesterol is actually necessary to prevent migraines because it holds the cell walls together and prevents the damage caused by having too much glutamate.[541] But our bodies also need cholesterol and fat to produce vitamin D, which also prevents glutamate toxicity.[542]

On the bright side, this ability to control glutamate may be the reason why diets rich in healthy fats reduce the risk of cognitive decline,[543] neurological disorders,[544] and migraine attacks.[545] Perhaps, when the brain is having trouble burning fuel from glucose and insulin, we should try the other fuel, ketones.

Ketogenic diets that are ultrahigh in protein pose another risk. They have been associated with kidney damage. There are many ways to get to ketosis that don't involve excessive protein, but there is still a risk with all of them. The first three days of cutting carbs can be excruciating for a headache sufferer, or just about anyone. And transitioning away from the chemical-packed Western diet could be deadly for those with unstable health.

If you're interested in trying a ketogenic diet, research thoroughly and only do it under the guidance of someone with extensive knowledge of it. While we don't know what the ketogenic diet will do for your personal health, the new information is looking good.[546]

Migraine Vitamins and Herbs

Vitamins are, basically, a crutch and cannot replace the nutrients you get from real foods. Even so, what vitamins can do for your migraines make the drug success rates look sad—very sad. And vitamins are the route you follow to bypass the migraine gene. That's right, if you inherited this painful genetic problem, vitamins could be the answer to your headaches and migraines, according to information from the leading migraine gene expert, Dr. Benjamin Lynch, who may have the "cure" to the majority of migraines and headaches.

A warning: The success I'm writing about here is based on real supplements. The FDA *does not* regulate supplements with strict rules and regulations.[547] In February 2015, the New York State attorney general accused four national retailers (Walmart, Walgreens, Target, and GNC) of selling fraudulent dietary supplements—this was nothing new in our unregulated market.[548] For example, they tested GNC's "Herbal Plus" brand and found five out of six samples contained unrecognizable ingredients or substances other than those described on the label. In many cases, brands in these stores contained "little more than cheap fillers like rice and house plants."[549]

Consider getting these vitamins by eating natural food sources as often as possible. The likelihood is high that you could stumble upon a false vitamin that contains allergens. So if you're going to purchase vitamin supplements, buy reputable brands as opposed to knockoffs or store brands.[550]

Your goal is to lower your overall inflammation so you don't push it over your headache threshold. The supplements listed in this chapter, depending on your body's needs, could be very helpful to that end. This is not a complete list of the vitamins and herbs that might help migraine sufferers. There are thousands of substances that can improve your headache health. However, there might not be studies to back these well-known remedies up in the migraine arena.

Take turmeric, for instance. It has incredible anti-inflammatory properties, yet it has no well-designed migraine studies to date that I'm aware of. The same can be said about green tea extract. Ginger has been used as a headache remedy for thousands of years. It wasn't until March 2014 that one study found that ginger (250 mg) is just as effective in halting a migraine in its tracks as sumatriptan, although the long-term side effects of ginger are the opposite of what sumatriptan will bring.[551] Unfortunately, this study of 100 migraineurs is not enough for a doctor to prescribe ginger over sumatriptan.

It's critical that we look into nutritional medicine before we take prescription medications that alter our brain chemistry.

Magnesium

If magnesium doesn't blow your mind, you haven't read what it does to stop a headache. Up to 50% of migraineurs are deficient in magnesium.[552] This problem could be much worse than we believe, considering that a routine blood test can only measure 2% of the body's magnesium since the vast majority of our magnesium is stored in the bones and intracellular space (inside cells).

A critical job of magnesium is keeping the body hydrated. Magnesium helps to regulate glutamate, serotonin, and calcium, which could be why a lack of magnesium may promote CSD.[553] It gets much worse. Magnesium helps relax the muscles, and a deficiency of magnesium will cause those muscles and their blood vessels to tighten, which is easier explained as high blood pressure. But this magnesium deficiency isn't the type of pick-me-up that you would expect from a vasoconstrictor, such as coffee. Your body often compensates for a problem by raising blood pressure to speed vital nutrients through the body—that's not always a good thing.

Magnesium is required for all energy production that takes place in the cells, and it is also needed to regulate a number of neurotransmitters (that conveniently carry your thoughts). How do you feel with a magnesium deficiency? You muscles are stressed, your blood pressure goes up, your energy levels drop, and your mind spins in various directions. It's a bad time.

Magnesium and the American Migraineur

Insulin gets magnesium out of the blood and into the cells where you need it. So what happens when we eat a diet that is responsible for a degree of insulin resistance? The insulin comes knocking at the door of the cells and says, "Let me in. I've got some sugar and magnesium."

The cells then say, "Get lost. You're high on aspartame or some other junk, and I don't see any sugar."

Now the cells don't have enough magnesium inside, which is a big problem for insulin. This is because magnesium supports the entry of insulin into the cells—the same insulin that's carrying more magnesium. Your body will pump out more insulin, because the insulin it currently has is doing a terrible job, which is another problem, because your body also needs magnesium to create insulin. Got it? Magnesium helps carry insulin, which contains more magnesium, and magnesium is also needed to create insulin.

Without magnesium, you will have high blood pressure, constricted blood vessels, and less insulin. That all adds up to less energy or glucose in the cells, defective tyrosine-kinase, and an overall downward spiral of your health.[554] Tyrosine-kinase is an enzyme that helps switch cell growth and division on and off. A defective switch results in uncontrolled cell division. Let me just write the definition of cancer: "The disease caused by an uncontrolled division of abnormal cells in a part of the body."[555] That says enough, I think.

Magnesium is critical in regulating the glutamate and calcium that may be responsible for a migraine, among other things.

Where to Get It

The minerals in fruits and vegetables, according to research from the University of Texas, have declined significantly in past years.[556] The good news is that organic crops may still contain the same overall mineral and magnesium content of the fruits and vegetables of the past.[557] [558]

These things are high in magnesium:

- Mineral water
- Coconut water
- Fish
- Nuts
- Beans

- Fruits and vegetables

These things are *really* high in magnesium:
- Sunflower seeds
- Pumpkin seeds
- Almonds
- Brazil nuts
- Green leafy vegetables
- Broccoli
- Beets
- Beans
- Avocados
- Bananas
- Watermelon
- Wild salmon
- Halibut
- Magnesium vitamins

Do You Need to Count Your Magnesium?

No. Natural foods are rich in magnesium, and you will have no problem getting enough. Also, don't look at white rice and enriched bread and think it's a good idea to eat those things because of their added magnesium. Anything that skyrockets your insulin levels is not going to help you absorb magnesium. You may need to take magnesium vitamins if you're currently eating a typical Western diet and have average or high insulin levels.

Are Magnesium Supplements Successful?

Several studies suggest that magnesium supplements reduce migraine frequency in those with low levels of it.[559] If you don't need it, it doesn't help. Magnesium supplements can cause low blood pressure and diarrhea. Think about how orchestrated the process is for cellular hydration. Do you think a pill will fix it all?

We don't even know how all minerals interact with each other. Too much of one mineral can lower another. Our bodies do the hard work for us by regulating the proper amounts of each. So let's give our bodies all the nutrients they need to do a good job from the natural foods and drinks mentioned previously.

Well, supplements actually "fix it" for some. One study found that 600 mg of magnesium resulted in a 42% reduction in migraine-attack frequency.[560] This nearly tripled the success rate of the placebo at reducing the amount of attacks per month, which is exactly what people want—fewer migraine attacks. It should be noted that 600 mg is more than the daily recommended allowance, which is around 400 mg for men and 310 mg for women, and 18.6% of the patients on 600 mg of magnesium ended up with diarrhea.[561]

Most Americans (68%) consume less than the daily recommended allowance of magnesium, and 19% of Americans consume less than half of what we are supposed to. These individuals are more likely to have elevated CRP levels (those markers of inflammation) that contribute to the risk of cardiovascular disease.[562]

Can you believe how important magnesium is? This isn't saying we need magnesium for headache prevention. It's saying we need magnesium for survival, and the migraineur may be the only one smart enough to realize it. Magnesium is wonderful.

Butterbur

Butterbur is a natural herb that's used as an anti-inflammatory for pain, stomachaches, migraines, asthma, and hay fever. The positive effects of butterbur have put it in the big leagues for migraine treatment. A German study of 289 children and adolescents with migraines found attack frequency was reduced by 63% and that 91% of patients felt substantially or at least slightly better, with no serious side effects from the use of butterbur. In addition, 77% of all patients reduced their migraines by at least 50%.[563]

A four-month study of adults taking 75 mg of butterbur twice per day found a 50% or greater reduction of migraines in 68% of patients.[564] That's a stunning success rate!

Just look at the numerous five-star reviews on Amazon for "Now Butterbur" vitamins. One reviewer who gave the product five stars said, "I've reduced my migraines from 9 or 10 a month to the occasional headache with weather changes."

It doesn't work for everyone, but with a success rate like that, this natural herb is certainly worth a try!

Coenzyme Q10

Coenzyme Q10 is also known as ubiquinone. That name is derived from the word "ubiquitous," which means "found everywhere." This is a fitting name for the substance found in every cell in the body. Coenzyme Q10 plays a crucial role in energy production with antioxidant properties. You can't go without it.

In theory, coenzyme Q10 could help to reduce the cellular stress (excitotoxicity) caused by a bump in glutamate and calcium. We don't want the cells to become excited to death, which is the result of oxidation. A 2012 study boosted this antioxidant theory by finding that coenzyme Q10 inhibits the release of glutamate through the suppression of a voltage-dependent calcium influx. Do you know what that means? This study is saying that coenzyme Q10 may halt that electrical brainstorm that starts the migraine aura.[565]

Remember that a migraine aura is a slow buildup of headache triggers until just one cell says, "Nope, I've had enough glutamate, calcium, and inflammation. I'm going to burst." It starts in one part of the brain and sweeps across to leave the migraineur with a head full of inflammation. This is the final straw that breaks the camel's back, and we need to stop it before it happens.

The anti-inflammatory effect of coenzyme Q10 also sounds like a good idea for the average person who gets headaches. We need it for our cells to survive, so it's a good idea to not run out. Is that possible?

A study in 2007, by the Cincinnati Children's Hospital, of over 1,500 children and adolescents with migraines found that a third were deficient in coenzyme Q10.[566] So they gave these kids coenzyme Q10 for three months and found that their headaches dropped by a third and headache disability went down by more than 50%—that's a lot of time back for the little ones who suffer from migraines.

An adult study out of Switzerland that involved 42 migraine sufferers with an average of 4.4 migraine attacks per month found that 48% of those who took coenzyme Q10 had half as many attacks after a three-month period.[567] Cutting the frequency of migraines in half is a big deal. More importantly, coenzyme Q10 was well tolerated, meaning that this top-of-the-line migraine treatment comes at little cost to your health.

Another study showed even better results, with 61% of users having greater than a 50% reduction in the number of days with migraine headaches. The average number of days dropped from a little more than seven per month to fewer than three per month. Again, this occurred with *no* side effects.[568] Can you imagine how happy those migraine sufferers are?

Remember how important cholesterol is for your cells? Cholesterol basically keeps your cells from bursting, which would not be fun. Well, cholesterol shares the same pathway that helps form coenzyme Q10. Statins (cholesterol-lowering medications) can reduce coenzyme Q10 by up to 40%.[569] Right now there are studies going on to find out if coenzyme Q10 can help with the adverse muscle reactions of statins, such as muscle fatigue and death—because your heart is a muscle and will die without coenzyme Q10.[570]

If you're taking one of the statin medications to lower your cholesterol, coenzyme Q10 supplements may help as the loss of coenzyme Q10 means the loss of energy production. This energy production does everything from making you feel livelier to allowing your heart to pump.[571]

Where to Get It

The richest source of coenzyme Q10 is in meats, fish, and nuts, followed by fruits and vegetables.[572] It's a fat-soluble product, so you need omega-3 fatty acids to absorb coenzyme Q10.

B Vitamins

I believe that metabolized B vitamins are going to be one of the top migraine treatments at some point in the near future. You can't just take the vitamins and expect them to work. They require knowledge of their brilliance. When taken the correct way, B vitamins have the power to control the migraine gene and produce energy—as in the energy that drives all human functions. I'm excited.

Vitamin B2 (Riboflavin)

Vitamin B2 is a water-soluble vitamin, so it easily mixes with blood, and unlike fat-soluble vitamins, whatever amount the body does not use is immediately urinated out. Because of this, we need a constant supply of fresh vitamin B2 and the rest of the B-complex vitamins.

Vitamin B2 helps break down proteins, fats, and carbohydrates. It plays a large role in producing energy for muscles. We're talking about metabolism here. If you want a slow metabolism that leaves you tired and fat, stop ingesting vitamin B2. Vitamin B2 can help a person maintain a healthy digestive system. It can also provide benefits with respect to a person's eyes, nerves, and ability to absorb iron and other B vitamins, among others.[573]

Vitamin B6 helps break down amino acids to create serotonin and dopamine, the happy brain chemicals. So it will be hard to stay positive if your body lacks the chemicals to make you feel positive in the first place. But you need vitamin B2 to absorb vitamin B6.

Let's put vitamin B2 to the migraine test. We know that anything that helps the cells create energy and balance neurotransmitters will help prevent the destruction of a headache.

One vitamin B2 study showed a 50% reduction of migraine frequency and a large reduction in acute drug use. Sounds great for migraine sufferers and not so hot for Big Pharma. They used 400 mg per day for six months—an ultrahigh dose.[574]

In another study, 25 mg of vitamin B2 was just as successful as the combination of 400 mg of vitamin B2, 300 mg of magnesium, and 100 mg of feverfew—which have all had substantial success individually.[575] This means that you do not need much vitamin B2 for great results. In fact, if you look at the recommended daily intake of vitamin B2, it's only 1.3 mg per day for men and 1.1 mg for women.[576] It's what happens with a water-soluble vitamin—the body discards what it doesn't need, so taking 364 times the vitamin B2 you need is probably *not* going to help you and may even be toxic.[577]

Unfortunately, more than a decade later, we still don't have a controlled study regarding vitamin B2 and migraines, which means doctors can't confidently prescribe it, despite the fact that it has as much potential to lower migraine frequency as many pharmaceutical drugs.

Where to Get It

- Mushrooms
- Green leafy vegetables
- Lean meats
- Eggs (Headache trigger)
- Seaweed
- Beet greens
- Broccoli
- Brussels sprouts

- Almonds
- Asparagus

Vitamin B12

Vitamin B12 plays a role in the metabolism of every cell in the human body, including the metabolism of fatty acids and amino acids. Metabolism is a great thing, isn't it? Vitamin B12 is the most complicated of vitamins, and its relationship to migraines isn't much different.

When you get a migraine, your body's level of the amino acid homocysteine rises. B12, B6, and B9 all work together to control homocysteine.[578] A rise in homocysteine was related to cardiovascular disease, but researchers weren't exactly sure why. It's not much of a surprise, because homocysteine regulates inflammation. Very recently, migraines have been linked to elevated homocysteine, but again, researchers aren't sure why.[579]

It would seem that we want to lower this amino acid called homocysteine, but it takes all three of these B vitamins to do it. In 2009 a six-month study by Griffith University tested this theory.[580] Researchers took 52 migraine sufferers and put them in two groups. One group received vitamin B6, vitamin B9, and vitamin B12. The other group received a sugar pill. The patients in the B vitamin group showed homocysteine levels lowered by 39% and their migraine disability dropped by 30%. Yes, get out of here, homocysteine! The placebo group had no reduction in headache frequency or pain severity.

What intrigues me about this study is how poor the placebo group did. Migraine patients have some of the most successful placebo effects, and this group stayed the same, with no placebo effect. In comparison to the placebo group, 400 micrograms of vitamin B12 was extremely successful when combined with 2 mg of B9 and 25 mg of B6.

This shouldn't discourage you from thinking that B vitamins are anything short of extraordinary. Pills, like food, may have a hard time becoming digested in the belly of a headache sufferer, but there is a way to bypass the belly and the migraine gene.

B12 Deficiency

You may be at risk of a B12 deficiency if you are vegan or if you have AIDS. B12 is the backbone of the argument held by carnivores. A French vegan couple verified the notion back in 2011 when they were convicted for the death of their baby—with a serious vitamin B12 deficiency.[581] You need meat or animal products to naturally gain vitamin B12. It's easy to take a vitamin, but vitamin B12 is complex, and you may not get optimum levels from its unnatural form.

Algae breaks the carnivore rule by containing B12, but studies show that it doesn't appear to be bioavailable, so consuming algae doesn't correct a vitamin B12 deficiency in any measurable way.[582] What happens when you don't eat meat products? Aside from the vegan baby, because that was truly a horrible circumstance, 92% of vegans and 47% of vegetarians are deficient in vitamin B12.[583] Carnivores, don't get excited just yet.

What's a migraine really protecting us from? B12 deficiency may result in anemia, impaired brain function, a whole list of mental disorders, and even a smaller brain.[584,585,586] It's also linked to Alzheimer's disease, which I consider a more painful outcome than death itself.[587] With all of this information, the migraine puzzle is becoming a clear picture.

Where to Get It

These things are high in B12:

- Fish
- Meats
- Poultry
- Eggs*
- Milk and milk products*

*Be careful when shopping for eggs and milk and milk products. They are top migraine triggers. Go organic and read the labels if you are going to take the risk.

These things are *really* high in B12:

- Clams
- Salmon
- Oysters
- Mussels
- Crab
- Liver
- Lamb
- Tuna
- Chicken
- Beef

Of course, these levels will vary depending on the source. In general, fish and lean meats are a favorable source.

Why Not Just Take a Pill?

Vitamin B12 is very complex and needs vitamins B2, B9, and B6 to support numerous human functions and to reduce migraines, so if you go the supplement route, be sure you are getting enough of all four of these B vitamins. A treatment that uses only one B vitamin is like driving a car with only one new tire.

A word of caution: Don't take the synthetic version of B12, cyanocobalamin. Though it's 100 times cheaper, your body has to convert the cyanocobalamin into methylcobalamin. That could be why one study suggested that 39% of the population is deficient in vitamin B12 despite fortified foods and widespread vitamin B12 supplementation.[588] Methylcobalamin is the good, bioavailable stuff you want.[589] Don't go cheap.

Vitamin B9: Folate or Folic Acid?

This may be the most exciting vitamin in migraine treatment. You already know vitamins B9, B12, and B6 reduce migraines in combination. The study referenced, however, had a critical flaw and used the cheap synthetic version of vitamin B9 called folic acid. The study could have had far better results with folate. Today, there is reason to believe that folate, not folic acid, is part of the solution that eliminates the genetic difference between migraineurs and nonmigraineurs.

Many health professionals will argue that there is simply no difference between the two, and for the most part that's true—after proper ingestion. But if you have headaches, migraines, hypothyroidism, or simply want to function at 100%, you should learn the difference between the two.

Folic acid is synthetic and was unknown to every species on earth before World War II when it was found that a lack of B9 resulted in neural tube defects (NTDs) in newborns.[590] NTDs may result in spina bifida and anencephaly and, interestingly, chronic headaches later in life.[591]

The nation wanted to prevent NTDs, so it made sense that the synthetic version of B9, folic acid, was added to processed foods. It is cheap and has a long shelf life. But we don't need folic acid: we need tetrahydrofolate (THF).[592] The natural version of B9, folate, is a derivative of THF and converts to THF quickly in the gut.[593]

Folic acid is a man-made oxidized version of vitamin B9 that cannot convert into the THF we need without an additional step that takes place in the liver. New research is showing that this process may be slow in humans, because the conversion of folic acid—that fake crap—is extremely low and limited by the availability of dihydrofolate reductase (DHFR).[594] When your body's not using it to break down unnatural folic acid, DHFR recycles folate for brain function. In other words, we created an underachieving vitamin (folic acid) that unnaturally depletes the very thing (DHFR) that protects us from folate deficiency in the brain. A DHFR or folate deficiency creates severe neurologic conditions that lead to Alzheimer's symptoms.[595]

How bad can folic acid be, considering it's in pretty much all of our processed food?

Studies on the implementation of folic acid on the general population have shown an end result of increased colon cancer, lung cancer, and a doubled risk of prostate cancer.[596,597] The studies are controversial. In a 2013 meta-analysis by the Norwegian Institute of Public Health that included over 50,000 people, researchers found no increased or decreased risk of cancer from folic acid.[598]

However, a year later, one study found that folic acid promoted the growth of breast cancer in rats, which is a concern for everyone eating government-mandated food with folic acid or taking folic acid vitamins. Some 30 to 40% of the American population take folic acid supplements, and they've never been proven to have health benefits.[599] The FDA has proposed that only "folic acid" should be allowed on a supplement label, making it impossible to differentiate natural folate from folic acid.[600] Thanks, FDA.

Researchers at Oxford University found that high levels of unmetabolized folic acid will lower the immune system and may even compete with folate by binding to folate enzymes and blocking the transportation of methylfolate to the brain. Methylfolate is metabolized folate, and it's necessary for normal brain function.[601][602][603]

Where to Get Natural Folate

These things are high in natural folate: [604]

- Dark leafy greens
- Broccoli
- Asparagus
- Cauliflower
- Beets
- Beans
- Peas

- Lentils
- Lettuce
- Avocadoes
- Papaya
- Numerous other fruits and vegetables
- Nuts
- Seafood
- Liver
- Poultry
- Meats

Folate comes from the Latin word "folium," which means "leaf." As you can see, the complex formula that keeps all of our B vitamins at proper levels is best solved by our natural diet, and a nutritionally deficient box of food with sprinkles of folic acid is not our "natural diet."

The Migraine Gene and B Vitamins

MTHFR is the migraine gene and takes folate and converts it to methylfolate. Migraine sufferers often have a mutation of the MTHFR gene that reduces the gene's ability to produce methylfolate.[605] Migraine triggers can also reduce the function of a healthy MTHFR gene.

Folate → Migraine Prevention

↓ ↑

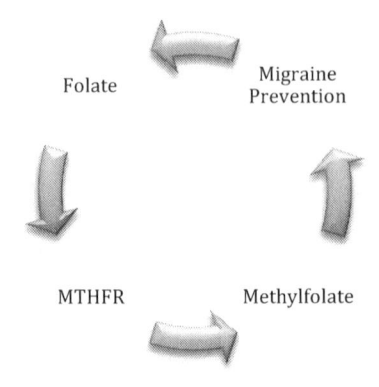

MTHFR → Methylfolate

Methylfolate production is 40% lower for those who have the gene mutation passed down from one parent. For those with the gene mutation from both parents, Methylfolate production is 70% lower.[606] This means that your body will only be able to produce 30% of the methylfolate that a normal person is able to.

The problem is that methylfolate is a vital component of a cycle called methylation. The cells lining the gut regenerate every five days, and methylation is responsible for regenerating those cells. This process produces energy, serotonin, dopamine, DAO, and stress hormones; controls stress, glutamate, hypothyroidism, weight gain, and biogenic amines; and cleans toxins out of the blood, such as acetaldehyde and ammonia.[607,608,609]

All migraine triggers are affected by low levels of methylfolate. Migraine triggers will also deplete methylfolate levels, which could cause you to break your headache threshold.

Want to Bypass the Migraine Gene with Methylfolate?

In order for methylfolate to bypass the migraine gene, it must first bypass the gut because the migraine gene may inhibit digestion. This is now possible with a dissolvable supplement called Active B12

Lozenges with L-5-MTHF from a company called Seeking Health. The supplement includes a premium form of vitamin B12 (methylcobalamin) that is required for the body to use methylfolate (L-5-MTHF). This supplement is the answer to the genetic problem passed down from one migraine sufferer to the next. Don't forget vitamins B2 and B6, which are also required for the methylation cycle and migraine prevention.

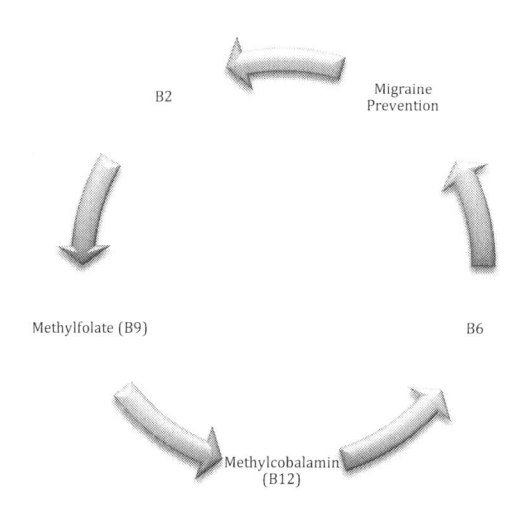

```
        B2  ⬅         Migraine
                      Prevention
         ⬇               ⬆
Methylfolate (B9)        B6
              ↘        ↗
              Methylcobalamin
                  (B12)
```

I recommend seeing a doctor before using any supplements because obtaining proper B vitamin levels is extremely complex. The MTHFR gene is also immensely complex.

Want to Learn More?

- www.mthfr.net – To learn more about how to successfully bypass the MTHFR gene
- www.seekinghealth.org/gift – An 80-minute video by the leading expert of the MTHFR gene, Dr. Benjamin Lynch

- www.3dayheadachecure.com, *The Migraine Gene: Curse and Cure* – A video that will make the entire headache threshold easier to understand

Vitamin D

"Despite many publications and scientific meetings reporting advances in vitamin D science,
a disturbing realization is growing that the newer scientific
and clinical knowledge is not being translated into better human health."

– A.W. Norman, from a study published in the *American Journal of Clinical Nutrition*[610]

There have been over 30,000 studies published on the benefits of vitamin D, which include lowering your risk of cancer, diabetes, autism, heart disease, rheumatoid arthritis, depression, pain, inflammatory bowel disease, and headaches.[611] Your body actually turns vitamin D into a hormone, which may be referred to as "activated vitamin D," "calcitriol," or just "vitamin D."

Vitamin D helps promote calcium absorption. Calcium is kind of like a light switch for your body, and if you don't have enough of it (a condition called hypocalcemia), that light switch starts to go haywire on your nerves. This calcium light switch is what inhibits that electrical thunderstorm of depolarization in the brain— the migraine aura. But too much calcium in the cells is bad because it can burst the migraine threshold, and not enough calcium is bad because it can burst the migraine threshold.

The bottom line is you need vitamin D to help regulate calcium. Researchers actually studied this in 2009. They exposed rats to high levels of glutamate,[612] and like clockwork, this exposure began to excite the cells in the brain to death. The rats they gave vitamin D to had significantly less brain damage. For a migraine sufferer, this is phenomenal news.

Vitamin D is classified as one of the primary biological regulators of calcium.[613] So migraineurs, look into this—have your doctor run a blood test to find out if you're deficient. You may need to add vitamin D to your bag of tricks.

A recent study of over 10,000 patients found that those with low levels of vitamin D were more likely to have diabetes, high blood pressure, and heart disease. Here's the scary part: *Those vitamin D–deficient patients were nearly three times more likely to die from any cause of death compared to those with normal levels.*[614] A lot of this book is based on controversial research. Vitamin D no longer falls in this category.

But wait. How can blood levels of vitamin D increase or reduce your risk of any cause of death? Seriously. Here's one way. In 2014 Cleveland Clinic researchers found that those with low blood levels of vitamin D are at increased risk of death after surgery.[615] Let's say you get into a car accident, the ambulance takes you to the hospital for surgery—your chance of survival is significantly altered based on the amount of vitamin D in your blood.

A ton of research is saying that people are dying without vitamin D, and information is not making it to our grandparents, friends, children, or even to many of our healthcare professionals. The study with over 10,000 patients found that more than 70% were deficient in vitamin D based on a level of under 30 ng/ml.

I had vitamin D levels under 30 ng/ml right before I quit my career as a firefighter. After a blood test, it was the only red flag that came up. I was experiencing headaches, stomach pain, and sleep deprivation. A slight vitamin D deficiency was the only problem shown from my medical evaluation, which is extremely embarrassing for the guy who tells everyone that "milk is for babies." Even so, recent research is showing that vitamin D levels of 30 ng/ml may be way too low, so I may have gotten off easy.

You know what that means? It means that anyone with a vitamin D deficiency could find relief by taking vitamin D supplements. It also means we don't know where to set the bar for what a deficiency is. This problem may be even worse. Experts are saying we need at least 40 to 50 ng/ml to be healthy.[616]

A 2007 study found that women who were given enough vitamin D to bring their levels to 40 ng/ml experienced a 77% reduction in all forms of cancer.[617] This is great, but we may see an even higher reduction in cancer rates if we raise those levels of vitamin D above 50 ng/ml. We just learned that something you can get for free (from the sun) might be just as powerful as every cent people spend on cancer treatment, which may be why it's not heavily advertised in places that make money off of sick people.[618]

Are You Vitamin D Deficient?

Probably. According to a 2009 study published in *JAMA* that involved a large number of people, 77% of Americans are vitamin D deficient.[619] In addition, black Americans are 97% vitamin D deficient, and Mexican Americans are 90% vitamin D deficient. Dark pigmentation reduces the entry of vitamin D.[620] This huge study was all based on that low level of 30 ng/ml, meaning that even more than 77% of Americans are in serious need of vitamin D. This problem seems to be getting worse and worse.

Your Happy Chemicals and Vitamin D

Researchers have just found that vitamin D is responsible for activating serotonin, oxytocin, and vasopressin. Vasopressin is a hormone that helps regulate water, glucose, salts, and blood pressure. Without vasopressin, you will not be headache-free. Nitroglycerin, nitrites, and nitrosamines—from smoke, calcium, and vasopressin—all interact with each other.[621][622] You probably already guessed that vasopressin relates to the adrenal glands and thyroid function, which will inevitably kick back to a poorly functioning MTHFR gene. We're talking about the most important functions of the human body, and without vitamin D, we are screwed.

Oxytocin is the love drug that monkeys and humans have a tough time surviving without. Serotonin helps to regulate toxic amounts of glutamate. Both of these happy brain chemicals stop stress and inflammation.[623] In a study of over 31,000 patients, researchers found that a lack of vitamin D correlates directly to high rates of depression—and it's no wonder.[624] As we know, depression and stress can lead to migraines and numerous other diseases.

Where to Get It

Taking a supplement won't solve everything. However, of the 10,000 patients who were vitamin D deficient, those who took supplements cut their risk of death in half. That's substantial. No, that's invaluable.

The best place to get vitamin D is still the sun. The human skin supplies about 90% of the vitamin D in the body from exposure to the sun's UV rays. This "sunshine vitamin D" is known as vitamin D3. Get some sun, and you will get your vitamin D3.[625]

Many doctors prescribe vitamin D2, but a 2011 study of over 90,000 people found that the risk of death was three times greater with vitamin D2 when compared to using vitamin D3.[626] Vitamin D3 is way more powerful, and that makes perfect sense when we understand that the human body creates 90% of its vitamin D from natural sunlight, that natural source of vitamin D3.

What About Eating It?

Vitamin D2 can be obtained from some types of mushrooms. Vitamin D3 is found in fatty animal-based foods, such as tuna, salmon, mackerel, sardines, fish oils, eggs, and fortified milk. But, as you know, you've got to be careful with eggs and milk. Many low-nutrient foods are fortified with vitamin D but may not raise vitamin D levels in the body without fats and other nutrients.[627] Food sources are thought to be less effective when compared to sunshine. Plus, sunshine makes you feel good.

Getting Proper Sunshine

Direct sun exposure is the best way to get vitamin D, and obviously, the more skin you have showing, the better. Sunshine between 10:00 a.m. and 3:00 p.m. will be most effective during non-winter months. Many places will not have enough sun during the winter to create enough vitamin D, and you'll need to take supplements or consume vitamin D–rich foods.

There are a couple of factors that can prevent vitamin D intake from the sun. Sunscreen blocks 99% of vitamin D synthesis from the sun.[628] Also, there's no way to effectively measure all the variables related to health and sunscreen use. Despite a few isolated studies that show sunscreen may actually increase the risk of the deadliest form of skin cancer, we can't determine if sunscreen is good or bad. It is possible that sunscreen can inhibit all the positive effects that would have come from the sunshine's ability to form vitamin D. There is also a massive number of sunscreens that contain potentially dangerous chemicals.

But of course I'm not suggesting you go in the sun and get scorched. For an online guide to healthy sunscreens that provide maximum protection, visit www.ewg.org. You can also visit www.mercola.com to find information on vitamin D testing, safer tanning beds, and when to get natural sun. There are no tanning beds that have been tested as completely safe, and older tanning beds have been linked to cancer, although Dr. Mercola makes the argument that "safe tanning beds" have fewer harmful UVA rays than the sun.[629]

Getting vitamin D from the sun or a tanning bed is a risk, but it also keeps humans happy and healthy. And because the body creates vitamin D from sun rays using fats and cholesterol, if you are deficient in both healthy fats and cholesterol, you are more likely to burn in the sun and more likely to get cancer.[630] You're going to get some sunshine at some point and will need that fat, unless you are a vampire, but even vampires still need healthy fats to digest the vitamin D from whatever animal they sink their teeth into!

How you get your vitamin D is a personal choice. Many people are against supplements, some burn too fast in the sun, sunscreen has pros and cons, the sun produces a cancer risk, and vitamin D deficiency increases a person's risk for certain types of death. I personally felt way better after taking vitamin D3 supplements to get my vitamin D back up to healthy levels, but I do prefer real sunshine. You may need to research the topic and consult with your doctor about the best way for you to get vitamin D, because everyone produces it at different levels.

Do you feel happy when you've been inside all day and haven't seen the sun? I don't. The cubicle lifestyle may be killing Americans. If you're stuck inside all day, remember to take breaks and step outside every chance you have. Happiness is stress leaving your body, so get some vitamin D and stay happy and headache-free.

Feverfew

"I started getting ocular migraines almost every day, I've been taking this once every night for the past three or four months and haven't had a migraine in WEEKS!!! It's fantastic! Waking up without a headache is AMAZING!!! THANK YOU!!!" This was an Amazon review for feverfew leaves by Nature's Way.

Another reviewer exclaimed, "I started having migraines at 35 and was prescribed Topamax right away… Horrified with its side effects, I started my own search for alternative treatment and came across feverfew and decided to try it. It basically got rid of all headaches, even if they started, they were VERY mild and went away without any painkiller. It is amazing! It is a miracle!!! It saved my life! I got back to jogging and all sorts of vigorous exercise and no headaches!!!"

Can you believe this? This really makes the world spin in another direction. There are a lot of migraine and headache sufferers who are ready to kill themselves. This is one of the many reviews that say in one way or another that "feverfew saved my life." Could you imagine taking medications for years with heavy side effects and then stumbling into a better life from consuming the leaves of a natural plant?

In a 16-week study of 170 migraine patients, those who used 6.25 mg of feverfew three times per day found a significant reduction in migraines compared to those who used a placebo. The average number of attacks per month prior to treatment was 4.76. After treatment, migraines went down by 1.9 attacks per month. That's a 40% reduction in migraines in exchange for swallowing a few pills of a natural herb.[631]

Other studies have shown that feverfew can reduce the severity of migraines when it's taken just before the onset of a full-blown migraine attack. It's both acute and preventative.[632]

Side Effects?

In one study by University Hospital in Nottingham of 59 migraineurs, researchers found no serious side effects associated with feverfew; however, one user reported stomachaches in a review on Amazon.[633] Herbs can be very powerful, they can trigger side effects, and they can interact with other medications and supplements. Make sure you buy from a reputable company and speak with your doctor before taking the herb risk, which seems minimal in the case of feverfew.

Omega-3

You would have to be mad as a hatter to consume less than enough omega-3 as a headache sufferer. The inflammatory meat chapter referenced a fish oil study that took adolescent migraine sufferers from 15 migraines per month down to two. That's almost a 90% drop in headaches. To be fair, this was a small group of just 23, and the placebo effect was incredibly high with the same reduction in migraines—from 15 down to two per month. But you're going to laugh when you read what the placebo was. They used olive oil.

It's crazy, right? You already know about olive oil's health benefits! In addition to that, olive oil contains oleocanthal, which provides similar anti-inflammatory benefits to ibuprofen.[634] And actually, many researchers (who clearly didn't do *all* of their homework) have made the same mistake time and time again of using olive oil as a placebo. It really wasn't until the middle of the first decade of the twenty-first century that studies started confirming that olive oil reduces inflammatory markers.[635] Before that, olive oil was just a well-documented health factor in the under-researched area of things that grow on trees. Twenty-three patients isn't much, but a nearly 90% success rate is.

Lucky for us, a 2013 study gave us numbers and adults to find out just how much omega-3 helps migraine sufferers.[636] This study took 56 adults with migraines and put them on a diet that lowered their omega-6 intake. Half of those 56 six adults also raised their omega-3 levels at the same time and had spectacular success. Headache days per month went from 23.3 to 14.5, and headache hours per day went from 10.2 to 5.6.

The study's graph of mean headache days plummeted all the way to the last day of the 12-week period, making us wonder what would happen after three months. These patients ended up using acute medications 37% less often. They were on an average of six medications each, which is why the study is so impressive. It tells us they were serious migraine sufferers that benefited despite the blending of medications that surely have the side effects of more headaches. I'm very excited about these results, and you should be too.

You already know omega-3 lowers the risk of high blood pressure, heart disease, and rheumatoid arthritis, and may help relieve pain, including back pain and headaches. But that's not why you want omega-3 fat. You want omega-3 fat because it helps you absorb your most important vitamins, like vitamin D.

Where to Get It

I think fish oil is the best thing on earth, but not all of the research is positive. Many vitamin supplements are fake, and a number of fish oil supplements are oxidized—inflammatory destruction as opposed to healthful help. The "hard" research is rather soft. One large meta-study pointed to a decreased risk of cardiovascular death,[637] and one of the longest-running studies pointed to an increased risk of cardiovascular death, but that study stated the result was "unexplained."[638] Chris Kresser believes the fish oil craze "highlights the danger of isolated nutrient studies." Anything isolated in large quantities has the potential to be harmful, especially if you choose a brand that sneaks in toxic ingredients.[639]

Make sure you know where your fish and fish oil came from. The fish swimming outside a city's waste facility or nuclear plant or within thousands of miles of a mercury-erupting coal plant may be questionable.

This is why krill oil is becoming a popular substitute for fish oil. Viva Labs Krill Oil is 100% Antarctic krill oil and supposedly 54 times more powerful than regular fish oil. The bioavailability of omega-3 and antioxidants in krill oil may lower triglycerides and glucose levels significantly more than fish oil, says one industry-sponsored study.[640] I would personally choose krill oil for the simple fact that Antarctica's water is cleaner than ours.

Omega-3 foods:

- Flaxseed
- Oregano
- Basil
- Broccoli
- Spinach
- Salmon
- Herring
- Tuna
- Wild game
- Free-range beef

Don't Forget to Avoid Omega-6

Soy oil has increased in production 1,000% from the year 1909 to 2000. These large increases of omega-6 inflammatory foods in the twentieth century may be responsible for lower levels of omega-3 in the average American. The inflammatory foods go up and our anti-inflammatory omega-3 levels go down.[641] Most grains, pastas, breads, rice, and cereals will be high in omega-6 and very low in omega-3.

5-Hydroxytryptophan (5-HTP)

The body uses 5-HTP to make serotonin. You already know from that sentence that 5-HTP is used as an antidepressant and anxiety reducer. Evidence also suggests that low serotonin may trigger migraines,[642] making this supplement a possible option for migraine treatment.

I'm not insinuating that 5-HTP is a problem, but you should definitely check with your doctor and proceed with caution. Anything that unnaturally plays with serotonin levels can be deadly when mixed with other medications. It also can have unknown long-term effects. That being said, let's see what's good about the happy drug booster.

The most successful 5-HTP study was done in the 1980s and found that high doses of 5-HTP (600 mg daily) were almost as effective as the drug methysergide, a standard migraine medication at the time that was discontinued for serious side effects. The study noted that 5-HTP was a more promising treatment, with 71% of patients showing improvement in the intensity and duration of migraines, rather than in the frequency of their attacks.[643]

Lower doses have not been so successful. In 2000 an eight-week study of 65 tension headache sufferers (mostly women) showed that taking low doses of 5-HTP (100 mg) several times a week did not significantly reduce patients' headaches but did reduce their need for pain medication.[644]

Perhaps the most promising results of 5-HTP lie within the effects of triptans, the expensive class of migraine drugs. Triptans work in part by boosting serotonin levels and have successfully aborted migraines in less than an hour.[645] Of course, these insanely powerful drugs can come with equally powerful side effects, including more headaches.

5-HTP may be a promising supplement at a fraction of the cost of medications. Of course, we can't say for sure, and I don't foresee a large, double-blind, placebo-controlled study running anytime soon, since it would be costly to prove that this $17 supplement is what doctors should recommend. Some of the WebMD user reviews claim that this cheap alternative is not only better at relieving pain than triptans; it may also take a chronic migraineur from 15 or more migraines per month to zero in just 90 days.

5-HTP is not commonly found in nature. For instance, the serotonin in a banana does not cross the blood-brain barrier. 5-HTP, on the other hand, is manufactured from the rare seeds of an African plant called Griffonia simplicifolia, and these 5-HTP molecules are small enough to cross the blood-brain barrier. They cross with ease in high doses. Once inside the brain, they convert to serotonin.

This should scare you. I'll say it again: The FDA doesn't strictly regulate herbs and supplements. Here we have a drug with the ability to significantly alter our entire brain chemistry. Serotonin regulates glutamate's rise and fall in a very complex way, meaning that taking 5-HTP could pose a high risk.[646] This means that 5-HTP could be advantageous or it could be detrimental. It is a Honda with a jet engine under the hood. If you want to take the risk, talk to your doctor about the common side effects, such as headaches and abdominal pain, and all the problems that come with this chemical's drug interactions. I know—it's a headache "cure" that might cause headaches. But look into it—the side effects may be less severe than other available medications,[647] so it may show promise as a last resort for migraineurs under the guidance of a doctor.

Where to Get It

Because 5-HTP isn't found in any foods, you have to get it from a store shelf or an online site. As the name suggests, the human body creates 5-HTP from tryptophan—you know, the turkey amino acid that's supposed to put you to bed. Tryptophan can be found in fish, sunflower seeds, eggs, and a number of meats, but eating these foods won't automatically increase your serotonin. If you want 5-HTP, go with the supplements.

The supplements come in doses of 100 mg. If you search for "Now Foods 5-HTP" on Amazon, you can see the reviews. Some people have headaches and bad gastric problems from relatively low doses. You would need to take six of these pills per day to get the results from the 1980s study.

We don't even know if that's a good dose. In fairness to the product, it also has many five-star ratings, mostly from people using it for sleep and depression issues. "Kate" writes, "I hate people, the American population for the most part repulses me. I have taken 200 mg as suggested by my therapist and this has helped me hate everyone less, or hold it in better. Yay!" And Julie from Florence, Mississippi, writes, "Great mood enhancer. Went from psycho to flowers and butterflies overnight. Can't recommend it enough!!!"

JEREMY OROZCO

Stress Less

"I am an old man and have known a great many troubles, but most of them never happened."

– Mark Twain

If you look back at the last 50 years of research, you'll learn that stress is the number one migraine trigger.[648] Stress led to the worst headache of my life. You would think that a firefighter's greatest source of stress would come from fire, but that's never the case. I thought I was happy as a clam with a world-class Santa Cruz surf break in our front yard, a three-day workweek, and a beautiful fiancé.

My four days off per week were consumed with surfing and developing understandmigraines.org with my fiancé, Sondra, who is now my wife. Bringing the best headache help to one place is kind of like attempting to build a car with a Ferrari motor, Lamborghini suspension, a Porsche transmission, and a BMW body. You'll end up with a gorgeous pile of junk that doesn't move or fit together. I realized that I wasn't going to help anyone, including me, until I understood the intricate parts of every headache trigger. Otherwise, we're just left with a lot of expensive help that doesn't fit together.

I began writing this book to find incredible studies that make sense of the headache mess. However, it started to require more time than I had. And I was starting to realize that, in writing this book, I was expressing views that the United States government, my employer, might not appreciate. I was at one of those crossroads in life when you know you need to make a change, but you just haven't admitted it to yourself. I had recently become an acting captain, taking on the heavy responsibility of two other firefighters' lives; I was running several fire programs; and I was juggling understandmigraines.org along with all of that.

Something had to give. I set in motion a headache that lasted three weeks before things deteriorated. My stomach had a constant tightness, I was losing sleep (more than just the usual night calls), I was having trouble concentrating, and my head had constant pressure within. Then the final straw broke. About 90 hours into a shift, I forgot my turnout pants on a night call for a fire.

Luckily, the night call was a false alarm. You may think that it's not a big deal to forget something after being sleep deprived. It is. It's not like I forgot a pen at a desk job. If the fire alarm had been for a real fire, someone could have died, which is a worst-case scenario way of thinking that often leads to stress. No one noticed, and even if someone had, accidents happen. But this wasn't a normal accident for me.

I immediately went to the doctor for the first time in 10 years. I told him that I was thinking of quitting the fire service. He stayed away from the stomach and headache symptoms to focus on the actual problem. He prescribed for me three weeks off and stress counseling, which was the best thing he could have done.

The therapist he recommended listened carefully as I explained that my life goals had changed. She inquired about the first company I co-founded, which now controls the largest crowd-sourced information of wildland fires. Eventually, she said, "You want to do something else, quit." While the first company was impressive, it was a free site, and it always will be.

I said, "It took more than a decade to get where I am. The odds of just landing a California firefighter job are 700 to one. My retirement is at age 50, the benefits are great—"

She interrupted and said, "Life's too short. Worst-case scenario, you make less money. Would you be OK with that?" I would, and I am.

And then I did it. I quit. I gave a six-month notice to transition the programs I was running and to save up some cash. I thought my stress level would go up, but I felt great. My stomach was back to normal in about three weeks, and within about two days, I was having far fewer headaches. Looking back, I was stressed out of my mind, of course. I had to make a life decision that I never thought was possible. But I discovered that thinking about a decision is far more difficult than making one.

Sondra jokingly told her boss that we could live anywhere now that I wasn't tied down to the Bay Area, and her boss approved. She is now working remote. We sold all of our stuff, gave up the plush beach condo, and hit the road (and the air).

I know you might be thinking, "OK, I can't quit my job. I've got bills, kids, car payments, and obligations." The funny thing is that quitting didn't actually fix my problem. I went to work happy for the next six months because I knew I was getting closer to my goal of completing this book. I worked even more hours at work and at home but with a completely different attitude.

This is a story of self-induced stress, which can trigger powerful migraines, but a single stress-induced headache or migraine is nothing compared to the physical and emotional stress that chronic migraines bring.

Here's one example of that intense stress. A Canadian man, Randy Janzen, ended the life of his teenage daughter in May of 2015 and then posted this on Facebook: "Emily had tried everything to get better but nothing seemed to help her. I took a gun and shot her in the head and now she is migraine-free and floating in the clouds on a sunny afternoon." Janzen continued, "I don't think anyone really knew how much pain Emily was in on a daily basis and the severe depression that these migraines caused."[649] Finding what triggers migraines will eliminate these hopeless acts.

And seriously, if the trigger is something as simple as a job, quit. Find another one. Search online for "Gary Vaynerchuk: Do what you love." In this video, he shows us that, as long as we're working toward our goals, the hours we work won't matter—we'll be happy. I should warn you not to watch this video unless you are prepared to start doing what you love. It may have been one of the turning points for me in deciding to end my career.

Life doesn't usually cause stress; it's the perception of life that causes stress. Watch the documentary *Burn* and you will see underpaid and overworked firefighters who are happy to risk their lives. Even the trailer is incredible. Many people, including some firefighters, would be traumatized under the same conditions.

What's the difference? One person would perceive the life-threatening exposure as a positive stress that will save a life or allow growth as a firefighter. The other person would see no positive outcome from the same situation. Fortunately, most firefighters welcome the stress with open arms. Your stress may be much worse than the stress of a firefighter. "No! My stress?" you say. A firefighter will leave 99% of all calls at the firehouse. Aside from evaluating the emergency to make stronger decisions, the stress comes and goes. Chronic stress is what you carry on your shoulders.

When I was the CEO of my first company, I was more stressed than any real emergency could ever make me. There are over 30,000 fire departments in the United States, and none of them has a world-class training program that is shared online for free with all other firefighters. It doesn't make sense, ethically or financially, that lifesaving information is available and is not distributed to everyone.

I wanted free education sharing for firefighters to be sustainable, and that was a very hard thing to do. It was a gut-wrenching transition to temporarily abandon free education to support free wildland fire information-sharing technology—which the company is now the nation's leader of. The problem is that a business may struggle even while you sleep. This drawn-out stress that is self-created by long-term business goals is chronic stress, and it does not help achieve those goals. I worried about things I couldn't change at 4:00 a.m., and it did not help the company get where it is today. Firefighters do not stress about the things they cannot change, and neither should you or I. Ask yourself if it will benefit the situation to stress. If not, change your perspective.

We know that stress causes a rise in glutamate and inflammation, which leads to migraines. But how bad can it be? Any monkey will tell you that stress can be calamitous. No one knows this better than Stanford University's Robert Sapolsky. Stop reading this book and find "Robert Sapolsky: The Psychology of Stress" on YouTube to learn about a lifetime's worth of work in just a few minutes.

At a time when an ulcer was the only condition related to stress, Sapolsky was in Kenya studying the stressful lives of low-ranking baboons. Sapolsky says that baboons only swing a three-hour workday to gather food, leaving "nine hours per day to make someone else just miserable." Sapolsky has spent more than 30 years observing these animals that are "quite awful to one another, constantly scheming and backstabbing."[650]

Collecting blood samples from baboons on the receiving side of aggression revealed high levels of stress hormones, elevated heart rates, and high blood pressure. This was the first time anyone had linked stress and deteriorating health to primates in the wild.

And this is the same stress hormone that helps you survive an attack by turning off all nonessential functions to survival, such as digestion, growth, reproduction, and many brain functions. This can lead to hardening of the arteries and a less than healthy immune system.

Today, Sapolsky's once loony stress hunch is a widely accepted fact in medicine and links the six leading causes of death. Forty-three percent of adults suffer adverse health effects from stress, and 75–90% of all physician-office visits are for stress-related ailments and complaints—with about half accompanied by headaches.[651]

Sapolsky's most interesting finding was that terrorizing baboons was not the cause of stress but a trigger of stress. Getting thrown out of a tree may be stressful for about three seconds, but the stress ends when the baboon lands on his or her hands or feet. The baboons with Type A personalities held serious grudges that made them agitated, even when seeing a rival peacefully sleeping 100 yards in the distance. Their anger is self-created.

The low-ranking Type A baboons were most susceptible to stress. However, up-and-coming baboons consistently tested the alpha male's short-lived rank. People experience similar stress; it's hard to watch everything you have worked for threatened by newly successful colleagues or overhanging businesses.

Ten years into Sapolsky's research, something terrible happened to his initial baboon tribe. They ate food that was tainted with tuberculosis from the open garbage at a nearby tourist destination. Nearly half of the males in the troop died, taking with them a decade of unfinished research.

The result, however, was "scientifically significant." Only the males that were aggressive and antisocial died. The tribe was left with twice as many females as males, and those males that survived were "good guys"—unaggressive and socially affiliated. Twenty years later, the same culture remains in the tribe and has contributed to a lack of high blood pressure, high levels of stress hormones, altered brain chemistry, and anxiety.

The research tells us two things. First, maintaining a strong social balance has tremendous benefits to our health. Second, the perspective of a threat is more important than the actual threat itself. Baboons that waited for theoretical fights had twice the stress levels as those that only took action on real threats. The calmer baboons were not weaker; they just spoke with fists and walked away from fights they couldn't win.[652]

Unfortunately, the more cognitively inclined of us make life so much more complicated than running from a lion or deciding on the appropriate time to punch a fellow monkey. Superior wisdom allows us to create a perceived stress from the color of our shoes—or things we have absolutely no control over. Our minds can have a meltdown from something that will not jeopardize our survival, so it will really benefit us all to learn to stress less.

Stress and Migraines

Stress sets up the perfect conditions for a migraine, and it makes those conditions last. Chronic pain is a slow buildup and a slow breakdown. It leaves us confused as we experiment with quick fixes for a slow problem.

There are countless studies that show the relationship between stress and migraines. Of most concern for a migraine sufferer is how stress affects the stomach in combination with widespread inflammation. A leaky gut may let nitrites and other biogenic amines slide past the stomach and the blood-brain barrier to the white matter of the brain that is currently struggling with stress-induced insulin resistance.[653]

A stress-inflamed gut may exacerbate vitamin deficiencies that can cause a significant decline in health. When you start trying to figure out what's causing your migraines, it's important to address the root problem. Those baboons can go gluten-free all day long and still have a number of stress symptoms, including depression. They won't be susceptible to heart attacks, but how grand of an achievement is it to live unhappily?

So first, identify the root cause of your problem. Next, work on changing that condition. I decided I couldn't work two full-time jobs forever. Life really is too short.

You may not be in a position to change the condition causing you the most stress—quitting a job you don't love, moving across the country, leaving a lover, whatever. That's OK; neither was I. The goal is to identify what's causing your stress so you can come up with a plan to eliminate it. It's not an easy move to make. You need to weigh your options and decide what's really important to you. I have friends who have decided that they could work toward a more enjoyable career, but they would rather spend time with their kids. It's the people who are stuck somewhere in the middle who have the most stress. You can start by changing how you think about your problem. Instead of constantly thinking, "I hate this job," try thinking, "I love this job because it is getting me closer to my goal."

We may be able to cure a migraine by eliminating food triggers, but we can't always avoid stress. Dr. Sapolsky, the stress master himself, is a self-proclaimed stress case. He works 80 hours per week to find the human pathway of stress, and of course he is stressed. Sapolsky differs from most people because he identifies exactly where his stress comes from, and like most great overachievers, he refuses to slow down. He emphasizes that stress is not a lost cause. If you don't have the weight of the world on your shoulders (and no one really does), there is a good chance you will be able to eliminate your chronic stress.

Attempting to "cure" the stress migraine is like a doctor trying to "cure" crying. Crying, a migraine trigger for many people, is an accumulation of stress with a breaking point. You wouldn't suggest drugs for someone who is crying, so why are people prescribed drugs for stress-related headaches? Find the stress and evaluate the resources you have available to eliminate or change that stress—and if you can't change it, change your perception of that stress. Fortunately for you, you're no different from any other human—we all have illogical stress responses—and there are multiple resources that are proven to help us in ways that drugs can only erratically mimic. Get ready for the happiness chapter to kiss stress goodbye.

Get Blissed on Your Own Chemicals

Do you know what makes you happy? I'm not asking about your friends, family, cat, car, or favorite spot under a palm tree. I'm asking if you know what chemicals in your brain make you happy. Your brain will never be content without all four of those chemicals. They are the chemicals that reverse stress and reverse migraines. Let's get you those happy chemicals.

The four happy chemicals are dopamine, serotonin, oxytocin, and endorphins. Case closed. Go to your local pharmacy and pick some up, right? You know it doesn't work that way. Do you know the problem with cocaine? Sure, it offers addiction, financial ruin, and destroyed relationships, but the real problem with cocaine is that you come down.

Anything that boosts dopamine, like cocaine or coffee, to unnatural levels will come with a rise and fall; the higher the rise, the harder the fall. You cannot trick your brain into thinking it's happy without the eventual reality of a downfall. What do the last 20 years of mass school murders have in common? It's not guns.

Thirty-four school shootings and other school-related acts of disturbing violence have had the common denominator of the use or withdrawal of psychiatric drugs.[654] Low levels of dopamine caused by prolonged antidepressant use are documented to cause aggression, depression, and suicidal tendencies. This is why the commercials say, "If you have thoughts of hurting yourself or others, you should stop taking this [awful] drug immediately and consult with a doctor."

If you would like to be happy, not just numb, give your body those four chemicals without any shenanigans or trickery. You can read a summed up version of what those chemicals do here, or read the fantastic book *Meet Your Happy Chemicals: Dopamine, Endorphin, Oxytocin, Serotonin* by Loretta Breuning.

Dopamine

Today we most identify dopamine as the reward "drug," but what was it intended for? Our ancestors got a rush of dopamine when they found a new berry patch, fishing hole, or hunting spot. Dr. Sapolsky elaborated on this effect during his class speech for the 2009 graduating Stanford class.

Researchers thought dopamine would flood a monkey's brain after a reward was given for completing a signaled task. What actually happened was the dopamine sharply inclined as soon as the monkey received the signal to work. The monkey began and finished the work while dopamine was at the top of a roller-coaster ride. It wasn't until the work was finished that the dopamine levels dropped back down to normal levels and the monkey enjoyed the reward. To the surprise of many, dopamine was not the reward, but the anticipation of the reward.

What happens if the monkey only gets the reward 50% of the time? The dopamine goes through the roof and drops back down whether the monkey receives the reward or not. This doesn't make much sense. Why would a monkey do the work if he were *not* to be paid half the time? This is known as the "gambling effect" that makes an addict go nuts, or bananas, until that card flips and anticipation is withdrawn.

Animals, including humans, have used dopamine for millions of years to hold on to the idea that food is nearby, and if we try hard enough and long enough, well, as the Stones say, "we might just find we get what we need." Dopamine connects neurons so it is released at the next possibility of food. If the food is not guaranteed, the body pushes you with euphoria to take that chance for survival. This also holds true for pursuing a mate, especially if that mate plays hard—but not impossible—to get.

Humans are unlike any other animal in the way we hold on to chance, sometimes for a lifetime. Dopamine is present if you work toward heaven and believe you'll make it, but it's abundant if you believe there's a chance you might end up in hell. Dopamine is the stuff that gets us through high school, college, and work.

Where to Get It

So how do we climb this dopamine mountain without getting to the top? As Dr. Breuning puts it, find that "I got it" feeling. Dopamine is based on learning or progress toward success. Whether you are designing the world's next big thing or picking blackberries for a pie, dopamine will connect the neurons toward your goal and even remind you of the path of least pricks.

Traveling and discovering new places releases tons of dopamine. You learn new roads, languages, foods, and cultural differences that all lead toward the goal of survival. Maybe traveling is not your thing. Learn or do anything new: surfing, writing, or crossword puzzles, for example. Work toward a promotion, find a new hobby, go back to school—take one step toward any goal.[655]

Serotonin

You learned what serotonin was as soon as you came into this world crying. Serotonin is the "important" feeling. It is the "I'm going to cry until you realize that I'm here and feed me" feeling. Boys, more than girls, carry on this behavior when they yell, scream, and hit others to get attention, which clearly means they are important. Serotonin is sought when someone posts on Facebook, "I hate my life."

While some look for serotonin in depressing and sometimes barbaric ways, serotonin is responsible for great things. It's the feeling a father gets when he knows he is the most important person in the world to his little boy or girl. Serotonin is what made Steve Jobs say, "I wanna put a dent in the universe."

Where to Get It

- Become important to someone. Anyone.
- Focus on what you are good at and on the good you do.
- Buy a cup of coffee for a friend. Giving makes you happy.
- Donate to charity. Helping others can give you purpose.
- Eat healthy fat! Essential fats are needed to produce serotonin.
- Avoid diet soda as it can lower serotonin levels and is associated with depression.[656][657]
- Workout! Serotonin makes you feel like you are an important, sexy beast after just one workout. Omega-3 will support this process, and studies show it will also help you lose weight!
- Sleep. Quality sleep makes you "serotonious"—my new word for the perfect amount of sleep. Too much or too little sleep can negatively impact serotonin levels, but researchers aren't sure how. In any case, people tend to feel better about

- Get some sun. Sunshine boosts serotonin! Serotonin was linked in February 2014 to vitamin D.[658] Serotonin and oxytocin are activated by vitamin D, which is fat soluble.[659] So get your sunshine and fat. Sounds like a perfect day.

- Be the person you want to be, whoever that person is, today.

Oxytocin, the True Love Drug

Oxytocin reduces stress while producing intoxicating love, giving people the drive to die for one another. Gandhi must have had a lot of this love drug. Oxytocin is also released after childbirth, fueling the feeling of unconditional love a mother has for her child. Oxytocin is also released during breastfeeding. Oxytocin is released during orgasms for both sexes. I'm telling you, it's good stuff!

Monkeys that are groomed by bond partners have high oxytocin levels, indicating that oxytocin helps form strong bonds for survival.[660] While other animal studies show that just being in the same area of a friendly face can increase oxytocin and lower anxiety.[661]

Oxytocin is involved with social recognition and trust. There is nothing like the feeling you get with family and old friends.

Where to Get It

- Visit your friends and family.
- Make new friends and build trust.
- Think about the love you have for people.
- Get intimate.

Endorphins

Endorphins mask pain and produce the runner's high. This is how a zebra escapes with force after a lion has ripped open its intestines. The endorphins will immediately raise antibodies that will help kill the violent exposure of foreign bacteria and viruses from the outside world.[662]

Endorphins also help motivate us to complete the physical tasks required for food, shelter, and reproduction. "Oh, you want me to come over? No, I wasn't asleep. It's only 4:00 a.m. Sure, I'll just peddle my bicycle in the rain with a broken foot to come and see you"—those are endorphins at work.

Where to Get Them

- Exercise, smile, and laugh. Exercise is proven to produce endorphins, and because it helps induce happiness, you could find yourself trapped a vicious happiness cycle.[663]
- It's common sense, but we must always remind ourselves that we need fruits and vegetables. This holds true for the production of happy chemicals and the nutritional happiness required in releasing those happy chemicals. Eat vegetables; be happy.

Make a Stop at Motivation Station

You probably already know which happy chemicals you have a surplus of and which ones you are sadly missing. These are our basic animalistic motivators, but what motivates us on a deeper level?

This question is best answered by the best-selling author Daniel Pink in his book titled *Drive: The Surprising Truth About What*

Motivates Us and his seriously entertaining YouTube video "RSA Animate – Drive: The surprising truth about what motivates us."[664]

Pink has us question our own intentions as he reviews the power of money. He cites a study done at the Massachusetts Institute of Technology where students were motivated by three monetary incentives, and as their performances increased, their pay increased.

Our basic understanding of the world was warped when the study introduced rudimentary cognitive skills. Completing a children's puzzle shouldn't pose a threat to some of the brightest minds on earth. However, larger rewards led to poorer performances when basic cognitive thinking was involved. Huh?

That didn't make sense, so they took the incentives the MIT students clearly didn't care about and brought them to India where the incentive was worth up to two months of salary. The same results applied. The highest incentive led to the worst performances.

In the end, he speculates that we can only be led by a carrot on a string if the tasks are mindless. This finding flies in the face of the vast majority of the leadership and management practices used by businesses today.

Once we surpass the basic funds for survival, there are three motivators in work and life: autonomy, mastery, and purpose.

Autonomy

Autonomy is the desire to be self-directed. It's the idea that employees will accomplish great things when management steps out of their way. Autonomy has helped to create an entire new workweek in the tech industry, as companies are allowing employees to spend a portion of their time working on whatever they want. This allows employees to show their skills and experience an increase in serotonin.

Can you imagine the things you would accomplish if people just got out of your way?

Mastery

Bruce Lee said, "I fear not the man who has practiced 10,000 kicks once, but I fear the man who has practiced one kick 10,000 times." Why would anyone practice a kick 10,000 times? For the same reason someone learns to master the guitar, knitting, or curling.

It's not what other people think that dictates the rush of dopamine and serotonin. You may have the time of your life perfecting the slide of a rock on ice or balancing stacks of rocks on top of each other at the beach—it doesn't matter. These happy chemicals of mastery have led to advances in technology by highly skilled people who choose to work thousands of hours for free. Wikipedia, Firefox, Linux, and hundreds of other open-source software companies are changing the world we live in—powered by people working for free and enjoying it.

Purpose

Purpose is the smile at the door, it's the mint on your pillow, it's the high five from a gym trainer, it's the compassionate bedside manner of a doctor, and it's the idea that someone cares about the service he or she is providing you.

Purpose is what makes people stay at a job for money that they would gladly do for free. It is the idea that, together, we can accomplish something great. Purpose utilizes the dopamine of progress, the serotonin of success, and the oxytocin of trust—validated time and time again by the commitment of people who share the same values. Add in a little elbow grease and a smile and you will finish the happiness package with endorphins.

What Motivates Your Life?

All I need is a million—no, a billion dollars, and then I'll be happy. A famous study was done in the 1970s that compared lottery winners to average people and paralysis victims. The study found that there was very little difference between the overall happiness of lottery winners and average people. In fact, even the paralysis victims found more enjoyment out of everyday pleasures.[665] According to happiness expert Shawn Achor, "We can only predict 10% of your long-term happiness. Ninety percent of your long-term happiness is predicted not by the external world, but by the way your brain processes the world."

How Powerful Is the Mind?

Achor's favorite happiness study is one in which Japanese researchers took 13 kids who were highly allergic to poison oak and had them rub a plant on their left arms. The kids were told that the plant was harmless, but it was actually poison oak. Surprisingly, only two of the kids had allergic reactions.

In another test, researchers told the students that they had rubbed poison oak on their right arms, which was another lie. They had actually used a harmless shrub. The students' right arms broke out with the boiling inflammation and itchy redness that occur when someone has an allergic reaction to poison oak. Don't be afraid. It's not witchcraft. It's just science.

The success rate of the placebo effect for migraine medications that reduce migraine pain and prevent migraines can be well over 50%.[666] Your mind has the power to create or eliminate inflammation in very specific ways that we do not fully understand today.

What Does All of This Have to Do with Headaches?

We know stress, inflammation, and glutamate trigger migraines and headaches. Happy chemicals reverse stress, inflammation, and glutamate, so you need happy chemicals!

And here it is in a nutshell: Simply find what makes you happy and do it. Positivity has proven to be more powerful than any drug. Stress is inversely as potent. Science, religion, and influential leaders are telling us that happiness is one of the best ways to immediately and continuously lower the very thing that triggers headaches.

Want to Learn More?

- "Class Day Lecture 2009: The Uniqueness of Humans," Dr. Robert Sapolsky, YouTube
- "The Happiness Advantage," Shawn Achor, TED Talk
- *Before Happiness: The 5 Hidden Keys to Achieving Success, Spreading Happiness, and Sustaining Positive Change* by Shawn Achor
- *The Happiness Advantage: The Seven Principles of Positive Psychology That Fuel Success and Performance at Work* by Shawn Achor

Exercise

A 2008 study took 20 migraine sufferers who didn't normally exercise and had them cycle in 40-minute sessions three times per week.[667] The last month of the 12-week study showed a significant decrease in the number of migraine attacks, the number of days with migraines per month, the mean headache intensity, and the amount of headache medication used. This study teaches us that workouts with proper warm-ups, cooldowns, and stretching are very beneficial to migraine sufferers.

Exercise or Drugs?

Ninety-one migraine patients in another study were broken into three groups: One group exercised three times per week for 40 minutes at a time, one group listened to a relaxation program, and one group was given topiramate daily.[668]

Topiramate is an antiseizure medication that works by blocking excitatory neurotransmitters and high-voltage-activated calcium channels. In migraine therapy, this translates to crushing the gun (glutamate) and taking out the bullets (calcium). Remember, we previously discussed that too much glutamate may initially trigger excitotoxic injury, and calcium continues through the cell like a bullet to start the aura associated with both migraines and seizures. Topiramate medications work well to prevent this electrical thunderstorm as a last resort for migraine sufferers, but they come with over 200 possible side effects that include everything from memory loss to drooling.

The relaxation group went to therapy once a week for six relaxation exercises that each lasted from five to 20 minutes. This included breathing and stress management techniques.

After three months, all three groups showed a reduction in migraine attacks, with no significant difference observed between the groups. That means that exercise, even minimal amounts, can be just as effective for migraines as medication. The same can be said about relaxation. We should consider regularly doing both meditation and exercise.

Since exercising three times per week for 40 minutes at a time isn't much, what does more exercise do? A 2003 study from at Dokuz Eylül University in Turkey involving 40 female migraine sufferers found that 60 minutes of aerobic exercise three times per week cut their migraine frequency and duration in half.[669]

Reducing migraines by 50% without side effects is exceptional. Increasing the frequency of exercise further may lead to greater benefits. Now add in meditation and the near 100% success rate of elimination diets, and you'll be unstoppable.

Don't Go Overboard

Nearly every time a runner collapses, it's near the finish line. It doesn't matter if the finish line is at one mile or 140 miles. Studies show that any type of finish line has psychological restraints. Many large races will position the majority of EMTs near the finish line. This is where dopamine can kill a runner. Dopamine increases when you see the finish line. When that possibility of success begins to physically diminish, the body's dopamine raises even more. Along with the endorphin rush, pain is completely masked. The last bicyclist heart attack emergency I responded to was about 100 feet from the finish line.

Here's the thing: You're not going to cure your headaches with exercise alone, so don't push your body beyond its limitations. It can actually be fatal. Remember that exercise won't automatically remove all of your other headache triggers. The Western diet may be clogging your arteries despite your body's pristine condition.

What's the best thing that can happen from exercise? I'll explain what surfing does for me. I sit atop my surfboard with my legs dangling underwater, watching for the next wave. Dopamine rises and falls as each wave in the distance has the potential to be the best wave of my life. As the perfect wave begins to form, I am fully focused. Some call this a state of meditation, "flow," or clarity. There is no time for thoughts of work or uncertainty about life. There is just a wave.

As the wave builds a wall as heavy as a house, a final push allows me to stand and receive the first rush of "progress dopamine." The dopamine continues to spike as the wave takes me to the end of the beach. I sling back up the wave and into the air. The dopamine rush is gone by the time I cannonball into the water.

A new drug seeps into my brain: serotonin. It feels good to be that person, the only one who was able to catch that particular wave. Endorphins are still racing as my heart continues to speed. I paddle back over to where my old surf buddy Jon is to get the oxytocin of a familiar face. Oxytocin is definitely good to have in some of the more territorial surf spots. Some surfers believe that all laws and morals are forgotten as soon as you enter the water.

The inflammatory cytokines (IL-6) repair my muscles as I finish the surf session. Shortly after, as I load my board on top of my car, the inflammatory markers lower and my overall stress is reduced. The workout has released a number of toxins from my muscles. The blood vessels are then better regulated with more of the "good" cholesterol.[670]

When I exercise, I get a better night's sleep, even if I sleep less. I have more energy and stamina during the day. My body feels toned and releases more positive serotonin. The physical relaxation creates a mental relaxation, so I don't care or stress about trivial problems.

A good day of surfing can be relived every time you think about the experience. You might get the same experience from a walk, a jog, a rock climb, or playing golf. Find a form of exercise you enjoy and do it.

The Dark Side: When Exercise Causes a Migraine

Yes, it's true. Exercise can either cause or cure headaches.

It's well established that exercise is responsible for an extremely long list of health factors, including an overall reduction of inflammation and an increase in immunity. So why do some people get migraines when they exercise?

Exercise will reduce inflammation, but not immediately. Let's say I stop writing this second and start sprinting for the ocean. What will happen? I hate running, so the muscles I rarely exercise will begin to tear as they adapt to this new behavior. I will make it about halfway up the block before the inflammation required for muscle repair convinces me that running hurts, and there is no need to run unless a lion is chasing me.

Theoretically, the immediately increased inflammation could trigger a migraine during exercise. If so, exercise would cause acute inflammation on a chronic problem. The successful 2008 study mentioned earlier was able to reduce that chronic inflammation, and the migraines that came with it, from exercise that included proper warm ups, cool downs, and stretching. During the 12-week study, exercise only induced one migraine for one patient. The benefits greatly outweighed the risk.

Electrolyte imbalances can trigger a migraine for those who were not hydrated before the exercise. Electrolyte imbalances can also be a problem during heavy exercise with profuse sweating. The solution here requires hydration with minerals well before a workout.

A third problem can come into play from exercise-induced allergies. This may occur when an allergenic food such as wheat or milk is consumed before exercise and a histamine response provokes adverse symptoms. Common prevention efforts include avoiding food triggers and refraining from eating at least 4 hours before exercising. The elimination of my breakfast of champions, a bowl of cereal, was enough to eliminate my exercise-induced headaches, which often were accompanied by nausea and vomiting—not fun, especially in a job that requires exercise while wearing a mask for breathing. Patients are also advised not to exercise outdoors during very cold, hot, or humid weather, or during pollen season.[671]

Meditation

Food eliminations helped reduce my headaches tremendously, but simple relaxation techniques were the final cure. I still find eliminating my food triggers necessary for living a headache-free life. My wife completely eliminated her migraines using relaxation techniques combined with eliminating top food triggers, especially milk.

Don't take my word for it—most studies show that meditation produces around a 40–60% reduction in headache pain and frequency, and one study showed meditation provided greater pain reduction than morphine.[672] Meditation has even led to a 48% reduction in the rates of heart attack, stroke, and death.[673]

A review of 47 studies by Johns Hopkins University found that "meditation appeared to provide as much relief from some anxiety, pain, and depression symptoms as…antidepressants."[674] A 2012 meta-analysis of 163 studies found that certain meditations help with negative emotion, anxiety, attention, learning, and memory.[675]

Harvard researchers recently found that meditation increases the gray matter in the brain that is responsible for learning, memory, and emotional regulation. The new study found that, in eight weeks, the brain *grew* in a positive way.[676] We can't begin to interpret how significant this is. We can only accept that meditation does change a person's thought process, and most people feel super-duper from developing a bigger brain.

While writing this book, I would often stare at a computer screen, researching dozens of confusing studies for up to ten hours at a time. I thought I would never "cure" the headache I got at the end of those days. Ten hours is too much work, right? Studying happiness, along with taking a meditation course in Ubud, Bali, changed my late-night headache.

Meditation Techniques

The first thing I learned from my teacher, Punnu Wasu Singh, about meditation is that you don't need to do anything to meditate. All you need to do is be aware of your body and your stress. It's essentially taking time to relax, and you can do this while sitting on the couch, lying down, getting some fresh air, or pretending to work.

So for the next 15 seconds, concentrate on how your body feels and don't think about anything else. Can you do it? I couldn't. My thoughts kept running, which is why I found one of the guided meditations I learned from Punnu so helpful. It's called "Ananda Mandala," and it requires inhaling deeply through the nose and then forcefully exhaling through the nose. You repeat this two-step process over and over. You don't have time to think about anything else because it's surprisingly a lot of work to breathe heavily and exhale quickly. If it's easy, you need to breathe harder and faster. The increased oxygen and blood flow gives you a heightened sense of clarity. The feeling is unexplainable.

Fortunately, you don't need to fly to Bali to do this meditation. You can download the guided meditation, "Ananda Mandala," by Sri Krishnaraj, on iTunes. However, if you do get the opportunity to go to Bali, I recommend going to the Yoga Barn retreat where Punnu teaches because it sits in one of the greatest places on earth, Ubud.

Punnu is not the leader of a cult or a multibillion-dollar meditation company. He is just a well-educated meditation instructor who teaches numerous forms of relaxation techniques. Many of these techniques are the same nonspiritual relaxation techniques measured in biofeedback—which is proven in over 55 studies to reduce migraine pain and frequency as well as medications.[677] Maybe it's getting high on oxygen, maybe it's true relaxation, maybe it's spiritual—whatever it is, meditation works. Practicing slow breathing and a calm serenity also helps you identify stress and let it go. It's just as beneficial as any other type of meditation.

While meditating, you can take an additional step to clear your mind by chanting a mantra. Mantras are especially helpful for those who have trouble focusing. A mantra is a sound or word that helps you concentrate on your body without a wandering mind, such as "om" or "aum." Any sound that doesn't inspire wandering thoughts will do.

Don't Want a Spiritual Meditation?

Sam Harris has a nine-minute guided meditation that is incredibly informative and comes from a purely scientific approach that stems from his PhD in neuroscience. This meditation has answered all of my original questions on how to successfully meditate.

This exact approach has led me to see a small glimpse of how powerful relaxation techniques are. I am able to work more hours by taking small meditation breaks that make me feel as if I just hit a reset button, which I find is the best way to prevent oncoming headaches. It will also help with severe headaches.

Over the course of writing this book, I've come a long way with meditation. For me, closing my eyes and attempting not to think has the opposite effect intended. Inside my mind, it's like watching TV, blasting music, and holding five conversations all at the same time. Somehow, just focusing on breathing turns this constant state of pandemonium off, like flipping a master switch, and there is silence. Only when you focus on relaxation are you able to realize just how restless the mind can be.

The Navy SEALs found they could increase their graduation rate in Basic Underwater Demolition (BUD) training from 25–33% by teaching a couple of simple relaxation techniques that include slow and deliberate breathing.[678] Four-second inhales followed by four-second exhales for just one minute can help you succeed in the most physically, mentally, and emotionally demanding conditions. Breathing techniques are used to reduce stress for all types of overachievers in the same way they are used to treat medical conditions.

Taking just one minute to relax and breathe during long hours of work will take me out of a restless and unproductive state. It maximizes the time I am able to do creative writing or any cognitive thinking. It stops my writing headaches and makes just about every part of my day better. The study on gray matter growth is what made me believe in the success of meditation. I don't know what it does, but it works. It's almost like waking up from a nap and feeling like you're starting the day off fresh, with no stress and no worries.

Binaural Beats

I swear by binaural beats. Binaural beats play two different frequencies in each ear at the same time. Your left ear hears a continuous sound, and your right ear hears a different continuous sound. But your mind hears something very different. It actually gives the illusion of a beat. You will take your earphones out in disbelief. How can two constant noises create a pulsing beat? The brain integrates the two signals and produces the sensation of a third sound called the binaural beat. You have to try it. A therapeutic binaural beat machine once had a price tag in the thousands, but now you can download binaural beats to your smartphone for free.

What's a Frequency Got to Do with My Brain?

Your brain runs on frequencies. You're practically a robot. Whether you're happy, sleepy, motivated, agitated, or focused, there is a frequency running through your brain. If you have a headache, you want to get off that frequency and relax.

The big question is, will a binaural beat change your brain frequency? Yes and no. Science has yet to prove that a binaural beat alone will change the brain frequency to that specific frequency being played. However, when people listen to binaural beats and are told what the frequency does, their brains will move toward that frequency with the expected placebo effect.

Frequencies for Headaches

Binaural beats don't have studies that prove a specific frequency will change the brainwave to that specific frequency. However, there are relaxing frequencies and sleep frequencies that most people benefit from. Mid alpha 10Hz or delta 2.5Hz are the most common headache relief frequencies that people are raving about.

A 2008 meta-analysis of 22 binaural-beat studies found that headache and migraine sufferers benefit from binaural beats.[679] This isn't so far-fetched since most people benefit from music therapy. We all have songs that help us relax, and most of the binaural beats come with relaxing background noise.

Placebo Effect or Relaxation Effect?

You're going to relax when you put in headphones and zone out all other noise. The placebo effect will be very strong because you're making an effort to stop your headache. Plus, if you know that thousands of headache sufferers have found binaural beats to be beneficial, it could trigger the placebo effect for you.

Could Binaural Beats Cause a Headache?

Absolutely. Before the tones go off at a firehouse, there is a set of pre-alerts that come over the radio to activate the bell. The bell lets us know there is an emergency. Some firefighters sleep with the radio on and will wake up when they hear their pre-alerts. This used to really impress me. There is a ton of chitchat on the radio, and other pre-alerts are running all night long, yet the firefighters will wake up when they hear their specific sequence of tones—before the alarm goes off.

Do these firefighters have super brains? No. Have you ever heard that gold fish only have a three-second memory span? A scientist put this theory to the test by ringing a bell with a certain tone before feeding his fish. Lo and behold, the lunch bell was the only tone that excited the goldfish, even after 3 months without hearing the bell—a bit longer than a three-second memory span.[680] Most organisms use sound for survival and could become excited or flooded with adrenaline by the sound of a certain tone.

All of this is based on your personal life experience. I've seen three-year-olds at the firehouse light up when the alarm goes off. The firefighters get excited too, but in a slightly different way. People react to a sound based on their experience with that sound. Try a few binaural beats or different types of relaxation music to see what gets your brain off the headache frequency.

Volume

If it's unpleasant to your ear, turn it down. The whole point is to relax. Studies have shown no benefit to turning up the volume on binaural beats. Some of the free programs have really low-quality music added and terrible static-like binaural beats. Find a binaural beat that is enjoyable and pleasant to the ears, but if you can't find one that works for you, find some good ambient music to relax to.

Apps

One study shows that binaural beats improve depression and decrease anxiety.[681] There are numerous positive studies on binaural beats, but again, there is no proof that they actually work to automatically adjust the brain to a desired frequency. Go to the reviews of these apps and you will find that many customers claim otherwise.

The binaural beat iPhone app called "Pain Killer 2.0" (also on Android) has 66 reviews, and nearly all are five stars. One reviewer wrote that "The standard hospital protocol barely puts a dent in it [a migraine]. I was in noticeably less pain in half an hour and asleep 15 minutes later." Another wrote the following: "Put it to the test with the kind of headache that leaves you in the fetal position—it worked! I am actually vertical today! Hurrah! Thank you too much!"

There are dozens of other five-star reviews that claim binaural beats help with insomnia, fibromyalgia, migraines, headaches, neck pain, and so much more. I decided to spend the three dollars on this high-end app and see for myself. I used it when I couldn't sleep, and I was unconscious in less than five minutes. Probably the placebo effect, even though I claimed there was no way something like this would work on me.

I played a binaural beat during a mild headache, and it went away as long as I kept the binaural beat going. Hundreds of reviewers of a binaural-beat app called "Brain Wave" reported similar responses to mine. I've used them for over a year now, and they seem to have a track record that goes past the standard placebo effect.

My favorite Android app is called "Relax Melodies Premium," which has been used by eight million people. This app also has a significant number of reviewers who are confused by how well binaural beats relieve pain. "Relax Melodies Premium" has a good bank of ambient noises that completely drown out unpleasant distractions. There are a number of free apps and also many binaural beats on YouTube. They are worth a try, even if you don't believe they will work.

Acute Pain Relief

Massage It Away

There are a few people making big massage claims based on small-scale studies. A 10-person study from 2012 found a 69% reduction of migraine pain after massage.[682] Another small study by the University of Miami School of Medicine in 1998 found that massage benefits migraines—which is touted by massage therapists across the country.[683] One of the largest studies was completed with a whopping 47 patients (read with a hint of sarcasm) and stated that massage does indeed decrease migraine frequency and also improves sleep.[684]

Of course studies are going to show a reduction in migraines from massages. Massages feel great. Those happy feelings we get from a massage are measured in dopamine and serotonin—the happy brain chemicals that stop inflammation. Massages are proven to do just that, raise dopamine and serotonin while dropping cortisol levels.[685] That's just one way massages raise the headache threshold.

Headaches raise inflammation and can cause tension in and around the face, scalp, neck, and back. The problem is that muscle tension may also raise inflammation, causing headaches. It's another cycle that turns into a spiral. Many wonder, "What came first: the migraine or the tension?" Is it a neck injury causing the migraine, or is a migraine causing neck tension? It doesn't really matter: We know that muscle tension aggravates and is aggravated by headache triggers. So why not relieve that muscle tension?

There are a number of face and neck massages specifically for migraines. Unfortunately, that's an entire book on its own. There are many types and styles of massages you can choose from, so massage is not a "one size fits all" solution. Headaches can cause tension in different areas for different people, and the massage must be catered accordingly with an intensity and a style that are preferred by the individual headache sufferer. However, an average massage seems to be a "one size fits most."

Want to Learn More?

- "CNWSMT Exceptional Neck and Shoulder Massage," YouTube – Learn how to give a safe and effective massage in just three minutes.
- "Shankara Skin Care – Neck and shoulder self massage," YouTube – Learn how self-massage for just a few minutes a day combined with stretching can do wonders.
- Watch YouTube videos on how to massage trigger points. Some methods are as simple as putting pressure on a specific muscle location, which can free up the tension around the blood vessels, and in many cases relieve all headache pain. This will make more sense after you read about the trigeminal and occipital nerves.
- www.triggerpoints.net – This site has excellent diagrams of the trigger points.

Sex—Cure or Curse?

Sexual dysfunction is found to be high among migraineurs, and while not related to migraines as a condition, its kinship lies in the high percentage of migraineurs who suffer from depression.[686] It may also be due to the fact that sex, like any physical activity, can cause migraines, although this is rare. A study of 200 migraine patients in Brazil revealed that sex was only a trigger in 2.5% of migraineurs.[687] Sexual activity measured as an exercise, including foreplay, is put somewhere in between a brisk walk and a jog; let's call it a power walk.[688] Power walking is good exercise and will benefit your health.

Sex will also do a number of things for your health, including raising your levels of oxytocin, endorphins, serotonin, and dopamine.[689] That's all of the happy chemicals released for the sake of procreation. More importantly, oxytocin can strengthen your relationship because it's the love drug.

One small study researched whether women and men with migraines were more likely to have higher levels of sexual desire than others. The researchers were exploring the relationship between people with low serotonin levels and sexual desire. People with high levels of serotonin have less sexual desire, and just as predicted, migraineurs—many of whom have low serotonin levels—were found to have higher sexual desire.[690]

This type of craving is not always a good thing. Many sexually abused victims with low self-esteem will look for serotonin—the feeling of importance—in unhealthy ways. The goal for anyone with low serotonin levels is to find natural ways to raise those levels back up to normal. Sex in moderation while in a healthy relationship may be one of those outlets.

Sex During a Migraine

A large 2012 study by the University of Münster (based in Germany) found that 60% of migraineurs reported an improvement of their migraine attacks (some with complete relief) during sex.[691] That puts sex up there with some of the best drugs. But about a third of migraineurs reported feeling worse during sex.

What's riveting is the effect that sex had on cluster headaches—37% found that sex improved their attacks (91% of them with moderate to complete relief). These aren't the greatest numbers, considering about half of the respondents felt worse from sex, but that's expected. Cluster headaches are nicknamed "suicide headaches" because they're so excruciatingly painful that they often lead people to suicidal thoughts. I'm impressed that, not only were the sufferers able to have sex, a good amount of them had "great success."

Headaches and Your Relationship

A lot can be said about the risks versus the gains of sex, but this isn't twelfth-grade sex education, so we'll stick to the headache relationship. There's a reason why there is an entire industry of sex therapists who only do one thing, and it's not all about sex. Sex therapists work to find the underlying problems that cause difficulties in relationships.

Headaches can easily be the cause of stress on your relationship. I know this because I am a terrible person when I have headaches. It's not that I want to be snappy, short, and negative, but it's hard to be personable to anyone when you can't even stand the broken thoughts running through your own mind. Who wants to hang out with that person?

It might be important for you to evaluate whether headaches are causing a deep problem in your relationship. And identifying the stress that's triggering those headaches will lead to improved health, relationships, and overall happiness. There is a risk of headaches from sex in a healthy relationship, but for the majority of people, the benefits are worth it.

Cannabis

Cannabis has been used for centuries as both an acute and preventative medication of migraines. Many prominent physicians prescribed marijuana until 1942, when marijuana was removed from the US pharmacopeia after a large campaign against "reefer madness," which was led by timber tycoon William Randolph Hearst, who, at the time, was also the most powerful newspaper owner in the world.[692]

An acre of cannabis or hemp produces four times more fiber than an acre of trees. This is accomplished in just a few months versus the 20 plus years it takes trees to grow. Hearst was able to use propaganda to make this eco-friendly product illegal and protect his largest investment, slow-growth timber. Hearst halted marijuana's use as a medication and its ability to efficiently stimulate the US economy without destroying our forests.

To this day, the literature on the effect cannabis has on diseases, including migraines, is very poor. Governments don't want to support such controversy, and no pharmaceutical company wants a cure that "grows on trees." To be more specific, the government labels cannabis a Schedule I drug—the same as heroin—that has no accepted medical use. However, in 1990, there were several studies published on the treatment of migraines in the serotonin receptors. Cannabis positively affects these very receptors.

The research led to the very first drugs that were active on the serotonin receptors, sumatriptan and ondansetron. Ondansetron prevented nausea, and sumatriptan treated migraines. Sumatriptan works well at temporarily stopping a migraine, but recurrence is typical, and triptans in general do zilch to reduce the frequency of headaches. In fact, they likely will cause more headaches due to heavy side effects, including the rebound effect.

Cannabis, on the other hand, comes with few side effects as it supports therapeutic efficiency on the serotonin receptors. Cannabinoids inhibit the production of glutamate and may reduce migraines that occur from excitotoxicity and/or antioxidant properties.[693][694][695]

Recent studies show that cannabis activates the CB1 receptor, which influences perception, and the CB2 receptor, which plays a crucial role in inhibiting inflammation. Cannabis is widely used in the treatment and self-medication of painfully chronic inflammation, such as rheumatoid arthritis. A large percentage of rheumatoid arthritis sufferers use cannabis in preference to all other drugs, with some saying it's the only thing that allows them to have normal movement and a normal life.[696]

As a combination of an anti-inflammatory and a glutamate regulator, it seems that cannabis may protect the brain against neurodegeneration at a fraction of the cost of triptans. Triptans are pricey, but since cannabis is natural, you could grow it in a garden. Cannabis may also ease the stomach symptoms that often come with migraines—it's well-known as an anti-nausea treatment.

Marijuana is relatively safe. Ingesting 10 times the "effective amount" of many drugs, like alcohol, could result in death. Conversely, it would take 1,000 times the effective amount of marijuana to possibly cause death.[697] The risks of side effects are also low, especially when compared with other migraine medications. However, you will need to become a self-administered guinea pig.

Cannabis Drawbacks

To begin with, it's not legal everywhere in the United States, so if you're in a state where you can't get a prescription for medical marijuana, this isn't a good solution—not just because it could get you arrested, but also because the variance in quality and type of street drugs is a virtual grab bag. On the other hand, if you are in a state where medical marijuana is legal, you will have safe dispensaries to go to where the staff are knowledgeable about the different strains of cannabis and the products made with it. Some are better for pain than others, some are better for sleep, and so on. In other words, it's less like a grab bag and more like a pharmacy, but with only one drug in various strains and forms.

Cannabis can be so effective as a pain reliever that it's often compared to opioids. I consider this an area of concern, as opioids are powerful drugs. Cannabis may seem like the best value drug, but it also carries substantial risk with little research behind it.

Another drawback is that smoking cannabis produces tar in your lungs. So you may want to look for alternative ways to ingest it. Using vaporizers can also reduce the smoking risk, but they won't eliminate it.

While dead asleep at the firehouse one night, my engine company was sent out to a drug overdose involving a 40-year-old female in an affluent neighborhood about 30 minutes from my firehouse. Bad things can happen in 30 minutes. When we arrived at the home, a fit woman who appeared to be in her mid-20s opened the door.

She walked us into the living room and stopped. I asked where the patient was.

She responded, "Who?"

I shot back, "Where is the 40-year-old who overdosed?"

She confidently replied, "That's me." She then explained that her doctor prescribed her cannabis for her anxiety. She had sad puppy-dog eyes as she pleaded, "Why the F would they tell me pot is good for anxiety? I'm freaking out!"

We assessed her vitals, and except for a slightly elevated heart rate, she was doing fine.

She was coherent and refused to go to the hospital but begged for help. All of her friends lived too far away to come take care of her. We suggested food, water, and sleep. She said, "I can't sleep. I closed my eyes, but you don't need eyes to see. I'm hungry and scared." I said, "OK. Have some cereal and watch a movie; you have nothing to worry about. There are no documented deaths from marijuana overdose."

"Cereal! Pshhh…I want eggs and bacon!" she yelled and laughed at the same time. She was in no condition to play with a stove. This put us in a tight spot. A patient is our responsibility even after we leave the home. She refused hospital care. We could have called law enforcement to force her to go to the hospital, but she wasn't technically in danger to herself or others. Plus, that's no way to treat a member of the public who was having a bad night. So what did we do? We cooked her bacon and eggs and let her sit cozy on the couch with a blanket, and I put on a comedy DVD of her choice. We gave it about 30 more minutes until we felt comfortable leaving her alone.

I still wonder if she woke up thinking, "Did the fire department really come to my house in the middle of the night and cook me eggs and bacon?" The point of this story is that cannabis is not for everyone. Some people have negative reactions to even small amounts of cannabis that include anxiety, increased heart rate, headaches, cottonmouth, drowsiness, and in some cases, very slow thoughts—maybe even stupid thoughts. I'll explain.

The best and worst of cannabis is in its ability to reduce glutamate transmission. I personally like my thoughts to fire rapidly. With marijuana, it's possible for people to slow their glutamate transmission down to a temporary state of "stupid high." I want more memory retention, not less. But I also don't have excruciating pain caused by the buildup of glutamate. I don't believe anyone can judge a migraine sufferer for finding his or her best treatment.

Cannabis Strains and Types

There are thousands of strains of cannabis—too many to mention here—and they may all come with varied "highs" and potencies, which would be a nightmare for someone attempting to prescribe you just the right amount (and that's probably why that doesn't happen). There are synthetic versions that can be prescribed with consistent confidence, but they don't come with beta-caryophyllene.

Beta what? Beta-caryophyllene is oil found in cannabis and many other plants, such as rosemary. In 2008, it was found that beta-caryophyllene binds with the CB2 receptor and may significantly reduce inflammation.[698] This tells us that the synthetic versions of cannabis may not work as well as the real thing. But that's OK, because we may not even need to get high to benefit from some of cannabis's anti-inflammatory effects. There are plenty of products available that don't include THC, which is the psychoactive portion of the plant.

Beta-caryophyllene doesn't bind with CB1 and therefore will not slow you down. If you're comfortable with being stoned, it may actually benefit you to include THC in your struggle with inflammation. In 2014, researchers found two new signaling platforms in THC that have anticancer properties, which will hopefully lead to the development of anti-inflammatories that don't require mind games.[699]

Despite the anti-inflammatory effects, large studies show no cancer benefit or risk from smoking cannabis. I would say that's a triumph for the heavy tar-producing "gateway" drug used by many.[700] Many migraine sufferers avoid the tar with a number of edibles, creams, and oils that don't require smoking for medical benefits. Some migraine sufferers say that creams can release both migraine pain and neck tension like magic.

Among the growing options are cannabidiol-based products that may inhibit glutamate release with a low affinity for the CB1 receptor—in other words, you don't get high. Cannabidiol (CBD) is a major component of cannabis and has been extremely successful in treating epilepsy—completely eliminating epilepsy in some cases—and is likely to produce similar results in migraine sufferers.[701,702]

Always consider eliminating headache triggers before resorting to any drugs. And before trying marijuana, make sure you're familiar with the relevant laws in your area. Finding the cannabis that benefits your condition the most will come with many risks and involve a process of trial and error. Where it's legal, talk to the people working in your local dispensary about your condition, and ask for suggestions that will help with your condition specifically. This will help take some of the guesswork out of it, but you'll still have to try the different medication types and strains to know what works for you—and to know what dose works for you. However, with legalization there will be huge steps forward in the next few years in categorizing the therapeutic effects of cannabis for headache treatment.

Top-Rated Migraine Products

The following is a list of top-rated migraine products that many migraineurs refuse to live without, most of which can be shipped to your door tomorrow. I picked these based on hundreds of recommendations from real migraine sufferers. While many migraine products claim a world of relief, most are crap. These might not "cure" a migraine, but they do have a good track record of helping migraineurs take the edge off of the most painful of days—which can be priceless. Take a close look at the reviews before making a purchase.

Disclosure: I have no affiliation with these products.

And the top-rated migraine products are:

- WellPatch Migraine Cooling Patches are cooling head patches that are lightly scented with menthol and lavender oil. They're a hit with migraine sufferers.

- The IMAK Eye Pillow is a best seller. This comfortable eye pillow molds to your face. It's great for blocking out light, especially while traveling. But I find that the oldest and cheapest headache remedy of wrapping a scarf around the head is the most comfortable way to block light without constricting the nasal passages, while some headache sufferers prefer to tighten the scarf to use the pressure to their advantage.

- Mygrastick is a roll-on stick that contains both lavender and peppermint. While some love this combo, others prefer using either lavender or peppermint.

- Nutravana Headache Relief is a top-rated mix of peppermint, spearmint, lavender, and fractionated coconut oil. While coconut oil is used to hydrate the skin, it may also help relieve inflammation.

- Peppermint Oil by Eve Hansen is pure peppermint oil that can be used during a migraine to relieve pain, tension, and sinus congestion. Most rub a little on the neck and temples to ease the pain, while others may put some in hot water to open up their airways. Mint oils are the alternatives to Vicks Vapor Rub or Tiger Balm—both popular headache remedies—and have been used as headache remedies since the birth of civilization.

- NaturEarth French Lavender Oil is very popular. Pure oils will be preferable to all the additives in perfumes that may trigger migraines. Most people know immediately if they love the scent or hate it. While lavender and peppermint are the most popular, any soothing scent can be a migraineur's best friend or worst enemy.

- The Gel'O Cool Pillow Mat keeps your pillow cool during hot headache nights. It can be refrigerated or frozen for maximum cooling effect. There is also a memory foam cool pillow available for purchase. Migraine sufferers are pillow connoisseurs. If you're not one now, you've got some pillow shopping to do.

- Cold and hot packs are the usual for migraineurs. They can numb and relax the muscles in the neck, face, and head that contribute to headaches. Many migraine sufferers put their hands and feet in warm water and sit comfortably with an ice pack on the neck. This is thought to work by constricting the pipes in the neck while pulling blood to the extremities. If it feels good, do it. Some migraine sufferers prefer a hot pack, as everyone's comfort is subjective. Here are a few hot and cold packs:
    - Ace Hot & Cold Compresses
    - English style hot or cold reusable ice packs
    - Elasto Gel Hot/Cold Therapy Sinus Mask
    - A bag of ice or frozen peas

- Acupressure mats can have the same relief as acupuncture. You can lie on them right before bed to help you get a great night's sleep.

- Sleeping products are essential for the sleepless migraineurs. Whatever makes sleep better can make migraines better too: comfortable mattresses, sheets, pillows, jammies, blackout curtains, mouth guards, sleep apnea machines, air purifiers, humidifiers, dehumidifiers, and air-conditioning units.

- BluBlocker products block out artificial light to help the sleep cycle: BluBlockers, Cocoons, and Theraspecs are the most popular blue blocking sunglasses for migraineurs. Also look into blue blocking computer screens and lights as well as lenses for your prescription glasses.

- Tragus and daith piercings have become overwhelmingly popular for migraine sufferers. Some migraineurs go as far as to say that these ear piercings can eliminate migraines completely. This is possibly due to pressure points, but sufficient research has yet to be completed on the phenomenon. Make sure this basic piercing is done at a reputable piercing or tattoo shop that has experience piercing the tragus and daith locations.

- Cefaly is an electronic device that looks like a headband out of *Star Trek*. The new device has been approved by the FDA to prevent migraines for an out-of-pocket expense of about $300. In a trial period of 58 days, about half of the 2,313 patients were satisfied enough to purchase the device—or too lazy to return it.[703] It's too soon to say whether the electric-impulse device will be effective in the long run. Some patients feel uncomfortable or even in pain while using the device. Others can't say enough about how great this product is. The buzz has been growing in online migraine communities with some happy customers. It's exciting to see electrical-stimulation devices on the market that come at a reasonable price. This will most definitely lead to advances in the treatment of migraines through trigeminal and occipital nerve relief.

- Saltstick capsules have the perfect mineral combination for migraines. They have been tested to reduce the time of triathletes in the ironman runs and happen to have all the critical electrolytes for migraine prevention—with no additives or sweeteners.

Pain Relief + Prevention

Acupuncture

The success of acupuncture for migraines was deadly for Hua Tuo. Hua Tuo was best known for his abilities in surgery, acupuncture, and herbal medicine. He was the first recorded surgeon in China to use anesthesia. Cao Cao knew him best for his abilities to disable headaches.

Cao Cao was a man in the second century that you did not want to piss off. He was an emperor who would later be known as the merciless tyrant and warlord of the Eastern Han Dynasty. He also had headaches that would leave him disabled—later identified as migraines. He summoned the best man for the job, Hua Tuo.

Hua Tuo used an acupuncture point on the sole of the foot known as Yongquan—look for it online because it's still used today. The procedure immediately alleviated the warlord's headaches. Cao Cao said, "Hey, dude, you're my new doctor," or something of that nature. Hua Tuo couldn't refuse. It was a direct order. He resented the fact that he would be waiting on one man, as he was a scholar first and foremost who could influence the course of medicine.

Tuo eventually made up the excuse that his wife was sick and went home. He lied to a warlord—a warlord with chronic headaches. Cao Cao sent men bearing gifts for Tuo's sick wife. If she were truly sick, they would negotiate a casual return date, and if she were not ill, the men would apprehend Tuo. Cao Cao had little option but to sentence Tuo to death upon his return.

As Hua Tuo awaited execution, he wrote down his surgical and medical techniques. Just before the end of his life, he handed the scroll over to the jailer, saying, "This can preserve people's lives." The jailer lawfully refused the scroll. Hua Tuo then asked for a fire in which he burned the only copy of his medical work, and so ended an era of Chinese surgery.

Cao Cao's migraines came back with force, and he ended up regretting the death of Hua Tuo. Worse, Cao Cao's son, a child prodigy, soon became sick and died. Cao Cao believed that the man he had sentenced to death was the only one capable of saving his son.[704]

Well, that was depressing. Let's look into something not depressing. And maybe say a little silent, "Thanks, dude" to Hao Tuo for coming up with acupuncture for migraines.

Acupuncture for Migraines

Before I get to the benefits of acupuncture, let me start by stating the following: The success of a treatment is compared to the placebo. Unfortunately, there is no real placebo for acupuncture. They call it "sham acupuncture." This means they put needles in areas of the body that aren't supposed to have an effect on headaches instead of using a placebo that does not have a medical effect.

The first problem is that science doesn't really know if pricking these areas will actually do anything or not. The second problem is that any time people are stuck with needles and told that they will help their migraines, it's likely to help their migraines. The placebo effect is very high. The results are very good.

This is not a good thing for well-designed studies that rely on a specific measure of success and start off with the statement, "In comparison to the placebo, x, y, and z were effective." The studies on acupuncture are saying, "Acupuncture is very effective, and so is the placebo for any type of acupuncture."[705] I don't really care if the placebo works as well or not. Give me the success. I'll take it. With that said, results on acupuncture are all over the place, but they do show promise.

Successful Acupuncture Study #1

The study "Acupuncture for migraine prophylaxis" used three different styles of acupuncture over a four-week period.[706] They also used the "sham acupuncture." The results were measured over a 16-week period for 480 patients.

Let's look at the results after four weeks, when the acupuncture therapy was finished. Acupuncture group one started with 6.3 headache days per month and ended with 4.2 headache days—not bad. Group two went from 5.6 to 3.7 headache days per month. Group three went from 6.1 headache days to 4.1. The "sham acupuncture" group went from 5.5 to 4.6 days per month. Overall, the acupuncture groups had a more than 30% drop in headache days, and the "sham acupuncture" group had around a 16% drop.

Here is where the magic happens. All the patients were also evaluated at 16 weeks—remember the acupuncture was only performed during the first month and the above results were taken at the one-month mark.

At week 16, acupuncture group one went from 6.3 to 2.2 headache days per month. Group two went from 5.6 to 2.1. Group three went from 6.1 to 2.4. The "sham acupuncture" group went from

5.5 to 3.3. These results are significant. The "real" acupuncture groups had an over 60% reduction in headache days.

Successful Acupuncture Study #2 – The Biggie

A 2012 meta-study of 17,922 patients measured the overall pain level of chronic headache sufferers as well as people with chronic back and neck pain.[707] The pain score of those who received the acupuncture was 15 for headache sufferers and 23 for those with neck and back pain. The headache sufferers who didn't receive the acupuncture had a pain level of 42, and those with neck and back pain had a pain level of 55.

What is this big study telling us? It tells us that the overall pain levels of the chronic headache sufferers for the month was about a third of the pain level of the group that had no acupuncture. It's a big difference, and 17,922 patients are enough to say, "Acupuncture might be onto something."

The study noted that acupuncture also showed moderate benefit when compared to "sham acupuncture." This is significant because any type of acupuncture is associated with a "potent placebo effect." This study provides "the most robust evidence to date that acupuncture is a reasonable referral option for patients with chronic pain." Those are strong words from one of the most prestigious medical journals, *JAMA*.

Does It Hurt? Does It Really Work?

"Not really," is the answer that most people give when you ask them if acupuncture hurts. Some say that they can't even feel it. Others say it is relaxing, and a few say that some needles can be slightly uncomfortable but not painful.

It won't work for everyone. But you will find an entire online community that says that acupuncture is the only thing that has worked for them. For example, Brittany from a popular women's blog called *XOJane* said: "After months of few or no migraines, I accepted that acupuncture actually works for me. It was also a scary thing to believe evidence that I might be better, that I might have the privilege of living a new fearless sort of way."[708]

Chiropractic Care

Let's start this neck manipulation off with a one-person case study involving "Stacy." Stacy was a 72-year-old woman with a 60-year migraine history. She had an average of one to two migraines per week, including all the terrible symptoms of nausea, vomiting, photophobia, neck pain, and phonophobia, and the migraines had an average duration of one to three days.

In Stacy's world, a migraine cure wasn't imaginable. She was taking a bag of meds, including pain relievers, codeine, sumatriptan, blood-pressure meds, and a few others. Her average pain was an 8.5 out of 10. Chopping the tip of my finger off was about an 8. The doctor who pried the tip of my thumb open for repair upgraded the temporary pain to a 10. Stacy was having this level of pain every week, sometimes every day.

Stacy's initial chiropractic treatment was twice a week for four weeks. She then lowered the treatment to once a week for eight more weeks. Stacy kept her visits down to just one treatment per month for the next seven years.

Her last migraine was immediately before her first chiropractic treatment. By 2008, at the time of this particular study, Stacy had been migraine-free for more than seven years.[709] All of those hospital visits, unnecessary medications, and years of pain had been completely wiped out with chiropractic care. All of those years of pain were halted in less than a week. She had also reduced her big bag of medicine down to, well, no bag of medicine.

While the link between the cervical spine and headaches is well documented, the connection between migraines and the cervical spine is not. This migraine case is still important for future research.

What the Big Studies Say

The most applauded study of chiropractic care was published in 2000.[7,10] The study had 127 participants and involved two months of chiropractic treatment. Twenty-two percent of patients reported more than a 90% reduction of migraines. Imagine going from 10 migraines a month to one. How about going from a migraine almost every month to just one a year? An additional 50% of patients found "substantial" or "noticeable" improvement. That's a victory for 72% of individuals with an average of more than 18 years of migraine pain.

While modern science is more comfortable with paralyzing the neck with Botox to reduce migraines than it is with chiropractic care, maybe we should look into working out the kinks. But don't go overboard with enthusiasm yet—there are numerous studies that show chiropractic care benefits migraines, but none are conclusive and research is limited, of course.

My Experience with Chiropractic Care

When I was a kid, I ran like a duck. My right leg was almost two inches lower than my left leg. I went to the hospital, and the doctor said, "You've got scoliosis, kid, a spine that's bent like a question mark. You need surgery." What did my mom say? "I'm a flower power child of the '60s, and my son is not having surgery."

I went to a chiropractor a couple of times a week, and my X-rays showed progress every month. Two years later, the chiropractor said, "Your back is straight as an arrow, and you don't need to come back." Back surgery is serious and can haunt you for the rest of your life, and medications can have equally heavy side effects. I am very thankful I had this option.

Is It Safe?

Chiropractors are not medical doctors, but they do receive the title of doctor by completing just as many years of education. In many cases, they actually get as much hands-on training as medical doctors, too. It's estimated that as many as 30 million Americans see a chiropractor every year, and that number is growing as more people continue to seek alternative forms of medicine and treatment.

Chiropractors are masters of the nervous system and inflammation, and they are typically educated with a heavier emphasis on nutrition than medical doctors.[711] They also have the ability to kill you. A 2010 study reviewed by Medscape found that a total of 26 fatalities from chiropractic care had been published since 1934, and it's believed that a great deal more have been swept under the rug with out-of-court payments. Over 140 vascular accidents have also been reported after chiropractic care.[712]

Many medical professionals have called quackery on the entire chiropractic profession. Even some chiropractors have come out to voice the need for a standardized approach to chiropractic care. There are a lot of studies that say chiropractic care is beneficial, but many have been inconclusive. Nutritional benefits and physical therapy are very hard to prove when time allows for so many variables. The multibillion-dollar medical industry has made this very clear in attempts to discredit chiropractic care. There is a war between these two professions, similar to most industries that share a lucrative market.

Let's look at the big picture. By 2010, there had been 26 fatalities associated with chiropractic care since 1934, many of which involved patients who had serious neck injuries to begin with, hence the need for spinal manipulation. Now let's multiply that number by 10 to account for any fatalities that didn't make it on the list for some reason.

A history of 260 possible deaths is not a bad ratio when you consider that 30 million Americans are treated each year by chiropractors. Not bad? Not bad if you are not the one dying, I suppose.

Now let's look at the "oops" rate from standard hospital care. A recent study in the *Journal of Patient Safety* increased the estimate for the number of preventable deaths in hospitals each year from 210,000 to more than 400,000.[713] That would make hospital mishaps the third-leading cause of death in the United States, falling just behind heart disease and cancer—all cancers. But I haven't seen any walks or ice-bucket challenges for "hospital goof-up awareness."

Here's one example of what a "mishap," "goof up," or "oops" could be. Surgeons operate on the wrong body part as many as 40 times per week, as noted in a great article in the *Wall Street Journal* that was subtitled "Medical errors kill enough people to fill four jumbo jets a week." You might be able to double those jumbo jets by now, because this article was published before the estimated preventable deaths jumped in 2013.[714]

None of this touches on the nonlethal side effects that our overmedicated population will incur. A history of 26 or even 260 possible chiropractic-related deaths does not compare to the annual death toll from preventable hospital deaths. In comparison to medication, a number of small studies have found chiropractic care to be just as effective as well-established migraine meds and favored for not causing serious side effects.[715]

Choose Your Doctor Carefully

If you take the chiropractic risk, you don't want to end up part of the small percentage that has a negative or deadly experience. Like finding a place to change your oil, some places are better than others. In fact, some places will forget to screw the oil plug back in, and a few miles down the road, you will hear the "clunk" that lets you know that your motor is blown. Make sure your chiropractor has a good track record and a wealth of knowledge.

Look, chiropractors spend nearly a decade learning how to help neurological conditions. They might have something to say about your headaches or migraines. You could be like Stacy and walk into a chiropractic office with a migraine and walk out a different person. The brain and spinal cord are your central nervous system. Taking steps to limit inflammation in our central nervous systems through nutrition and physical therapy seems like a good way to lower the inflammation that causes headaches and migraines.

You might say that I'm preaching quackery and promoting unproven, fraudulent medical practices. Sure, a poor diet and mangled spine can lead to headaches or migraines, so if it's quackery to suggest that nutrients and spinal health may reduce or eliminate migraines, I guess that makes me a certified quack. We must acknowledge, though, as with any profession, there are going to be a large number of chiropractors who are not good at their jobs and don't base their work on monitored results. Some chiropractors are actual quacks and send people to the hospital on a regular basis. Finding a good spine manipulator is critical, because one jolt in the right or wrong direction could change your life.

Nerve Blocks and Surgeries

Nerve blocks and surgeries are risky options, so always consider these a last resort. What's great about these types of procedures is that headaches caused by nerve pain are getting some real medical attention, which gives me hope for even better long-term solutions for the headaches triggered by nerve inflammation.

Nerve Blocks

Most migraine medications are either acute or preventative, but nerve blocks are different. Nerve block injections can immediately stop a headache and, at the same time, can continue to prevent migraines for up to a year, but they typically last from a few days to a few months. A patient can walk into the hospital with a migraine that even opiates can't tame, get a big needle in the neck, and walk out of the hospital without any pain. How's that for a quick fix?

Nerve blocks are the latest and greatest in migraine studies. Their success rates are almost too good to be true. The novice migraineur probably won't have the opportunity to feel the ease of this new treatment since it is considered a last resort when medications fail. The treatment involves the injection of either a steroid or anesthetic or both.

These treatments work to block pain and lower inflammation that's usually in the neck. A pain in the neck is a circling drain for some migraine sufferers. The inflammation can trigger a migraine by influencing inflammation in the brain. Once triggered, the brain may send stress signals through the occipital nerve to the upper neck. So the neck produces more inflammation that goes back to the brain, and a painfully repetitive cycle is set forth.

Headache sufferers with neck pain are good candidates for occipital nerve blocks. The exact mechanism of success for the popular nerve block injection is unknown. Stopping inflammation in the neck doesn't fully explain how this procedure can limit other forms of head pain. What about all of the headache pain around the forehead, eyes, face, and jaw?

That would be the trigeminal nerve that has long been associated with migraine pain. Your nervous system is a closed loop of sensation and reaction. All of those nerves from the face and the neck are connected to the brainstem and spinal cord. One explanation is that limiting the sensation of initial pain can reduce the pain created by the trigeminal nerve that would spiral a headache into a full-blown migraine.[716]

How Successful Are Occipital Blocks?

The studies are small and undoubtedly funded by the medical industry that will profit from their success, but many of them are quite impressive. A 2011 occipital block study found that 37 patients with chronic migraines had rapid relief of headaches, neck pain, photophobia, and phonophobia after the treatment.[717] One study found up to six months of pain relief in more than half of migraine patients.

Hey, that's pretty great. What if we inject more? In a 27-patient study, patients received up to 10 blocks of the greater occipital nerve and supraorbital nerve.[718] Twenty-three patients (85%) had a significant reduction in headache intensity, duration, and frequency for up to six months.

The occipital nerves run on each side of your upper neck to the back of your scalp. Sometimes doctors will focus on the side with pain or they will do injections on both sides to reduce the inflammation you might not feel. The supraorbital nerve is above the eye sockets. That's part of the trigeminal nerve, and just like with Botox, more injection sites on more pain receptors can lead to less pain.

All of these treatments work best for patients who have pain in the areas that are to be blocked of pain, of course. In a study of 47 patients with cervicogenic headaches (headaches caused by pain in the neck), 87% had six months of significant pain relief from multiple occipital nerve blocks.[719]

Lower neck injections have also been successful in the emergency room setting for a variety of serious headaches, including migraines. In one study, 417 patients received lower neck injections of bupivacaine—a common anesthetic in nerve blocks—and complete relief was observed in 65% of patients. Another 20% had significant relief. That's 85% of patients finding headache relief for many of the common migraine symptoms.[720]

A number of trigeminal nerve blocks on the face are showing confident results. One study with 26 migraine patients found that three treatments of lidocaine nerve blocks around the eyes brought on six months of pain relief. Patients went from a mean of 10 migraines per month to just two.[721] This type of relief is more than just a placebo effect.

Other studies are not so successful on nerve blocks. The "neck headache" answers a big part of that puzzle. Studies will have the most success by selecting patients that have pain in those areas—no pain, no gain. Many headache sufferers in migraine support groups have had no luck, yet some say occipital nerve blocks have given them a second shot at life. Many doctors use this as a quick fix, but not too many doctors envision the temporary blockade of your body's information roadways (nerves) to be a long-term goal.

Let's ask Dr. Khorsandi why there's so much variability. He performs nerve blocks weekly for the Migraine Relief Center (with locations in Houston, Vegas, and Beverly Hills) and is one of the few occipital nerve surgeons that specialize in migraines. He says the reasons for variability are: "(1) Site placement of the injection. The injector should know the location of the nerves. Many do not. (2) The medication injected. I use a combination of anesthetic and steroid (usually Depo-Medrol). (3) Quantity of medication injected."[722] That's a word to the wise: If you think you're a good candidate for this procedure, find an experienced, reputable doctor to perform it.

How exactly do these injections into the lower neck muscles work for migraines? No one knows. The lower neck is not directly part of the occipital nerves. Some doctors are calling it the placebo effect taken too far.[723] Others speculate that pain relief in any area of the shoulders, neck, and head may be helpful for headache relief.

Side Effects

The short-term side effects are very mild, and despite the fact that nerve block injections require a huge needle, most patients feel minimal pain. We don't know what the long-term side effects are. Rare side effects have a long list that will be different for each medication and procedure. Death is listed as a side effect, but the initial groundwork and positive track record have labeled this procedure as "very safe." There is always the possibility of infection.

The worst side effect I've read about was a temporarily paralyzed neck—"Oops, I used too much numbing medication in the wrong place." The largest complaint by far has been that it has no effect at all—which is the largest complaint for most migraine treatments.

Cost

Here's where you might have some pain. The cost for a five-minute nerve block injection can be over $3,000. Prices are generally not made public. If insurance picks up the majority of the tab, you could be left with no fee, or a $200 to $600 co-pay. However, a medication that is labelled by many studies as a last resort will require a paper trail before most insurance companies approve the cost. Prices vary widely depending on the hospital, insurance company, and procedure. You might not want to go with the cheapest option on this one, as a big needle in the wrong place can hurt more than your wallet.

But then, if the nerve block is super successful, you will be recommended for surgery. Yeah. In marketing, they call this strategy "the bait."

What if you don't want surgery? Any of the measures in this book that lower inflammation will reduce this neck pain. The medical "cause" of a headache from neck pain is "stress around your neck and spine."[724] This can be caused by poor posture, office work, problems sleeping, disc problems, injuries, poor diet, and just about any kind of stress buildup.

Surgeries

Dr. Khorsandi's nerve blocks last from seven to 14 days, and he does not expect them to be long-term solutions. He uses occipital nerve blocks as a diagnostic tool. If the block works, there is a high probability the patient has compression on those nerves. Dr. Khorsandi is an expert of the surgery that corrects this nerve suffocation problem.

The surgery, nerve decompression surgery, involves freeing the nerves from tight muscle and putting a cushion layer of fat around the nerve so it cannot be compressed. He believes that it's not the nerve causing all the trouble, but the pressure on the nerve. Nerve decompression surgery, although controversial, has been successful in a small number of rare patients who have migraines triggered by specific locations.[725]

The other option for surgery is to have a stimulator implanted that delivers electrical impulses to ease the pain from those nerves. This surgery has a lower success rate, a price tag of $75,000, the need for battery replacement, and a high percentage of patients—71% in one study—have had adverse results, including the migration of the stimulator, ineffective stimulation, and infection.[726,727,728] But there are patients who have had complete remission of their migraines.

Any surgery is an extreme risk that you should only consider after all treatments have failed. The success of nerve decompression surgery has proven that we need to address inflammation on the nerves. I love this, because it gives hope for a diet that lowers inflammation and for muscle relaxation exercises that aim to reduce the muscle tension that is responsible for nerve compression. This may result in a permanent solution, or we can temporarily stick a needle in it.

Visiting Your Doctor

Your Doctor, Your Partner in Research

If you're trying to figure out why you get migraines so you can truly heal them, you're on the research mission of your life, so you need your doctor to be your research partner. But since you've been a student of your own migraines for time untold, you're going to have to bring your doctor up to speed. The greatest tool you can provide your doctor is a headache diary. The doctor will also need a detailed history of your health, even the things you don't think relate to your headaches. The doctor may be able to put together the pieces of your puzzle that are currently an unorganized mess floating around somewhere inside your thoughts.

The slightest hints of symptoms of another ailment may explain the headache problem you're trying to solve. For example, if a good doctor can identify that you have a thyroid problem, he or she will immediately look into what time of month you get headaches. Estrogen and progesterone are directly tied to thyroid production. In 2013, a study made the link between hypothyroidism and migraines clear.

This is going to blow your socks off: Hypothyroidism is 3.5 times more likely in migraine sufferers. Hypothyroidism occurred after the onset of migraines in 96.7% of patients requiring hormone therapy, which suggest that migraines may be a warning sign of the potentially fatal condition. Migraines also became significantly worse after the onset of hypothyroidism.[729]

It's been known since the 1980s that 90% of underactive thyroids stem from autoimmune diseases.[730] The prevalence of celiac disease is so high in hypothyroidism that researchers recommend all autoimmune thyroid disease patients be screened for celiac disease.[731] Even the best doctor will not be able to identify all of these links without a clear understanding of all your signs and symptoms.

When I was a firefighter, every medical call would consist of gathering as much history as possible from a patient before we sent that patient off in an ambulance. Even if the patient was dying, we would ask for his medical history and medications. Most family members don't understand why we want to know what the patient ate for breakfast, the day's activities, and the list of medications the patient is on. But the more information we have, the more effectively we can treat the patient, and the higher the chances are we could save that life.

Those medications and events will often be the reason for the patient's deteriorating condition and part of the answer to his or her successful treatment. It doesn't matter if it's a scheduled appointment or a life or death visit to the ER; information is invaluable. The same goes for your doctor visit. The more clues you can give doctors, the more effectively they can treat you.

You should share the following with your doctor:

- Your detailed migraine diary
- The Headache Help Checklist from this book
- Your family's history of migraines
- Your medications and their side effects
- Your medical history
- How often your migraines occur
- How long they last and the pain scale
- How migraines affect your life

- The symptoms of your migraines
- Any recent changes in your migraines
- What has helped your migraines
- Any information that affects your well-being

Questions you should ask your doctor:

- Do you believe migraines can be triggered by foods?
- What tests do you recommend to assess migraines?
- What is your experience with migraines?
- How do you typically treat migraines?
- How successful are those treatments?
- Do you have experience in this type of treatment, or should I see a specialist?

If you expect a level of care that will lead to an elimination of headaches and your doctor only has experience in prescribing migraine drugs, the relationship may need to terminate. If your doctor does not have the time, patience, or empathy to help you, you should find another doctor. There are too many great doctors out there to continue a relationship with one who doesn't value your health goals.

You're not looking for a thyroid problem. You're looking for any symptoms that may affect your headaches and an objective mind to interpret those documented links. Many of those links, like the thyroid-migraine link, were just discovered. So not only will you need an incredibly smart doctor, you will need one who's up to date on the latest migraine studies. You may need to shop around, as a doctor can be a jack-of-all-health-fields and a master of none. Healthcare is a business and there is no excuse for being a repeat customer of a business that doesn't help you.

The Medical Evaluation

Migraine sufferers will often go through a number of tests only to be told, "Good news—there is nothing wrong with you!" It can almost be a disappointment when headache sufferers hear they don't have some rare and deadly tumor. Unfortunately, this is where many medical evaluations end and a lifetime of drug prescriptions start.

I'll Have the Usual Migraine Tests, Please!

When you go to the doctor, here are the typical tests to consider asking for.

Blood Tests

Blood tests can rule out anemia, allergies (IgE, IgG, or ALCAT), infections, blood clots, immune system problems, arthritis, diabetes, and much more.

Urine Tests

Urine tests can find infections, kidney diseases, thyroid conditions, urinary tract infections, and liver damage.

CT Scans

A CT scan—which is also referred to as "X-ray computer tomography" or a "CAT" scan—uses multiple X-rays to produce two-dimensional images that are virtual slices of the brain, without actually slicing open the skull. The multiple X-ray scans also mean more exposure to radiation—100 to 1,000 times more than a single X-ray, as explained in a recent *New York Times* article titled "We Are Giving Ourselves Cancer."[732] The *Times* article noted a study that predicts 29,000 excess cases of cancer from 2007 CT scans alone. While this is debatable and the risk is low, it is a risk to consider *not* taking. With an MRI, there is no radiation. MRIs can show the common brain lesions found in the white brain matter of migraine sufferers. While this is not something that can be "fixed," it can give you inspiration to take evasive actions to limit further brain damage through diet and prevention efforts.

EEGs

EEGs have been used since the 1940s to record abnormalities during a migraine; they cannot accurately diagnose a migraine sufferer who is not under attack. They can, however, help diagnose conditions associated with migraines, such as epilepsy, brain inflammation, sleep disorders, memory loss, and dementia.

Eye Exams

Eye exams are given to migraineurs because they often suffer from visual disturbances, light sensitivity, and concentration problems that can both trigger or be triggered by vision problems. Eye exams can rule out glaucoma, cataracts, nearsightedness/farsightedness, and eye injuries.

Sinus X-Rays

Sinus X-rays will often identify migraine sufferers before they are known as migraineurs. Many migraine sufferers will have surgery that opens up the inflamed sinus passage but does nothing to remove the root cause of the inflammation. Sinus X-rays should be used as a tool to work toward finding the cause of the sinus pressure. Sinus X-rays can also be used to detect bone structure abnormalities, tumors, obstructions, and fluid in the sinuses. All of these conditions could trigger migraines.

Spinal Taps

A spinal tap, which is also referred to as a "lumbar puncture," is used to check for bleeding in the brain or spinal cord, nervous system disorders, meningitis, MS, and a number of other problems that may stem from the interaction of the brain and spinal cord. The length of the needle is disturbing, but the diameter is actually quite small. Most people are far more afraid of the severe headaches they may experience afterward as a side effect, which can last for several days.[733]

Tests Your Doctor Might Not Tell You About

Metabolic Panels

A comprehensive metabolic panel is a group of blood tests that provide an overall picture of the body's chemical balance and metabolism. It can provide information regarding how your kidneys and liver are functioning, as well as your blood sugar, cholesterol, protein, and electrolyte levels. You may have had this check for abnormalities done with your annual physical. However, you want to compare each individual measure with optimum levels as opposed to what's "normal," because pre-diabetic is now considered normal. A glucose level that is within normal range could give you a splitting headache.

CBCs

A complete blood count (CBC) is part of a common blood test that can help discover blood diseases and disorders, infections, and immune system disorders.

Thyroid Function Tests

A thyroid function test can check for optimum levels of thyroid hormones before the thyroid takes a dump and initiates a downward spiral of sluggishness. The thyroid-headache link will only grow in the years to come. Look up the *Vice* article titled "A Contaminated Lake Is Poisoning a Thai Village."[734] You will never forget how the migraine trigger fluoride can directly affect the thyroid. Fluoride, bleach, and soy may impair thyroid function and are also migraine triggers.[735][736] A thyroid function test could help you find your personal headache triggers.

Micronutrient Tests

A micronutrient test measures your body's ability to absorb numerous vitamins, minerals, antioxidants, and other essential nutrients.

Stool Tests

A stool test can be done to evaluate the health of your gut. We know that the more headaches you suffer, the more likely you are to have gastrointestinal problems.[737][738][739] We also know that stomach problems can lead to the high rates of allergic reactions that are common in migraine sufferers. Companies such as EnteroLab offer advanced tests that can be ordered online and discretely shipped.

Inflammatory Marker Blood Tests

An inflammatory marker blood test will show all the levels of inflammation that you don't want. These inflammatory markers are associated with just about any disease and may raise the levels of glutamate in the brain. You also want to check for elevated homocysteine levels that can cause inflammation in the blood vessels, leaving us at risk for strokes and headaches.

The MTHFR gene regulates homocysteine levels, and if the gene is mutated, you may have an inflammation problem.[740] There are actually two migraine gene mutations: MTHFR C677T and MTHFR A1298C. You can have your doctor test you for MTHFR C677T and MTHFR A1298C or you can get it done on www.23andme.com. For a hundred bucks, they mail you a DNA kit, you spit on some cotton, and mail it back in the prepaid envelope. They email the results back, but for legal reasons, it needs to be interpreted by a different company. Try sites like www.mthfrsupport.com or www.geneticgenie.org. They take the file, interpret it for a small donation, and let you know if you have the migraine gene or any other cool DNA problems.

Histamine Tests

Elevated histamine levels have been found in patients with migraines, both during headache periods and during symptom-free periods. A histamine test can alert patients of simple ways to avoid allergic conditions while monitoring headache occurrence.[741]

TMD/TMJ Tests

Temporomandibular joint disorders (TMJ or TMD) are hot items in migraine treatment. TMD disorders arise when there is a problem with the jaw that creates inflammation around the jaw and surrounding facial muscles, affecting the trigeminal and occipital nerves.[742] Those nerves cause the pain of migraines as well as cluster headaches, which are described as "probably the worst pain that humans experience," by multiple neurologists.[743] Guess what the likelihood of headaches and migraines is with TMD? In one study, 85.5% of those with TMD had migraines or headaches—55.3% had migraines, 30.2% had headaches, and 14.5% were headache-free.[744]

Sleep Tests

A sleep test can be very important. It certainly was for Percy Harvin—the football player who was able to cure his migraines after a near-death sleep apnea diagnosis by using a CPAP machine.[745] One small study found that CPAP use in sleep apnea migraineurs lowered attacks from 1.2 migraines per week to 1.2 migraines every three months. Researchers observed this in 18 people over the course of two years.[746] A CPAP machine could be the answer to your dreams.

Drugs

Drugs are on the brink of a paradigm shift. Until recently, the human brain was thought of as a bag of "chemical soup" that needed a splash of medication to offset the recipe. Neurobiologist David Anderson unfolds the story in the TED Talk "Your brain is more than a bag of chemicals." [747] He compares treating brain chemistry to changing the oil in your car by opening the hood and pouring oil all over the engine block. Some of it will get into the right spots, but a lot of it is going to do more harm than good.

Unfortunately, this translates to side effects in just about any drug that's currently on the market. However, Anderson also gives hope with new research that is pinpointing exactly where chemical imbalances are, leaving rapidly growing technology able to start categorizing the billions of neurons in the human brain. In the very near future, this will result in a better understanding of migraines and the development of drugs that are able to pinpoint the problem without side effects.

Today, we need to know what drugs are on the market, how they work, and what their risks are. This knowledge will improve the success rates for anyone who requires medication.

Beware of Money Drugs

Many drugs are prescribed to migraineurs that have shown zero success for migraines, and I call them "money drugs." In 2009, the pharmaceutical company Pfizer had to pay the largest healthcare fine in history ($2.3 billion) for fraudulently marketing several drugs, including the use of Lyrica for migraines. A 2013 study found that Lyrica (pregabalin) has no published trials for successful use in migraines. Lyrica was designed as a more potent successor to gabapentin, which the study found should not be prescribed for migraines. Basically, the research is saying there is no reason to take this drug for migraines.[748]

So why then is Lyrica prescribed to many migraine sufferers today? That's how the largest healthcare fine in history became so. "The civil settlement also relates to allegations that Pfizer paid bribes and offered lavish hospitality to healthcare providers to encourage them to prescribe four of the company's drugs." Lyrica was one of those.[749]

Pharmaceutical companies spend $4 billion marketing to us, but $24 billion marketing to doctors. Nine out of 10 pharmaceutical companies spend more on marketing than they do on research and development.[750]

Drug companies have started to release the amounts they pay doctors, mostly because of legal settlements, and you can see your doctor's incentive for helping you by searching for your doctor on a site called Dollars for Docs (www.projects.propublica.org/docdollars/).[751] You will find Dr. William Jay Binder as a top recipient of this hospitality from the company Allergan, taking in over $10 million in 2013 for royalties, licenses, and business expenses, such as lunch (must have been lobster and Dom Pérignon). What does Allergan make? Botox. Dr. Binder is the Beverly Hills plastic surgeon who pioneered the use of Botox for migraine sufferers. He was experimenting with Botox to cure migraines in patients who had been administered the drug for wrinkles.

If you receive Botox for migraines, you will be thanking Dr. Binder with royalties. How do you feel about that? I personally am thankful for this doctor's work, because it has led to migraine research that will ultimately find a "cure." Plus, this treatment has allowed many chronic migraine sufferers to live without migraines and the heavy side effects of other drugs. However, I do accept that a large portion of doctors will promote drugs in unethical ways in hopes of a large payday, or at least a free lunch.

But all of this is to say that, if you choose to keep some migraine drugs on hand, look into what your doctor prescribes. Read all you can about it, including the insert from the pharmacy. If you don't understand why your doctor prescribed it to you, ask.

Want to Learn More?

- "John Oliver: Marketing to Doctors," YouTube

Drugs for Acute Pain Relief

Now that you've been warned, let's get down and dirty with some drug information. Acute drugs are any prescription, over-the-counter, or recreational drugs that immediately improve the symptoms of a headache or migraine. They are not intended to prevent headaches.

Ergotamines

Ergotamines come from the ergot fungus used in the sixteenth century to save mothers from bleeding to death after childbirth. In the 1920s, ergotamine was isolated from the fungus and has been used as an acute migraine medication ever since. Despite the long run, the prices for most of the ergotamines have not fallen with age, leaving you to wonder how a little pill could cost so much. Triptans have since become more popular, but they have not replaced the need for this powerful drug.[752]

Ergotamines work, in part, by stimulating serotonin while constricting blood vessels. Ergotamines double down on more serotonin receptors by blocking the pain signals of the trigeminal nerve—those painful facial nerves that amplify migraine pain.[753] Ergotamines deliver serotonin to block inflammation/glutamate and stop the pain that many Botox treatments attempt to paralyze.

Unfortunately, more than half a century of documented migraine use has delivered a list of heavy side effects, which include a change in taste, diarrhea, headaches, nausea, vomiting, numbness, tingling, itching, weakness, or a blue color in the extremities.[754]

Blue extremities? Historical accounts of ergotamine-contaminated grain have caused blackened extremities known as St. Anthony's Fire.[755] Ergotamine is a mycotoxin (mold) that often contaminates wheat, corn, barley, sugar, coffee, soy, and cheeses.[756] Mycotoxins in large doses or prolonged exposure are a problem for many migraine sufferers and should be avoided, unless you're thinking of joining the Smurfs.

Most chronic migraine sufferers know ergotamine best as dihydroergotamine (DHE), which is commonly given in the emergency room by injection. Other ergotamines include Migranal, Cafergot, Migergot, DHE 45, Cafatine, Cafetrate, Ercaf, Ergo-Caff, and Wigraine.[757] Despite the side effects, according to research from the Glostrup Hospital in Copenhagen, ergotamine is the "drug of choice in a limited number of migraine sufferers who have infrequent or long duration headaches and are likely to comply with dosing

462

restrictions."[758] Perhaps this small target market of infrequent and severe migraines has contributed to the lofty cost of ergotamines.

Cost

Sufferers have claimed a $150 to $300 price tag on a single dose of some ergotamines, which may or may not work and may come with the possibility of a rebound headache. You won't find the varying prices slapped on any migraine menu, either. I've heard of sufferers paying between $6,000 and $12,000 for 20 vials, which is 40 doses. Fortunately, insurance frequently picks up the tab, but not without a fight. Forty doses may seem like a lot, but at one dose per hour and a max of three per day or six per week, the small fortune may not last seven weeks. You can see how the math doesn't add up for a chronic migraine sufferer who needs 15 or more treatment days per month. You certainly wouldn't want more treatments than recommended, since the possibility of rebound headaches for a drug this strong could initiate a vicious cycle of constantly taking medication on top of having chronic migraines.

There are doctors prescribing ergotamines, such as Methergine, for three months at a time as a preventative. These doctors may be attempting to cure migraines by way of death. Ergotamines have not been tested for long-term use, and we should avoid them for short-term use as well because lots of people have lots of heavy side effects.

Ergotamines may seem like the worst drug ever, but they aren't. Opiates will take that first-place medal. Ergotamines have been a lifesaver for many migraineurs in the ER. If this drug becomes your lifesaver, be sure you are aware of the risks.

Triptans

Drug companies are going to state that triptans are up to 70% effective. What that really means is the drug will provide some pain relief for up to 70% of patients when promptly taken in ideal conditions with handpicked candidates. Larger studies show that temporary pain relief is closer to 55% for patients, and complete pain relief comes at the two-hour mark for about 33% of patients.

We hear that and think, "Well, that sounds OK. A third of patients became pain-free. That's not as good as 70%, but it's worth a try." Wrong. That pain relief is temporary, and within 24 hours, there is up to a 40% chance that the pain will come back. So that leaves us with about 20% of patients becoming pain-free in ideal conditions.[759] The most successful study found that 54% of migraine sufferers immediately experienced complete pain relief with eletriptan and that relief continued for more than 24 hours.[760]

What the studies don't tell us is that the headaches may come back in a few days or a few weeks or that they may double within the next year. Many migraineurs take these powerful drugs and feel great when they do. Then one day they realize that, not only are the drugs providing less relief, their headache frequency is higher than ever, a scenario proved in countless studies that have had a significant number of chronic migraineurs revert to episodic migraines after the discontinuation of acute medications.

Triptans work in part by increasing serotonin and constricting blood vessels. This may lower inflammation and glutamate in the brain.

The triptans are:

- Sumatriptan (Imitrex, Sumavel DosePro, and Treximet)
- Rizatriptan (Maxalt)

- Naratriptan (Amerge)
- Zolmitriptan (Zomig)
- Eletriptan (Relpax)
- Almotriptan (Axert)
- Frovatriptan (Frova)

Why are there so many? There are slight differences in their ability to become absorbed by the body and the time they remain in the body, which amounts to minor differences in how successful they are. The individual side effects are going to be slightly different for each triptan as well. For these reasons, it's advised that sufferers give one type of triptan several tries and then move on to the next until they find one that works.[761]

WebMD has a great user review section to help you find the top-rated migraine drugs.[762] At the time this book was published, Imitrex (sumatriptan), a first-generation triptan, is still one of the most popular. However, Relpax, a second-generation triptan, has the highest user ratings, followed by Zomig. They work so well that one of the largest complaints is that many doctors will only prescribe six per month and for good reason.

Side effects of triptans include feelings of tingling, heat, pain, tightness in the chest or throat, dizziness, weakness, drowsiness, vomiting, and dry mouth. These side effects aren't that bad compared to a migraine. The reason doctors don't want to prescribe more than six or nine pills per month is because of their likelihood to cause rebound headaches. The long-term concern is the unknown effect of serotonin manipulation.

Cost

Triptans come in different forms: a nasal spray, pills, injections, and needleless pressure injections. Imitrex is about $450 for nine pills, Relpax is the same, and a Sumavel air injection is about $1,800 dollars for six pens. Of course, if your insurance accepts your prescription, the co-pay can be anywhere from nothing to a few hundred dollars. Sites like www.goodrx.com will give cash coupons for your local pharmacy that could knock those prices in half. Manufacturers will often have discounts and offer insurance help.

Triptans are among the best acute medications on the market, but they are just that, acute. Any acute medications are strong and fast, and provide temporary relief. They do not reduce the number of headaches patients get.

Who Shouldn't Take Triptans?

People with heart disease or uncontrolled high blood pressure, as well as people who have had a heart attack or stroke, are prohibited from taking triptans. Of course, that doesn't stop doctors from mistakenly (or negligently) prescribing them. In a study of more than 120,000 migraineurs presented at the annual meeting of the American Neurological Association, more than one in five patients with serious heart conditions were prescribed triptans.[763] Triptans were approved by the FDA after less than 1% of patients developed life-threatening cardiovascular problems—which is a very low risk. However, the risk becomes much higher with people who already have heart problems.

Over-the-Counter Drugs for Acute Pain Relief

Even over-the-counter medications can have serious side effects and drug reactions, especially when used frequently. When taken at the onset of a migraine, over-the-counter drugs can be just as powerful as some of the most expensive prescription drugs. They can also cause just as much damage. The general advice is to consult a doctor if you are using over-the-counter drugs more than twice per week, but some doctors recommend not using any kind of acute medication more than twice per month. What lovely, pain-free lives those doctors must lead! But really—those guidelines are there to help keep you safe from side effects, so if you can heal your pain in some other way, say with food maybe, then do it when you can instead of taking some form of medicine.

Nonsteroidal Anti-Inflammatory Drugs (NSAIDs)

NSAIDs can provide pain relief and anti-inflammatory effects without causing a steroid or narcotic addiction, however they can cause problems. NSAIDs may block two enzymes, COX-1 and COX-2. Those enzymes are involved with the formation of inflammation and pain, and they also help to form the mucous membrane that protects us from the outside world. In addition, the enzymes help produce hormones that aid with digestion and lower acid in the stomach. In short, destroying these enzymes can lead to a destroyed gut with common NSAID symptoms of nausea/vomiting, dyspepsia, gastric bleeding, ulcers, inflammation, and diarrhea.[764]

A few NSAIDs:

- **Naproxen (Aleve):** This drug is often used by migraineurs as both an acute and preventative medication. Women with severe menstrual migraines regularly move on to powerful prescription medications without trying this "godsend" of a migraine prevention drug. It's typically taken several days before menstruation begins and during the first couple of days of the menstrual cycle.

Aleve is favored as a migraine preventative for having fewer side effects than many NSAIDs. However, you should become familiar with the list of over 100 naproxen side effects.[765] It has a 7.7 out of 10 user rating on www.drugs.com.

- **Ibuprofen (Advil):** Use ibuprofen for short-term relief because it has a number of side effects to the gut, affecting up to 25% of patients. Ibuprofen is often suggested for children, because there's a link between the use of aspirin and Reye's syndrome.[766] There is also a liquid-filled ibuprofen for faster ingestion that's marketed as Advil Migraine. Studies show ibuprofen as an effective migraine treatment, but between the limited usage and rebound headaches, most migraineurs prefer other meds.[767]

- **Acetaminophen (Tylenol):** What acetaminophen lacks in gastric side effects, it makes up for in liver damage. Acetaminophen is by far the largest cause of liver failure in the United States and contributes to more overdose hospitalizations than any other single drug in the Western world. It has a narrow window for overdose and is not recommended for people who have more than a couple of drinks per day.[768,769] While most people don't think of Tylenol for migraine relief, acetaminophen is a main component in many popular headache medications, such as Excedrin Migraine.

- **Aspirin (Bayer):** When taken promptly during the onset of migraines, 1000 mg of aspirin is still one of the most successful drugs on the market.[770] Its anti-inflammatory effects can stop a migraine in the same way this nineteenth-century drug is used to save the lives of heart attack patients. Still, many patients who don't appreciate the stomach pain side effects completely avoid aspirin. Gastric mucosal lesions—stomach-lining holes—occur in most patients who receive a single dose of aspirin.[771]

- **Aspirin and caffeine (Anacin):** The combination of aspirin and caffeine is preferred by many migraineurs because of the speed of ingestion. Caffeine is often the only difference in drugs marketed for migraines, but it may increase the likelihood of rebound headaches from overuse.

- **Excedrin Migraine:** This combination of aspirin, acetaminophen, and caffeine will forever be remembered by many after the nationwide recall of 2012. While few remember why the recall happened—years of pills ending up in the wrong bottles—they do remember the chaos that arose from the shortage. People were paying as much as $100 for Excedrin Migraine.

    Excedrin Migraine is the first over-the-counter, FDA-approved migraine medication. While it has exactly the same active ingredients as Excedrin, one box is labeled with the word "migraine," and the other is not. In 2014, 100 migraine sufferers filed a lawsuit for the only real difference in the two medications: the price. Although some people believe that the inactive ingredients somehow make the medication magical, the manufacturer only responded to the suit by saying the difference is in "their indications for use and the clinical studies conducted to support those indications." While those sufferers lost about a buck for every 200 pills, they believe $5 million will make the situation all better.[772]

- **Mix Your Own "Cocktail":** Taking one part aspirin, one part Tylenol, and a cup of coffee's worth of caffeine (Excedrin Migraine) is still one of the top-rated migraine medications. It hits a migraine from multiple levels with the speed and vasoconstrictive nature of caffeine. For some, lowering the amount of aspirin and acetaminophen will reduce the side effects. For others, it will increase them, so you have to find the amounts that work for you. Rebound headaches are always a concern from drugs with added caffeine.

    Cocktails with numerous other OTCs—such as Benadryl—are often used to avoid prescription medication overuse. OTCs are also added to prescription medications because they are extremely powerful. And of course, it is imperative you speak with an experienced migraine doctor before you mix any OTC or prescription medication.

Anti-Nausea Medication

Migraineurs are more likely to have stomach disagreements when migraines hit and even when migraines are in hibernation. A number of over-the-counter anti-nausea medications are used every day by migraine sufferers, including Benadryl, Dramamine, Pepto Bismol, Pepcid, and Tums.

Here are the current most successful prescription anti-nausea medications available:

- **Chlorpromazine (Thorazine):** This medication treats nausea as well as mood disorders, such as schizophrenia. Thorazine makes your tummy feel better by changing your brain chemistry and comes with over 1,000 drug interactions—which should give an indication of how vast the side effects are.[773] Consider yourself warned. One article describes patients on Thorazine like this: "They would run their hands over their heads over and over, and open and close their mouths while sticking their tongues out…with stiff legs dragging their feet along, all the while seeming about to topple. We called this the 'Thorazine shuffle.'"[774] Numerous side effect observations, like the one just detailed, are bringing down the popularity of this longstanding anti-nausea drug.

- **Metoclopramide (Reglan):** This medication increases muscle contractions in the digestive tract to speed up the rate at which the stomach dumps into the intestines, thereby speeding up the digestion of medications. Metoclopramide comes with an increased risk of a serious movement disorder called tardive dyskinesia that is often irreversible. Tardive dyskinesia was just described above as the "Thorazine shuffle." Over 12 weeks of use is typically avoided.[775] Reglan currently has a user-review rating on www.drugs.com of 6.6 out of 10.

- **Prochlorperazine (Compazine):** This is another antipsychotic medicine used for stomach discomfort that has over 1,000 drug interactions and an extensive list of side effects that include uncontrolled lip smacking, gastrointestinal issues, and nightmares.[776] It has a user-review rating of 6.3 out of 10 on www.drugs.com.

- **Ondansetron (Zofran):** This is a blockbuster drug that blocks the serotonin in the intestines from communicating to the rest of the body that the stomach is ready to vomit. This is a common drug that we use in emergency medicine because it's well tolerated and takes action just minutes after it's dissolved under the tongue—perfect for preventing a patient from throwing up on you in the back of an ambulance. It has an 8.8 out of 10 reviewer rating on www.drugs.com. "I thank God every day for this drug," was the response of a woman in a migraine support group. Despite the positive reviews, we don't want a serotonin blocker in the long run, and a small portion of people experience headaches, confusion, weakness, anxiety, and stomach difficulties, among other side effects.

- **Promethazine (Phenergan):** This is a strong antihistamine; a moderate neurotransmitter blocker of the involuntary movement muscles, such as the stomach; and a weak to moderate blocker of the serotonin transmission.[777] This means that it stops the histamine pain, relaxes multiple muscles, and may also block the serotonin signal of pain from the stomach to the brain. While the largest side effect is unusual tiredness, it's a favorite among migraineurs who desperately need sleep as much as stomach relief. Any time you mess with your involuntary movements, you run the risk of having difficulty breathing, an irregular heartbeat, irregular blood pressure, muscle fatigue, and all the side effects that come from your body not functioning properly. It also increases the prospect of seizures. Despite the risks, the drug has a user-review rating of 8.7 out of 10 and a host of positive customers. One affectionate reviewer wrote, "Promethazine, you are my hero and I love you."[778]

- **Trimethobenzamide (Tigan):** This is one of the few effective drugs for nausea that doesn't alter the serotonin, dopamine, or histamine levels, which means far fewer side effects. But it's not as effective as the others, nor as popular.[779]

Other Meds

There are several medications that migraineurs have found helpful, but with some of them, the drawbacks may outweigh the benefits.

Diphenhydramine (Benadryl)

Benadryl is one of the most underestimated drugs used for migraines. It is a first-generation antihistamine and significantly more potent than newer generations.[780] Benadryl is powerful enough to treat life-threatening allergic reactions. By successfully blocking histamine, it may also have preventative benefits to blocking the triggers of migraines. It's also a go-to drug for many experienced migraineurs. Despite its successful use in emergency room "migraine cocktails" throughout the United States, many sufferers go a lifetime without trying Benadryl. Its acute action may help lower sinus pressure and change something in the histamine response of a migraine that is not yet understood by scientists.

Side effects are considerably lower than with other NSAIDs and only come with the possibility of mild gastrointestinal problems that may include nausea and a dry mouth. The small number of negative side effects will come primarily from its hypnotic effect of sleepiness.[781] It should be noted that a recent *JAMA* study found that over three years of heavy Benadryl use is associated with a higher risk of dementia.[782]

Pseudoephedrine (Sudafed)

This decongestant shrinks blood vessels in the sinus passages to give a number of headache sufferers, including me, powerful relief. You don't need a prescription, but you will need to sign for the drug at the pharmacy. This lets the government know who is buying pseudoephedrine pills and lets you know that some people buy pseudoephedrine pills to make methamphetamine.

Pseudoephedrine can make you feel like a drug addict—perhaps meth-head is the correct terminology. Side effects include nervousness, restlessness, trouble sleeping, a pounding heartbeat, increased sweating, headaches, itching, loss of appetite, and other drug-addiction symptoms.[783] For me, the symptoms increase dramatically over the period of two weeks.

While it's not ideal to take this powerful medication, more and more migraine sufferers are finding that pseudoephedrine works very well. I believe that pseudoephedrine will become a very popular short-term migraine medication as the link between sinus headaches and migraines become well known. I don't believe long-term use will fare as well. If you think coffee can cause rebound headaches, try becoming addicted to pseudoephedrine.

Corticosteroids

Corticosteroids are made from a synthetic version of cortisone, a natural steroid hormone produced by the body to suppress the immune system, thus reducing inflammation and pain. If you ever pick up a bad case of poison oak, a corticosteroid shot can seem like the best thing that has ever happened to you. It works so well at suppressing the immune system that the most dangerous side effect is an immune system that is susceptible to bacteria, germs, and infection. For this reason, it's usually administered to abort migraines in emergency situations if the patient has withstood other forms of preventative and acute medications.

Some patients who have tried just about every medication to little avail are willing to accept the side effects of steroids, which include increased hunger, weight gain, aggression, difficulty breathing, stomach ulcers, abdominal pain, abnormal fat deposits on the neck, acne, glaucoma, diabetes, and osteoporosis.[784] Because corticosteroids may cause calcium loss and poor calcium absorption, long-term use could lead to an uncontrollable battle with migraines.[785]

One of the most popular prescription corticosteroids is dexamethasone, which is typically given for two days at 8 mg per day to break a long migraine or cluster-headache cycle. There are a number of others, such as Solu-Medrol, and most come with terrible side effects, such as trouble thinking, speaking, or walking.[786] Corticosteroids should be a last resort medication for migraines.

Rescue Medications

The unofficial term "rescue medication" is often given to the drugs that don't necessarily stop a migraine but ease the pain after all other options fail. Opiates fall in that group. Muscle relaxers, such as Soma, Skelaxin, and Zanaflex, also provide migraineurs with temporary relief and high addiction rates. Butalbital is another highly addictive substance that is not the first line of defense for migraines. There are heavy NSAIDs, such as Demerol, that are used in the ER to abort a migraine, but they should not be taken on a regular basis.

Many people view a migraineur who gets one of these counterintuitive medications as a junkie. Those people (including some doctors) do not understand that a pain level of 10/10 can exist for a migraine, and it can last indefinitely—with fluctuation. A strong treatment may be the only thing that prevents a sufferer from jumping off a cliff.

Opiates

When you think of opiates, heroin probably comes to mind. Watch the film *The Basketball Diaries* to understand the severity of that destructive drug. A heroin addict becomes sick from withdrawal. And people actually die from the withdrawal of prescription opiates, such as methadone. In 2008, the number of prescription drug overdoses surpassed fatal motor vehicle accidents—a number higher than both the yearly cocaine and heroin deaths combined.[787]

Opiate-based drugs cause nearly three out of four prescription overdoses. For every death, there are 10 treatment admissions for abuse, 32 emergency room visits, 130 people who are opiate dependent, and 825 nonmedical users.[788] In 2010, enough prescription painkillers were prescribed to medicate every American adult every four hours for one month straight.[789]

In 2007 in the United States, the cost of opioid abuse was $55.7 billion.[790] Those American losses constitute large profits for the drug companies. In fact, this opiate "epidemic" of 259 million painkiller prescriptions per year—that's more painkiller prescriptions than there are people in some states—has led to the development of an at-home naloxone injector called Evzio. Naloxone is the drug that stops the damage from opiates (or wheat) in seconds flat.

After the CDC had mentioned an opiate "epidemic" in 2008, naloxone jumped from $3 to $30 per dose. However, if you want the Evzio at-home version, you can purchase a two-dose box from Walmart for about $600.[791]

Doctors are often not hesitant to prescribe these drugs for migraines—I do mean, *not hesitant at all*. A 2014 study looked at prescriptions written in 13 clinics for about 17,000 headache patients. Thirty-six percent of migraine patients received opiates while only 19%

received triptans.[792] The more hospital visits, the more likely it was for patients to be prescribed opiates.

Opiates, opioids, and narcotics don't really eliminate pain; they just make you not care about the pain. For many migraine sufferers, this simply doesn't work because the perception of pain within the brain can be magnified by migraines. Overuse of opiates can also make pain relief medications nearly useless. I remember a 911 call from a woman who had broken her leg. She was screaming in pain even though we had given her enough morphine to relax an elephant. When I explained we had given her the maximum dose, she yelled, "I used to shoot that for breakfast!"

The tolerance effect may explain why the efficacy in opioid treatment of chronic pain has yet to be proven—yes, the most dangerous drugs are not proven for long-term pain relief. Could you imagine trying to get pain relief from lavender oil or a natural remedy after being accustomed to opiates? Addicts refer to using opiates as getting well, as opposed to getting high. Furthermore, if you thought a barometric drop in pressure was a headache trigger, try a drug that could kill you from withdrawal. The body's chemical fluctuation will have a significant impact on long-term headache health.

Common side effects are sedation, dizziness, nausea, vomiting, constipation, addiction, and respiratory depression.[793] According to the *The Basketball Diaries*, which was based on a true story of addiction, you will do things you never could have imagined for opiates. The actual side effects will vary with each type of opiate, however, none of them mention anything about the possibility of destroying your life.

Many opiates are combined with typical over-the-counter drugs to improve their effectiveness for migraines and other conditions. Tylenol with Codeine #3 is a mix of acetaminophen and codeine;

Percocet is oxycodone and acetaminophen; Empirin is aspirin and codeine; Nurofen Plus is ibuprofen and codeine; Darvon is a mix of propoxyphene, aspirin, and caffeine; and there are many more.

If you are following the direction of your doctor, you are probably not going to turn into a basketball-playing poet who becomes a complete drug addict. Dr. Alexander Mauskop is the founder of the New York Headache Center and has found that limiting patients to four doses of narcotics a month can provide safe relief. If more treatments are necessary, he moves on to other treatments, such as preventative medications.[794]

While some doctors believe that headache recurrence isn't a problem for a patient taking opioids just a few times per month, estimates of the rebound headache range from 23–71%.[795] This means we have no clue if your headache will rebound within hours of leaving the hospital, and we aren't sure how opioids will affect your long-term headache health.

Propofol

"Refractory migraine" is the term applied to a migraine patient who typically has years of frequent headaches (over 15 per month) or a continuous headache that, according to Medscape, has "defied all pharmacological treatment attempts, including multiple drugs from multiple classes—both FDA approved and off-label."[796] This definition, which plays a large part in the overall medical perception of what a migraine is or could be, isn't written in stone. There is one doctor who understands this problem better than anyone. He's found something that's 98% effective at stopping a migraine.

Initially, I was skeptical of this success rate. My opinion changed after I read that Dr. John Claude Krusz was achieving these extraordinary results. Back in 2000, Krusz led a study that reduced headache intensity by 95.4% in 20 to 30 minutes, with complete abolition of headaches in 63 of 77 patients.[797] His next study was 98% successful. The drug used was propofol, also called "milk of amnesia."

You've heard of this powerful sedative drug. It was the drug used before the death of Michael Jackson and for Joan Rivers' routine surgery.[798] Aside from being powerful enough to knock you out permanently, I believe that any drug that can wipe out the memories of your day will have a strong effect on reducing the rapid buildup of glutamate in the brain and headache pain. Joan Rivers may have had an overdose of propofol—they didn't even weigh her to get the correct dosage. Michael Jackson was a walking drug bottle, and clearly this drug didn't help his situation or the doctor who served it (the doctor served two years behind bars for Jackson's death). Propofol can be administered safely, as Krusz and many other doctors have proven.

What's more astonishing than the 98% success rate is the fact that the percentage came from the treatment of over a thousand patients.[799] Before you get too excited, here's how the success rate was defined: Success was achieved when patients reported more than a 50% reduction in pain or the ability to return to work or daily activities. The study's approach was not standard, and that's a large portion of its success.

One or more of the following drugs were used in the study:

- Magnesium sulfate
- Dexamethasone (Decadron)
- Valproate sodium (Depacon)
- Droperidol (Inapsine)
- Metoclopramide (Reglan)

Drugs

- Dihydroergotamine (DHE 45)
- Promethazine (Phenergan)
- Lidocaine
- Propofol
- Tramadol (Ultram)
- Levetiracetam (Keppra)
- Ketamine

The approach used was incredibly logical for the patient and practitioner. They used one drug at a time and documented the success or lack thereof. The treatment was then repeated, combined, or changed based on those findings as well as the combinations that had been successful for similar patients.[800]

But wait—did you catch that first drug on the list? It was one of the most successful drugs they tried: magnesium sulfate. That's right—Epsom salt or magnesium salt. And that leads us to the other rescue medications.

Saline IV

One of the benefits of seeking medical attention for a migraine is the ability to immediately hydrate with salt water, which can help flush out any of the inflammation the body is battling. Hydration is one of most underrated factors of headache health and may play a large factor in the success of any drugs that are also administered by IV.

Oxygen

Don't forget to consider oxygen therapy as a naturally powerful drug with few side effects. The very simple administration of high-flow oxygen has a success rate of more than 75% for complete or near complete cessation of cluster headaches within 15 minutes and is now strongly recommended for migraine therapy.[801][802][803] Oxygen tanks retail for about $100, with $20 refill costs, and most people feel immediate relief. You can also purchase 95% oxygen on Amazon without a prescription in a product called Boost Oxygen. For $10, why not give it a try? Deep breathing is the free option.

Preventative Medications

Dr. Buchholz's famous three steps to "Heal Your Headache" included removing your triggers, avoiding acute medications, and preventative medication use (as a last resort).[804] Preventative medications are the daily meds that reduce frequent headaches. They are typically prescribed for two or more headaches per month, but they can also be prescribed based on the severity of headaches and reactions to acute medications.[805]

Antiseizure Medications

Antiseizure medications may target four migraine pathways: sodium channels, calcium channels, GABA, and glutamate.

Many antiseizure medications attach to sodium channels to block their transmission. You can feel this happen when you become dehydrated and your mind begins to slow down or become confused as your mineral levels are depleted. Sodium channels tell the neurons when to send messages, which sounds like a good idea until those messages are sent too fast from unbalanced sodium and cause an overexcitement of electrical activity.

Calcium channels, much like sodium channels, send electrical messages through the brain. Calcium has been described as the bullet of the migraine/seizure aura. By blocking the bullet, these antiseizure medications can halt the start of a migraine or seizure.

Antiseizure medications can result in an increased amount GABA. As we know from earlier studies, an increase in GABA can result in a decrease in glutamate. More GABA = fewer electrical messages firing toward a growing migraine detonator.

Glutamate is the primary neurotransmitter and helps the movement of calcium and sodium ions into the cells. While antiseizure medications don't target the glutamate receptors, their effect on the rest of this complex system slows down the transmission of glutamate messages.[806]

These four targets are involved with migraines and seizures, but science has yet to understand the exact pathophysiology of migraines or how these drugs affect migraines. It's an ongoing science experiment with millions of people.

There are two antiseizure medications often prescribed for migraines: topiramate (Topamax) and valproic acid (Depakote). Topamax can make you skinny and Depakote can make you fat. Guess which is more popular.

Topamax

Topamax is the most popular antiseizure medication for migraines and chronic migraines. It's also one of the most disliked migraine medications with nicknames of "Stupamax" and "Dopamax."

Antiseizure drugs aim to slow down your brain activity and may come with the following side effects: memory problems, delayed reactions, speech or language problems, and trouble concentrating. Many people have claimed that these memory problems don't go away, but there is no way of knowing for sure, since poor memory is "normal" with aging and migraines.

Hair loss is one of the most disturbing side effects for Topamax. I am scared of going bald and becoming cognitively slow, so I can't imagine how women feel about these side effects. Just ask the Migraine Support Group on Facebook. These side effects are not just words listed as legal protection.

Other side effects include fatigue, cold feet and hands, fever, chest pain, dizziness, psychomotor slowing, nervousness, tremors, headaches, tingling sensations, red eyes, eye pressure, abdominal pain, mental changes, aggression, agitation, depression, hypertension, dehydration, and the list goes on and on.

The "Topasoda" effect is the strangest. Many Topamax users say that the taste of soda changes to "a disgusting flat mix of sweetened chemicals," which may be a good thing if it makes people quit drinking the stuff. A few of the "rare" side effects are discussed by migraineurs as if they were very common, such as hallucinations.

Suicidal thoughts and attempts have been reported from Topamax use. A lot of the problems are dose related. Unfortunately, the dose that is significant enough to reduce migraines is often just the right dose to start immediate memory problems, although some patients find a dose that gives them a new life with very few side effects—or side effects they can live with.[807]

It's risk versus gain. Sadly, Topamax is a better option than the overuse of acute medications, even OTCs.[808] There is a chance that

Topamax could completely eliminate your migraines. One study by the University of Texas Medical School found more than a 50% reduction in migraines for half the patients using antiseizure drugs— taken at a maximum dose.[809] Many migraine patients confirm this study by saying the migraines go away if you can handle the side effects.

A study by the Jefferson Headache Center found that 54% of patients on 100 mg of Topamax per day exhibited a 50% or more reduction in migraine frequency. This is a very high success rate for a medication, however the total reduction in migraines for the entire group was only 39%. A large chunk of patients—19.2%—discontinued treatment due to adverse events that included paresthesia (sensation of pins and needles), fatigue, nausea, anorexia, and altered taste. It's hard to say how effective a drug is when we don't know how the side effects are making those successful patients feel.[810]

A migraineur must weigh the acute side effects and immediate benefits. Furthermore, the migraineur must project what those warning signs will do for his or her future headache health. The final step, whether you take the Topamax risk or not, is to work on a plan that naturally improves your mineral, glutamate, and serotonin levels as part of your long-term headache health. Maybe salt is a good idea to keep those sodium channels self-regulated.

Antidepressants

Antidepressants are often used to prevent migraines. Emotions, such as crying, can trigger migraines, so removing the ups and downs of life can help. Migraine treatment's most successful antidepressant is amitriptyline.

Amitriptyline (Elavil) has an advantage over many of the other antidepressants. It blocks the sodium and calcium channels that can trigger a migraine, just like the antiseizure drugs that were already discussed.[811] In addition, it does what most antidepressants do and raises serotonin levels in the blood.[812] Those serotonin levels keep you happy, or eventually numb, and can fight off glutamate, inflammation, and sadness.

Amitriptyline is going to have two major complaints: weight gain and sleepiness. Nearly all antidepressants will cause a reduction in the overall amount of REM sleep per night. Not only does it steal your dreams, a side effect that many migraineurs experience is nightmares. Up to 84% of patients will experience anticholinergic effects, such as dry mouth, blurry vision, constipation, and urinary retention—which is no laughing matter and goes far beyond electrolyte problems. Antidepressants will double your risk of GI bleeds. Just like with Topamax, messing with the body's ability to transmit thoughts may cause delirium, cognitive impairment, movement disorders, hallucinations, suicidal ideation, and mental changes.[813]

A large amitriptyline study by the University of Oklahoma College of Medicine found that 50% of migraine patients reduced headache frequency, and 46% of chronic, daily headache sufferers reduced headache frequency by more than 50%. However, amitriptyline was not significantly superior to the placebo by the end of the study.[814] In another study, a group of 331 migraine sufferers with three to 12 headaches per month reduced their headaches on average by about 2.5 headaches per month. Not impressive, but some sufferers may completely eliminate migraines.[815]

There are many other antidepressants with fewer side effects than amitriptyline, but none has been thoroughly successful for migraine treatment. As with any drug, some migraineurs love amitriptyline and some hate it. Remember that weaning off antidepressants can be extremely difficult. In fact, the FDA has reported 444 homicides involving antidepressants in an eight-year period. However, only 1% of incidents are reported to the FDA, leaving the numbers closer to 40,000 psychoactive homicides.[816] These actions and disturbing feelings cannot be understood from reading a drug's side effects.

Botox

In 2010, Botox was approved to treat chronic migraines. In large studies of chronic migraines, Botox has been associated with a small to modest benefit for chronic daily headaches and chronic migraines. "Small" actually translates to great when compared to the strong placebo effects of injections. Botox studies have cut the number of migraines per month in half for 54% of episodic migraine sufferers and 55% of chronic migraine sufferers, but the placebo can be just as powerful.[817]

Botox has not been approved to treat episodic migraines (under 15 per month) because it hasn't been proven successful against a placebo, which doesn't tell us much, considering that the placebo success for 31 injections is about as high as a placebo can get.[818][819]

Two well-designed studies of chronic migraine sufferers found 7.8 to 9.2 fewer headache days from Botox and 6.4 to 6.9 fewer headache days from placebo injections.[820] The results were "approximately 2.3 fewer headache days compared to the placebo group."

In reality, this is a jumbo-sized success. It means that a chronic migraine sufferer will have up to nine fewer migraine days every month (technically every 28 days) with 134 fewer hours of pain.[821] That's 33.5 hours a week. According to Obamacare, which states that over 30 hours a week is full time, that is a full-time job of pain that could be eliminated. How would you spend those pain-free hours every week?

But you can't ignore that placebo effect, either! If I tell you that you won't be able to move your face muscles and neck muscles, you're probably going to believe those muscles are relaxed. You actively relax those muscles with your mind, because that's a pretty easy thing to do. And we know that relaxation techniques lead to results.

What Is It?

Botox (botulinum toxin A) comes from the Latin word *botulus*, meaning "sausage." Botox is derived from the bacteria Clostridium botulinum—which does cause botulism. This is where "sausage" comes into play. Improperly handled meat products, such as sausage, can produce the bacteria Clostridium botulinum that will essentially create Botox. Gross, right?

But Botox, thankfully, acts differently in the body than botulism. With botulism, the bacteria will spread throughout your body to places you don't want it, such as your arms, legs, chest, and respiratory tract. Botox injected into your face muscles won't spread like bacteria. What it does instead is paralyze the muscles that influence a headache and minimize the pain around the skull from the onset of a headache.

How It Works

Botox is injected into several typical injection sites on the forehead, temple, scalp, upper neck, and shoulders. There are many other areas, also, that specialists will use.[822] You can search for "Botox 31 migraine injections sites" to see images of the sites.

The success of using Botox to paralyze these muscles is not understood, just as with nerve blocks. Somehow relieving the pressure on nerves in the face and neck relieves the inflammation that triggers and further deteriorates migraines and headaches.[823]

Does It Hurt?

A typical needle used in an emergency situation or a blood donation is 18 gauge. Higher-gauge needles have a bigger number and a smaller needle size. A very small needle used in emergency service is 22 gauge, reserved for little old ladies with tiny veins. Botox needles can be 30 gauge, which is extremely small and painless for most people. The after effects of soreness and discomfort are usually more painful than the procedure itself.

How Long Does It Last?

Botox may paralyze muscles for three to five months, but migraine headaches may only disappear for one to three months. Many migraine sufferers complain about the period between the diminishing effects of Botox and their next scheduled Botox appointment.

Side Effects

The studies are painting Botox as a very safe treatment for migraine sufferers. In a meta-study involving 2,309 patients, BTX-A (another brand of botulinum toxin) showed only moderate side effects in 25% of patients compared to 15% in the control group.[824] Focal weakness (weakness of a muscle group) was the only side effect that occurred more in the Botox group than in the placebo group. But this is exactly what is supposed to happen—the muscle you intentionally paralyzed is not going to lift your eyebrow with ease.

If you want to know what patients are saying, there are a ton of blogs and chat groups on this topic. The biggest complaint I saw was stiffness in the neck. Any migraine group will have a number of people who say it completely eliminates their migraines or reduces pain significantly, while other sufferers will just be angry that they paid for a product that had no effect. The worst side effect I read about was from a woman who needed a neck collar because her Botox dose was too large.

Cost

In 2015, the cost of Botox ranged from $350 to $500 per area of injection.[825] Many people post that their co-pays are around $300. But you may be able to get the full 31 injections for that price. The cost is going to vary from place to place, as all medical procedures do.[826] You may be eligible for Botox at no charge if you are uninsured. Visit www.botoxreimbursment.us.

It's a really pricey procedure. Botox has annual sales of $1.6 billion, with about half for migraine treatment. But, with respect to side effects, Botox looks like a drug from the heavens when compared to most medications.

Beta Blockers

The beta blockers propranolol, metoprolol, timolol, atenolol, and nadolol have proven to reduce frequency in about half of migraine sufferers.[827] That's quite good. They also have a history. A 1991 meta-study of over 2,000 migraine patients found that, on average, propranolol yielded a 44% reduction in the total number of patients' migraines.[828]

Propranolol is the recommended beta blocker for migraines[829] and is the most successful migraine beta blocker, with one study finding up to 80% of migraine sufferers cutting their migraine frequency in half.[830] That is incredible, but take it with a grain of salt. Another study from 2013 by the Norwegian University of Science and Technology found that 40% of migraine sufferers cut their migraine frequency in half, which is still nice.[831]

There are two cautions with these terrific results: No successful long-term studies have been completed, and companies that will profit from the data they choose to include or disregard are the same companies funding the majority of the studies. That's part of the game, and beta blockers are very effective within the realm of that game.

How They Work

Beta blockers block the beta receptors from receiving the stress signals of epinephrine—pure adrenaline. While this drug is thought of as blocking the stress response to the heart, lungs, and arteries, it is also part of the larger stress system that Americans know all too well. The anxiety of the flight-or-fight response, which includes a pounding heart rate, increased respiration, sweating, and worrying yourself to death, is all reduced by beta blockers.

While modern science can't explain how this system is intertwined, musicians, public speakers, Olympic athletes, businesspeople, and actors have used beta blockers for over 30 years to stop self-induced stress from creating self-sabotage. It seems that more than 30 years is ample time to understand the drug, until you understand the impact it plays on a galaxy-sized system.[832]

A recent study found that the success of beta blockers on migraines might be linked to the ability to control neural excitability from inflammation and glutamate.[833] Beta blockers may reduce stress and glutamate in the entire human body, a system composed of 100 billion neurons (or more) and 125 trillion synapses (or more).[834][835] Those are incomprehensible numbers. Manipulating stress in a system of such magnitude will come with a number of side effects.

Side Effects

Depression symptoms alone can be found in 50–74% of propranolol patients—propranolol is the recommended beta blocker for migraines.[836] Propranolol patients on WebMD's user review section complain of extreme weight gain, fatigue, numb hands and feet, confusion, glucose spikes, permanent tachycardia, permanent nerve damage, and more. One patient wrote, "Worked beautifully as a migraine prevention, however caused a drug-induced lupus that nearly killed me," and another wrote, "I have been on this medication 6 days and gained 12 pounds." Heart medications all come with serious side effects, and those side effects are often treated with more medication.

The more medications you are on, the more likely you are to have negative drug interactions, and the more likely you are to call 911. One cardiac study found that patients were on an average of six medications, with 68% having potential negative drug-to-drug interactions at the time of a hospital check-in. When they left, patients were on an average of eight medications with a potential drug-to-drug interaction of 88.8%.[837] Heart medications are serious drugs that should only be reserved for patients in dire need.

The Future of Migraine Drugs

The first human genome sequencing, which was accomplished in 2003, took 13 years and cost $3 billion. Today's price for personal genome sequencing is under $1,000, and you can have the results back in a few days.[838]

In 2010, researchers made the first genetic breakthrough for migraines, finding the DNA variant between the genes responsible for regulating glutamate.[839] In 2013, the mutated MTHFR gene was discovered, explaining the migraine threshold and offering a vitamin that could bypass this mutated gene.

In 2006, an excitotoxicity study detailed the relationship between inflammation, glutamate, and migraines.[840] Just three years later, a study detailed how the human body is capable of reversing this excitotoxicity through the ketogenic diet.[841] Today, there are multiple proven ways to naturally lower inflammation and glutamate.

In Silicon Valley, this boom in medical technology and nutritional understanding is referred to as "exponential innovation." It will result in thousands of new tools to monitor your individual health, making it possible to accurately prescribe a targeted combination of drugs, supplementation, and nutrition. Drowning the entire body in drugs doesn't work. New drugs will treat the specific problems without side effects, while technology will monitor exactly how to support that treatment with nutrition.

The Best Pill—the Placebo

Now that I've quite possibly successfully destroyed any hope you may have had in all mainstream medications, we need to bring it back up with the placebo effect. You've already read how powerful the placebo effect can be in studies. The more expensive or painful the treatment, the more likely you are to be healed. The incredible poison oak study proved that our minds could create real and visible pain or make it disappear.

I've seen this magic happen in the fire service multiple times. My last placebo patient thought he was going to die during a heart attack—a reasonable time to panic. We hooked him up to an IV and prepared a drug called adenosine. Adenosine can be used when a patient's heart rate is through the roof, and his was climbing above 190 beats per minute. This drug can temporarily stop the heart—almost like a reset—and then dramatically slow it down.

Before we gave him the adenosine, he asked me if he was going to die. I told him, "You can try to stop breathing if you want to, but I've got a bag of oxygen here that will breathe for you. You can try to stop your heart, but we've got a state-of-the-art machine for that too, and we can fly you to one of the best hospitals in the world in just a couple minutes. We're all going to die eventually, but you are going to have a very hard time doing so in the next few minutes." At this time, his heart attack was not detectable. He replied, "Oh, thank you. The drugs are really helping."

His heart rate dropped from 190 to 160 to 140 to 120, and then we had to tell him, "We actually didn't push any drugs yet, but your heart rate has gone way down and your color is coming back. Does your wife tell you that you stress yourself out?" He started laughing, and his heart rate returned to normal. His heart attack was minor, and he was released from the hospital the next day. It's incredible what your mind can do.

This man turned one of the worst-case scenarios into a positive outlook. I probably wouldn't have even remembered this call, but he came back to the fire station the next day to thank us with a 12-pack of beer. I told him we couldn't accept that, and he said, "I thought you would say that. Don't look in the back of your truck." He then drove away. The man truly thought that we saved his life, but all we did was talk to him. The placebo is more than just an acute thought; it physically alters the chemistry of your body for better or worse.

The placebo effect is an accepted medical fact, yet we brush positive thinking off as some sort of quackery committed by unrealistic flower children or larger-than-life characters, like Sir Richard Branson. We see an old widower pass within a year of his wife and we say that he died of a broken heart. We see stress as a top killer of Americans, but we don't believe attitude can change outcomes. Relaxation techniques produce the pain reduction of morphine and the prevention success of blood pressure medication—without the side effects—and we call it "just the placebo effect."

The more we think about the placebo effect, the stronger it becomes. The medical community can only document this effect without the technology to understand it. A recent study found that a placebo shot reduced more than 50% of migraine days in 67% of migraine sufferers.[842] The placebo is a world-class treatment. What if this placebo effect only happened for the people who truly believed in it? What if the placebo effect was 100% successful for those with positive attitudes? Why not accept that we don't understand the success and use it to our advantage every day? I did not believe in the power of meditation, relaxation, happiness, elimination diets, nutrition, and exercise until I read all of the studies detailed in this book.

There is no going back now. What was once a nice thought is now a fact in my mind. Whether you take your placebo as a pill, injection, yoga, natural food, mineral water, or mental technique, you need to truly believe in it. If your current condition requires medication, believe in that medication and believe you can one day get off that medication.

The placebo effect is similar to the headache threshold: there are multiple factors that contribute to your success. A person who eliminates multiple headache triggers and believes that the lack of those triggers will bring success is correct. The person who has tried individual treatments and doesn't believe that those treatments affect overall headache health is also correct. The placebo effect is wonderful, if you want it to be.

Want to Learn More about Medications?

One of the best places to get detailed answers about migraine medications is the Migraine Support Group on Facebook. Many experienced migraineurs and health professionals are willing to share their stories. Of course, only a doctor can provide medical advice for you specifically. Others include:

- www.drugs.com (**User Reviews** section)
- www.webmd.com (**User Reviews** section)
- www.migraine.com
- www.wikipedia.com (As a starting point)
- www.scholar.google.com
- www.ncbi.nlm.nih.gov/pubmed/

Conclusion

The acute drugs that reduce the pain from headaches and migraines have around a 50% success rate and will likely come with side effects and rebound headaches. Preventative drugs reduce migraine frequency by around 50% and come with heavy side effects. One study found that the natural herb butterbur cut migraine frequency in half for 77% of patients and 91% of patients improved. The 1979 elimination diet was 100% successful at reducing migraines, and the 1983 elimination diet completely eliminated migraines in 89% of patients.

The migraine gene (MTHFR) taught us that we could completely bypass the genetic predisposition to migraines with the bioavailable vitamins B9 and B12. The gene mutation also explained why a headache threshold exists and how lowering levels of stress, inflammation, and glutamate will reduce headaches and migraines. Relaxation techniques such as breathing like a Navy SEAL—slow, four-second inhales and slow, four-second exhales—may reduce migraine pain as much as the strongest medications. Studies show that meditation increases the size of your brain; reduces heart attack, stroke, and many other causes of death; provides as much relief as antidepressants; and lowers headache frequency and pain by 40–60%. Any measure to lower inflammation and glutamate will raise the headache threshold and reduce headaches and migraines.

But where do we start? How do we remember all this information? And what do we do with it? The Headache Help Checklist includes all of the ways proven to reduce inflammation and glutamate that my research revealed. The free guide at www.3dayheachecure.com will help you remember what all those checkboxes mean so you can create a checklist that is just for you. You will also have articles and videos at the www.3dayheadachecure.com that expand on the concepts in this book. You now have the tools you need to be headache and migraine-free.

Please share this information to help other headache sufferers. Helping people may increase your serotonin, reduce your headaches, and make you feel great!

Citations

[1] "Frequently Asked Questions." *Migraine Awareness Group (facts)*. Web. 8 Sept. 2015. http://www.migraines.org/commfaqs/commfaqs.htm

[2] Steiner, T., Stovner, L., & Birbeck, G. (2013, January 10). Migraine: The seventh disabler. Retrieved September 16, 2015, from http://www.ncbi.nlm.nih.gov/pmc/articles/PMC3606966/

[3] Farooq, K. (2008, January 1). Headache and chronic facial pain. Retrieved May 1, 2015, from http://ceaccp.oxfordjournals.org/content/8/4/138.full

[4] Frequently Asked Questions. (n.d.). Retrieved September 8, 2015, from http://www.migraines.org/commfaqs/commfaqs.htm

[5] Cure. (n.d.). Medical Definition Retrieved May 4, 2015, from http://medical-dictionary.thefreedictionary.com/cure

[6] Cure. (n.d.). Retrieved May 4, 2015, from http://www.merriam-webster.com/dictionary/cure

[7] American Diabetes Association. (2009, November 1). Diabetes Care. Retrieved May 4, 2015, from http://care.diabetesjournals.org/content/32/11/2133.full

[8] Taylor, F. (n.d.). Migraine Headache | American College Physicians. Retrieved May 15, 2015, from https://store.acponline.org/ebizatpro/images/productimages/books/sample chapters/Headache_Ch04.pdf

[9] Mauser, E. (2014). So many migraines, so few subspecialists: Analysis of the geographic location of United Council for Neurologic Subspecialties (UCNS) certified headache subspecialists compared to United States headache demographics. Retrieved May 15, 2015, from http://www.ncbi.nlm.nih.gov/pubmed/24942840

[10] IHS Migraine definition. (n.d.). Retrieved September 9, 2015, from http://ihs-classification.org/en/02_klassifikation/02_teil1/01.01.00_migraine.html

[11] ICHD-II Full Text Search | International Headache Society. (n.d.). Retrieved May 15, 2015, from http://ihs-classification.org/en/02_klassifikation/02_teil1/01.00.00_migraine.html

[12] NIH. (2015, February 5). Estimates of Funding for Various Research, Condition, and Disease Categories (RCDC). Retrieved May 15, 2015, from http://report.nih.gov/categorical_spending.aspx

[13] Steiner, T., Stovner, L., & Birbeck, G. (2013, January 10). Migraine: The seventh disabler. Retrieved September 16, 2015, from http://www.ncbi.nlm.nih.gov/pmc/articles/PMC3606966/

[14] Burch, R. (2015). The prevalence and burden of migraine and severe headache in the United States: Updated statistics from government health surveillance studies. Retrieved May 15, 2015, from http://www.ncbi.nlm.nih.gov/pubmed/25600719

[15] Deshpande, L. (2007, August 1). Activation of a novel injury-induced calcium-permeable channel that plays a key role in causing extended neuronal depolarization and initiating neuronal death in excitotoxic neuronal injury. Retrieved May 7, 2015, from http://www.ncbi.nlm.nih.gov/pubmed/17483292

[16] Signs and Symptoms | UM. (n.d.). Retrieved May 15, 2015, from http://www.understandmigraines.org/migraine-topic/signs-and-symptoms

[17] Migraine Research Foundation. (n.d.). Retrieved May 15, 2015, from http://www.migraineresearchfoundation.org/

[18] History of Migraine. (n.d.). Retrieved May 14, 2015, from http://www.understandmigraines.org/migraine-topic/more/history

[19] Terrell Davis backs Mike Shanahan. (2013). Retrieved May 14, 2015, from http://www.washingtonpost.com/blogs/dc-sports-bog/wp/2013/01/22/terrell-davis-backs-mike-shanahan/

[20] Famous People with Migraines. (n.d.). Retrieved May 14, 2015, from http://www.understandmigraines.org/migraine-topic-summary/famous-people-migraines

[21] Egger J. (1983, October 15). Is migraine food allergy? A double-blind controlled trial of oligoantigenic diet treatment. Retrieved May 4, 2015, from http://www.ncbi.nlm.nih.gov/pubmed/6137694

[22] Tfelt-Hansen P. (2000, December 1). Triptans in migraine: A comparative review of pharmacology, pharmacokinetics and efficacy. Retrieved May 4, 2015, from http://www.ncbi.nlm.nih.gov/pubmed/11152011

[23] Winkler AS. (2010, May 30). Prevalence of migraine headache in a rural area of northern Tanzania: A community-based door-to-door survey. Retrieved May 4, 2015, from http://www.ncbi.nlm.nih.gov/pubmed/19735479

[24] Ferrante T. (2012, January 27). The PACE study: Past-year prevalence of migraine in Parma's adult general population. Retrieved May 4, 2015, from http://www.ncbi.nlm.nih.gov/pubmed/22287564

[25] Grant, E. (1979, May 5). Food allergies and migraine. Retrieved May 5, 2015, from http://www.ncbi.nlm.nih.gov/pubmed/87628

[26] ROWE, A. (1932, September 10). ALLERGIC MIGRAINE. Retrieved May 8, 2015, from http://jama.jamanetwork.com/article.aspx?articleid=283361

[27] Alpay, K. (2010, January 3). Diet restriction in migraine, based on IgG against foods: A clinical double-blind, randomised, cross-over trial. Retrieved May 8, 2015, from http://www.ncbi.nlm.nih.gov/pmc/articles/PMC2899772/pdf/10.1177_0333102410361404.pdf

[28] Hernández, A. (2007, August). Food allergy mediated by IgG antibodies associated with migraine in adults. Retrieved May 8, 2015, from http://www.ncbi.nlm.nih.gov/pubmed/18693538

[29] Eysink, P. (1999, May 1). Relation between IgG antibodies to foods and IgE antibodies to milk, egg, cat, dog and/or mite in a cross-sectional study. Retrieved May 8, 2015, from http://www.ncbi.nlm.nih.gov/pubmed/10231319

[30] Wilders-Truschnig, M. (2007, December 10). IgG antibodies against food antigens are correlated with inflammation and intima media thickness in obese juveniles. Retrieved May 8, 2015, from http://www.ncbi.nlm.nih.gov/pubmed/18072008

[31] Cole, J. (2006, September). Migraine, fibromyalgia, and depression among people with IBS: A prevalence study. Retrieved May 8, 2015, from http://www.ncbi.nlm.nih.gov/pubmed/17007634

[32] Lau, C. (2014, September). Association between migraine and irritable bowel syndrome: A population-based retrospective cohort study. Retrieved May 8, 2015, from http://www.ncbi.nlm.nih.gov/pubmed/24838228

[33] Aydinlar, E. (2013, March 1). IgG-based elimination diet in migraine plus irritable bowel syndrome. Retrieved May 8, 2015, from http://www.ncbi.nlm.nih.gov/pubmed/23216231

[34] Pascual, J. (2010, March 26). IgG-mediated allergy: A new mechanism for migraine attacks? Retrieved May 8, 2015, from http://cep.sagepub.com/content/30/7/777.full

[35] Vader, W. (2002, June 1). The gluten response in children with celiac disease is directed toward multiple gliadin and glutenin peptides. Retrieved May 8, 2015, from http://www.ncbi.nlm.nih.gov/m/pubmed/12055577/

[36] Kim, S. (2002). Transglutaminases in disease. Retrieved May 8, 2015, from http://www.ncbi.nlm.nih.gov/pubmed/11738475

[37] Kwon, J., Kim, J., Cho, S., Noh, G., & Lee, S. (2013, April 1). Characterization of food allergies in patients with atopic dermatitis. Retrieved May 8, 2015, from http://www.ncbi.nlm.nih.gov/pmc/articles/PMC3627928/

[38] Davidson, I. (1979). Antibodies to maize in patients with Crohn's disease, ulcerative colitis and coeliac disease. Retrieved May 8, 2015, from http://www.ncbi.nlm.nih.gov/pubmed/371884

[39] Buret, A. (2006). How Stress Induces Intestinal Hypersensitivity. Retrieved May 8, 2015, from http://www.ncbi.nlm.nih.gov/pmc/articles/PMC1592668/

[40] Cross-Reaction between Gliadin and Different Food and Tissue Antigens. (2012, December 13). Retrieved May 8, 2015, from http://file.scirp.org/Html/5-2700516_26626.htm

[41] Longoni, M. (2006). Inflammation and excitotoxicity: Role in migraine pathogenesis. Retrieved May 19, 2015, from http://www.ncbi.nlm.nih.gov/pubmed/16688611

[42] Medical News Today. (n.d.). Common food allergies. Retrieved May 8, 2015, from http://www.medicalnewstoday.com/articles/8624.php

[43] Kimmel, J. (n.d.). Pedestrian Question - What is Gluten? Retrieved May 4, 2015, from https://www.youtube.com/watch?v=AdJFE1sp4Fw

[44] Davis, W. (2011, September 20). On the evils of wheat - Macleans.ca. Retrieved May 4, 2015, from http://www2.macleans.ca/2011/09/20/on-the-evils-of-wheat-why-it-is-so-addictive-and-how-shunning-it-will-make-you-skinny/

[45] Davis, W. (n.d.). WheatBelly Lifestyle Institute. Retrieved May 4, 2015, from http://www.wheatbelly.com/articles/WBFAQs

[46] Soares FL. (2012, December 17). Gluten-free diet reduces adiposity, inflammation and insulin resistance associated with the induction of PPAR-alpha and PPAR-gamma expression. Retrieved May 4, 2015, from http://www.ncbi.nlm.nih.gov/pubmed/23253599

[47] Dohan, FC. (1980). Hypothesis: Genes and neuroactive peptides from food as cause of schizophrenia. Retrieved May 4, 2015, from http://www.ncbi.nlm.nih.gov/pubmed/6994444

[48] Kraft. (2009, February 26). Schizophrenia, gluten, and low-carbohydrate, ketogenic diets: A case report and review of the literature. Retrieved May 4, 2015, from http://www.ncbi.nlm.nih.gov/pubmed/19245705

[49] Unger, A. (1952, September 1). Migraine is an allergic disease. Retrieved May 5, 2015, from http://www.sciencedirect.com/science/article/pii/0021870752900075

[50] Hadjivassiliou, M. (2001, February 13). Headache and CNS white matter abnormalities associated with gluten sensitivity. Retrieved May 5, 2015, from http://www.neurology.org/content/56/3/385.short

Citations

[51] Dimitrova, A. (2012, November 5). Prevalence of Migraine in Patients With Celiac Disease and Inflammatory Bowel Disease. Retrieved May 5, 2015, from http://onlinelibrary.wiley.com/doi/10.1111/j.1526-4610.2012.02260.x/abstract

[52] University of Chicago Celiac Disease Center. (n.d.). Retrieved May 5, 2015, from http://www.uchicago.edu/research/center/university_of_chicago_celiac_disease_center/

[53] Celiac Disease Causes, Symptoms, Treatments, Tests, & More. (n.d.). Retrieved May 5, 2015, from http://www.webmd.com/digestive-disorders/celiac-disease/celiac-disease

[54] Catassi, C. (2013, September 26). Non-Celiac Gluten sensitivity: The new frontier of gluten related disorders. Retrieved May 5, 2015, from http://www.ncbi.nlm.nih.gov/pubmed/24077239

[55] University of Maryland Medical Center. (n.d.). School of Medicine Researchers Identify Key Pathogenic Differences Between Celiac Disease and Gluten Sensitivity. Retrieved May 5, 2015, from http://umm.edu/news-and-events/news-releases/2011/school-of-medicine-researchers-identify-key-pathogenic-differences-between-celiac-disease-and-gluten-sensitivity

[56] Christou, N. (2004, September 1). Surgery Decreases Long-term Mortality, Morbidity, and Health Care Use in Morbidly Obese Patients. Retrieved May 5, 2015, from http://www.ncbi.nlm.nih.gov/pmc/articles/PMC1356432/

[57] OECD. (2014). OBESITY AND THE ECONOMICS OF PREVENTION: FIT NOT FAT. Retrieved May 5, 2015, from http://www.oecd.org/italy/Obesity-Update-2014-ITALY.pdf

[58] Frequently Asked Questions About Food Triggers, Migraines, and Headaches. (n.d.). Retrieved May 5, 2015, from http://www.webmd.com/migraines-headaches/guide/triggers-specific-foods

[59] Diet and Headache - Foods | National Headache Foundation. (2007, October 25). Retrieved May 5, 2015, from http://www.headaches.org/content/diet-and-headache-foods

[60] Migraine Triggers | University of California, Berkeley. (n.d.). Retrieved May 5, 2015, from http://uhs.berkeley.edu/home/healthtopics/pdf/triggers.pdf

[61] Maleki, N. (2012, July 28). Her versus his migraine: Multiple sex differences in brain function and structure. Retrieved May 15, 2015, from http://brain.oxfordjournals.org/content/135/8/2546.abstract

[62] Gold, E. (2000, August 16). Factors Associated with Age at Natural Menopause in a Multiethnic Sample of Midlife Women. Retrieved May 15, 2015, from http://aje.oxfordjournals.org/content/153/9/865.full

[63] Migraine in Children | Migraine Research Foundation. (n.d.). Retrieved May 15, 2015, from http://www.migraineresearchfoundation.org/Migraine in Children.html

[64] Migraine in Children | Migraine Research Foundation. (n.d.). Retrieved May 15, 2015, from http://www.migraineresearchfoundation.org/Migraine in Children.html

[65] Rates of A.D.H.D. Diagnosis in Children. (2013, March 30). Retrieved May 15, 2015, from http://www.nytimes.com/interactive/2013/03/31/us/adhd-in-children.html?ref=health

[66] Use of Medication Prescribed for Emotional or Behavioral Difficulties Among Children Aged 6–17 Years in the United States, 2011–2012 CDC. (2014, April 24). Retrieved May 15, 2015, from http://www.cdc.gov/nchs/data/databriefs/db148.htm

[67] Keyes, K. (2013, November 1). Association of hormonal contraceptive use with reduced levels of depressive symptoms: A national study of sexually active women in the United States. Retrieved May 15, 2015, from http://www.ncbi.nlm.nih.gov/pubmed/24043440

[68] America's State of Mind Report | World Health Organization. (2015). Retrieved May 15, 2015, from http://apps.who.int/medicinedocs/documents/s19032en/s19032en.pdf

[69] Migraine in Children | Migraine Research Foundation. (n.d.). Retrieved May 15, 2015, from http://www.migraineresearchfoundation.org/Migraine in Children.html

[70] Maker of Children's Tylenol Pleads Guilty | ABC News. (2015). Retrieved April 15, 2015, from http://abcnews.go.com/Health/wireStory/maker-childrens-tylenol-plead-guilty-recall-29531769

[71] Anttila, V. (2010, August 29). Genome-wide association study of migraine implicates a common susceptibility variant on 8q22.1. Retrieved May 5, 2015, from http://www.ncbi.nlm.nih.gov/pmc/articles/PMC2948563/

[72] Anttila, V. (2010, August 29). Genome-wide association study of migraine implicates a common susceptibility variant on 8q22.1. Retrieved May 5, 2015, from http://www.ncbi.nlm.nih.gov/pmc/articles/PMC2948563/

[73] Lauritzen, M., Dreier, J., Fabricius, M., Hartings, J., Graf, R., & Strong, A. (2011). Clinical relevance of cortical spreading depression in neurological disorders: Migraine, malignant stroke, subarachnoid and intracranial hemorrhage, and traumatic brain injury. Retrieved September 9, 2015, from http://www.ncbi.nlm.nih.gov/pmc/articles/PMC3049472/

[74] Tanaka, K. (1997, June 13). Epilepsy and exacerbation of brain injury in mice lacking the glutamate transporter GLT-1. Retrieved May 5, 2015, from http://www.ncbi.nlm.nih.gov/pubmed/9180080

[75] Zlotnik, A. (2011). The effects of estrogen and progesterone on blood glutamate levels: Evidence from changes of blood glutamate levels during the menstrual cycle in women. Retrieved May 15, 2015, from http://www.ncbi.nlm.nih.gov/pubmed/20980684

[76] Zlotnik, A. (2011). The effects of estrogen and progesterone on blood glutamate levels: Evidence from changes of blood glutamate levels during the menstrual cycle in women. Retrieved May 15, 2015, from http://www.ncbi.nlm.nih.gov/pubmed/20980684

[77] Sang-Hwan, D. (2012). Progesterone increases the activity of glutamate transporter... : European Journal of Anaesthesiology (EJA). Retrieved May 15, 2015, from http://journals.lww.com/ejanaesthesiology/Fulltext/2012/06001/Progesterone_increases_the_activity_of_glutamate.471.aspx

[78] Martin, V. (2006). Ovarian hormones and migraine headache: Understanding mechanisms and pathogenesis--part 2. Retrieved May 15, 2015, from http://www.ncbi.nlm.nih.gov/pubmed/16618254

[79] Martin, V. (2006). Ovarian hormones and migraine headache: Understanding mechanisms and pathogenesis--part 2. Retrieved May 15, 2015, from http://www.ncbi.nlm.nih.gov/pubmed/16618254

[80] Adult Obesity Facts | CDC. (2014, September 9). Retrieved May 12, 2015, from http://www.cdc.gov/obesity/data/adult.html

[81] Bariatric Surgery May Alleviate Migraine. (2011, June 20). Retrieved May 12, 2015, from http://www.medscape.com/viewarticle/744932

[82] Peterlin, B. (2013, October). Episodic migraine and obesity and the influence of age, race, and sex. Retrieved May 12, 2015, from http://www.ncbi.nlm.nih.gov/pubmed/24027060

[83] Gold, E. (2000, August 16). Factors Associated with Age at Natural Menopause in a Multiethnic Sample of Midlife Women. Retrieved May 15, 2015, from http://aje.oxfordjournals.org/content/153/9/865.full

[84] Rakoff-Nahoum, S. (2007, October 1). Why Cancer and Inflammation? Retrieved May 12, 2015, from http://www.ncbi.nlm.nih.gov/pmc/articles/PMC1994795/

[85] Greenberg, A. (2006, February 1). Obesity and the role of adipose tissue in inflammation and metabolism. Retrieved May 12, 2015, from http://ajcn.nutrition.org/content/83/2/461S.full

[86] Yan, J. (2012, January 24). Sensitization of dural afferents underlies migraine-related behavior following meningeal application of interleukin-6 (IL-6). Retrieved May 13, 2015, from http://www.ncbi.nlm.nih.gov/pubmed/22273495

[87] Humans Carry More Bacterial Cells than Human Ones. (2007, November 30). Retrieved May 13, 2015, from http://www.scientificamerican.com/article/strange-but-true-humans-carry-more-bacterial-cells-than-human-ones/

[88] Human Microbiome Project. (n.d.). Retrieved May 13, 2015, from http://genome.wustl.edu/projects/detail/human-microbiome-project/

[89] Rapid and unexpected weight gain after fecal transplant. (2015, February 4). Retrieved May 13, 2015, from http://www.sciencedaily.com/releases/2015/02/150204125810.htm

[90] How Gut Bacteria Help Make Us Fat and Thin. (2014, June 1). Retrieved May 13, 2015, from http://www.scientificamerican.com/article/how-gut-bacteria-help-make-us-fat-and-thin/

[91] Barrett, E. (2012, June 15). γ-Aminobutyric acid production by culturable bacteria from the human intestine. Retrieved May 13, 2015, from http://www.ncbi.nlm.nih.gov/pubmed/22612585

[92] Abou-Donia, M. (2008). Splenda alters gut microflora and increases intestinal p-glycoprotein and cytochrome p-450 in male rats. Retrieved May 13, 2015, from http://www.ncbi.nlm.nih.gov/pubmed/18800291

[93] Scott, K. (2014). Prebiotic stimulation of human colonic butyrate-producing bacteria and bifidobacteria, in vitro. Retrieved May 13, 2015, from http://www.ncbi.nlm.nih.gov/pubmed/23909466

[94] Gao, Z. (2009, April 14). Butyrate Improves Insulin Sensitivity and Increases Energy Expenditure in Mice | ADA. Retrieved May 13, 2015, from http://diabetes.diabetesjournals.org/content/58/7/1509.full

[95] Ozturk, A., Degirmenci, Y., Tokmak, B., & Tokmak, A. (2013, April 1). Frequency of migraine in patients with allergic rhinitis. Retrieved May 6, 2015, from http://www.ncbi.nlm.nih.gov/pmc/articles/PMC3809225/

[96] Nakanishi, Y. (2008, February 1). Monosodium glutamate (MSG): A villain and promoter of liver inflammation and dysplasia. Retrieved May 6, 2015, from http://www.ncbi.nlm.nih.gov/pubmed/18178378

[97] Greenberg, A. (2006, February 1). Obesity and the role of adipose tissue in inflammation and metabolism. Retrieved May 6, 2015, from http://ajcn.nutrition.org/content/83/2/461S.full#ref-3

[98] ScienceDaily. (2015, March 23). Association between migraine, carpal tunnel syndrome found. Retrieved May 6, 2015, from http://www.sciencedaily.com/releases/2015/03/150323130853.htm

[99] Kister, I. (2010). Migraine is comorbid with multiple sclerosis and associated with a more symptomatic MS course. Retrieved May 15, 2015, from http://www.ncbi.nlm.nih.gov/pubmed/20625916

[100] Simons, F. (2011, February 1). World Allergy Organization Guidelines for the Assessment and Management of Anaphylaxis. Retrieved May 6, 2015, from http://www.csaci.ca/include/files/WAO_Anaphylaxis_Guidelines_2011.pdf

[101] Coyle, J. (2012). Inflammation, Cytokines and Glutamate | American Society for Neurochemistry. Retrieved May 6, 2015, from http://www.elsevierdirect.com/companions/9780123749475/boxes/Chapter_060.pdf

[102] McNally, L. (2008, June). Inflammation, glutamate, and glia in depression: A literature review. Retrieved May 6, 2015, from http://www.ncbi.nlm.nih.gov/pubmed/18567974

[103] Erhardt, S. (2013, January 9). Connecting inflammation with glutamate agonism in suicidality. Retrieved May 6, 2015, from http://www.nature.com/npp/journal/v38/n5/abs/npp2012248a.html

[104] Uzar, E. (2011, October). Serum cytokine and pro-brain natriuretic peptide (BNP) levels in patients with migraine. Retrieved May 6, 2015, from http://www.ncbi.nlm.nih.gov/pubmed/22165670

[105] Deans, E. (2011, March 31). Depression - Caused by Inflammation, Thus Like Other Diseases of Civilization. Retrieved May 6, 2015, from https://www.psychologytoday.com/blog/evolutionary-psychiatry/201103/depression-caused-inflammation-thus-other-diseases-civilization

[106] Tepper, S. (2004). New thoughts on sinus headache. Retrieved July 1, 2015, from http://www.ncbi.nlm.nih.gov/pubmed/15176492

[107] Kirthi, V. (2013, April 30). Aspirin with or without an antiemetic for acute migraine headaches in adults. Retrieved May 6, 2015, from http://www.ncbi.nlm.nih.gov/pubmed/23633350

[108] PubMed: Effects of chronic dietary exposure to monosodium glutamate on feeding behavior, adiposity, gastrointestinal motility, and cardiovascular function in healthy adult rats. (n.d.). Retrieved September 9, 2015, from http://www.ncbi.nlm.nih.gov/pubmed/?term=monosodium+glutamate+treated

[109] Youssef, M. (2010). Enhanced Platelet Aggregation, Hyperinsulinemia and Low Testosterone Level in monosodium glutamate obese rats. Retrieved May 5, 2015, from http://academia.edu/584834/Enhanced_Platelet_Aggregation_Hyperinsulinemia_and_Low_Testosterone_Level_in_monosodium_glutamate_obese_rats

[110] Hirata, A. (1997, May 1). Monosodium glutamate (MSG)-obese rats develop glucose intolerance and insulin resistance to peripheral glucose uptake. Retrieved May 5, 2015, from http://www.ncbi.nlm.nih.gov/pubmed/9283637

[111] Morrison, J. (2007, November 14). Sensory and autonomic nerve changes in the monosodium glutamate-treated rat: A model of type II diabetes. Retrieved May 5, 2015, from http://onlinelibrary.wiley.com/doi/10.1113/expphysiol.2007.039222/full

[112] Diabetes Health Center. (n.d.). Retrieved May 5, 2015, from http://diabetes.webmd.com/guide/insulin-resistance-syndrome

[113] MSG Use Linked To Obesity. (2008, August 14). Retrieved May 5, 2015, from http://www.sciencedaily.com/releases/2008/08/080813164638.htm

[114] Migraine. (2013, June 4). Retrieved May 5, 2015, from http://www.mayoclinic.com/health/migraine-headache/DS00120/DSECTION=causes

[115] Tang-Christensen, M. (1999, April 26). The arcuate nucleus is pivotal in mediating the anorectic effects of centrally administered leptin. Retrieved May 5, 2015, from http://www.ncbi.nlm.nih.gov/pubmed/10363921

[116] Martin, S. (2008, October 7). Leptin resistance: A possible interface of inflammation and metabolism in obesity-related cardiovascular disease. Retrieved May 5, 2015, from http://www.ncbi.nlm.nih.gov/pubmed/18926322

[117] FDA MSG. (n.d.). Retrieved September 9, 2015, from http://www.fda.gov/Food/IngredientsPackagingLabeling/FoodAdditivesIngredients/ucm328728.htm

[118] MONOSODIUM GLUTAMATE. (n.d.). Retrieved May 5, 2015, from http://www.truthinlabeling.org/MonosodiumGlutamate_DefinedForTheWeb.htm

[119] Hidden Sources of MSG. (n.d.). Retrieved May 5, 2015, from http://www.truthinlabeling.org/hiddensources.html

[120] Food and migraine: A personal connection - Harvard Health Blog. (2011, April 5). Retrieved May 11, 2015, from http://www.health.harvard.edu/blog/food-and-migraine-a-personal-connection-201104052222

[121] Tuormaa, T. (1994). The Adverse Effects of Food Additives on Health: A Review of the Literature with Special Emphasis on Childhood Hyperactivity. Retrieved May 11, 2015, from http://www.orthomolecular.org/library/jom/1994/pdf/1994-v09n04-p225.pdf

[122] Huthman, I. (2009). Monosodium Glutamate: A Good Replacement For Hydrogen Peroxide In Bone Preparations. Retrieved May 5, 2015, from https://ispub.com/IJBA/4/1/10469

[123] Glutamic acid. (n.d.). Retrieved May 5, 2015, from http://wholefoodcatalog.info/nutrient/glutamic_acid/

[124] OLNEY, J. (1972, July). GLUTAMATE-INDUCED BRAIN DAMAGE IN INFANT PRIMATES. : Journal of Neuropathology & Experimental Neurology. Retrieved May 5, 2015, from http://journals.lww.com/jneuropath/Abstract/1972/07000/Glutamate_Induced_Brain_Damage_in_Infant_Primates.6.aspx

[125] Kruit, M., Buchem, M. (2011, December 16). Migraine is associated with an increased risk of deep white matter lesions, subclinical posterior circulation infarcts and brain iron accumulation: The population-based MRI CAMERA-study. Retrieved September 16, 2015, from http://www.ncbi.nlm.nih.gov/pmc/articles/PMC3241741/

[126] Body Fortress | Super Advanced Whey Protein. (n.d.). Retrieved May 5, 2015, from http://images.vitaminimages.com/cdn/sd/pdf/L044320-AE.pdf

[127] MSG PDF. (n.d.). Retrieved May 5, 2014, from http://www.cornellcollege.edu/chemistry/cstrong/512/msg.pdf

[128] Jury convicts Shaneka Torres of firing gun at drive-thru window. (n.d.). Retrieved May 5, 2015, from http://www.wzzm13.com/story/news/2015/03/25/drive-thru-shooting/70444680/

[129] Liou, S. (2011, June 26). About Glutamate Toxicity. Retrieved May 5, 2015, from http://www.stanford.edu/group/hopes/cgi-bin/wordpress/2011/06/about-glutamate-toxicity/#excitotoxicity-theory

[130] Glutamine | University of Maryland Medical Center. (n.d.). Retrieved May 5, 2015, from http://umm.edu/health/medical/altmed/supplement/glutamine

[131] U-King-Im, J. (2010, November 18). Acute Hyperammonemic Encephalopathy in Adults: Imaging Findings. Retrieved May 5, 2015, from http://www.ajnr.org/content/32/2/413.full

[132] Mort, D. (2001, August 1). Effect of Acute Exposure to Ammonia on Glutamate Transport in Glial Cells Isolated From the Salamander Retina. Retrieved May 5, 2015, from http://jn.physiology.org/content/86/2/836.full

[133] Mort, D. (2001, August 1). Effect of Acute Exposure to Ammonia on Glutamate Transport in Glial Cells Isolated From the Salamander Retina. Retrieved May 5, 2015, from http://jn.physiology.org/content/86/2/836.full

[134] Anderson, J. (n.d.). How Untreated Celiac Disease Causes Malnutrition. Retrieved May 5, 2015, from http://celiacdisease.about.com/od/commoncomplicationsofcd/a/Untreated-Celiac-Disease-Can-Cause-Malnutrition.htm

[135] USDA Foods List. (n.d.). Retrieved September 9, 2015, from http://ndb.nal.usda.gov/ndb/foods

[136] Egger J. (1983, October 15). Is migraine food allergy? A double-blind controlled trial of oligoantigenic diet treatment. Retrieved May 4, 2015, from http://www.ncbi.nlm.nih.gov/pubmed/6137694

[137] Foods highest in Glutamic acid. (n.d.). Retrieved May 5, 2015, from http://nutritiondata.self.com/foods-000093000000000000000.html

[138] Masic, U. (2013, May 27). Does monosodium glutamate interact with macronutrient composition to influence subsequent appetite? Retrieved May 5, 2015, from http://www.ncbi.nlm.nih.gov/pubmed/23531472

[139] Yang, W. (1997, June 1). The monosodium glutamate symptom complex: Assessment in a double-blind, placebo-controlled, randomized study. Retrieved May 5, 2015, from http://www.ncbi.nlm.nih.gov/pubmed/9215242?dopt=Abstract

[140] Adult Obesity Facts CDC. (2014, September 9). Retrieved May 5, 2015, from http://www.cdc.gov/obesity/data/adult.html

[141] Barański, M. (2014, September 14). Higher antioxidant and lower cadmium concentrations and lower incidence of pesticide residues in organically grown crops: A systematic literature review and meta-analyses. Retrieved September 10, 2015, from http://www.ncbi.nlm.nih.gov/pubmed/24968103

[142] Carman, J. (n.d.). A long-term toxicology study on pigs fed a combined genetically modified (GM) soy and GM maize diet. Retrieved May 11, 2015, from http://www.organic-systems.org/journal/81/8106.pdf

[143] Dr. Don Huber Talks about Genetically-Engineered Foods. (n.d.). Retrieved May 11, 2015, from http://articles.mercola.com/sites/articles/archive/2011/12/10/dr-don-huber-interview-part-1.aspx?e_cid=20111210_DNL_art_1

[144] Séralin, G. (2014). Retraction notice to "Long term toxicity of a Roundup herbicide and a Roundup-tolerant genetically modified maize" Retrieved May 11, 2015, from http://www.ncbi.nlm.nih.gov/pubmed/24490213

[145] Séralin, G. (2014). Retraction notice to "Long term toxicity of a Roundup herbicide and a Roundup-tolerant genetically modified maize" Retrieved May 11, 2015, from http://www.ncbi.nlm.nih.gov/pubmed/24490213

[146] Hammond, B. (2004, June 1). Results of a 13 week safety assurance study with rats fed grain from glyphosate tolerant corn. Retrieved May 11, 2015, from http://www.ncbi.nlm.nih.gov/pubmed/15110110

[147] Soffritti, M. (2006, June 29). 3. CANCER PREVENTION: THE LESSON FROM THE LAB. Retrieved May 11, 2015, from

http://www.academia.edu/1617769/3._CANCER_PREVENTION_THE_LESSON_FROM_THE_LAB

[148] Criticism: Séralini used too few animals to draw any conclusions. (n.d.). Retrieved May 11, 2015, from http://www.gmoSéralini.org/criticism-Séralini-used-too-few-animals/

[149] H.R.933 - Consolidated and Further Continuing Appropriations Act, 2013113th Congress (2013-2014). (n.d.). Retrieved May 11, 2015, from http://beta.congress.gov/bill/113th-congress/house-bill/933

[150] Anger over 'The Monsanto Protection Act' (n.d.). Retrieved May 11, 2015, from http://stream.aljazeera.com/story/201303282113-0022643

[151] 'Monsanto Protection Act': 5 Terrifying Things To Know About The HR 933 Provision. (2013, March 27). Retrieved May 11, 2015, from http://www.ibtimes.com/monsanto-protection-act-5-terrifying-things-know-about-hr-933-provision-1156079

[152] Sean Poulter for the Daily Mail. (2012, September 26). Russia suspends import and use of American GM corn after study revealed cancer risk. Retrieved May 11, 2015, from http://www.dailymail.co.uk/news/article-2208452/Russia-suspends-import-use-American-GM-corn-study-revealed-cancer-risk.html

[153] Séralini, G. (2011, March 1). Genetically modified crops safety assessments: Present limits and possible improvements. Retrieved May 11, 2015, from http://www.enveurope.com/content/23/1/10

[154] Finamore, A. (2008, December 10). Intestinal and peripheral immune response to MON810 maize ingestion in weaning and old mice. Retrieved May 11, 2015, from http://www.ncbi.nlm.nih.gov/pubmed/19007233

[155] Magaña-Gómez, J. (2009). Risk assessment of genetically modified crops for nutrition and health. Retrieved May 11, 2015, from http://www.ncbi.nlm.nih.gov/pubmed/19146501

[156] D'Andrea, G. (2004, May 25). Elevated levels of circulating trace amines in primary headaches. Retrieved May 5, 2015, from http://www.ncbi.nlm.nih.gov/pubmed/15159465

[157] Schwalfenberg, G. (2011, October 12). The Alkaline Diet: Is There Evidence That an Alkaline pH Diet Benefits Health? Retrieved May 5, 2015, from http://www.ncbi.nlm.nih.gov/pmc/articles/PMC3195546/

[158] D'Andre Dell'Aglio, D. (2009, April 29). Acute Metformin Overdose: Examining Serum pH, Lactate Level, and Metformin Concentrations in Survivors Versus Nonsurvivors: A Systematic Review of the Literature. Retrieved May 5, 2015, from http://www.annemergmed.com/article/S0196-0644(09)00486-7/abstract

[159] Schwalfenberg, G. (2011, October 12). The Alkaline Diet: Is There Evidence That an Alkaline pH Diet Benefits Health? Retrieved May 5, 2015, from http://www.ncbi.nlm.nih.gov/pmc/articles/PMC3195546/

[160] Gastritis | University of Maryland Medical Center. (n.d.). Retrieved May 5, 2015, from http://umm.edu/health/medical/altmed/condition/gastritis

[161] Patterson, A., Yildiz, V., Klatt, M., & Malarkey, W. (2013, August 6). Perceived stress predicts allergy flares. Retrieved May 5, 2015, from http://www.ncbi.nlm.nih.gov/pmc/articles/PMC4120667/

[162] Alpay, K. (2010, July). Diet restriction in migraine, based on IgG against foods: A clinical double-blind, randomised, cross-over trial. Retrieved May 5, 2015, from http://www.ncbi.nlm.nih.gov/pmc/articles/PMC2899772/

[163] Asthma and Allergy Foundation of America - Information About Asthma, Allergies, Food Allergies and More! (n.d.). Retrieved May 5, 2015, from http://www.aafa.org/display.cfm?id=9&sub=20&cont=728

[164] Tappy, L. (2010). Metabolic effects of fructose and the worldwide increase in obesity. Retrieved May 5, 2015, from http://www.ncbi.nlm.nih.gov/pubmed/20086073

[165] Choi, H., Willett, W., & Curhan, G. (2010, November 24). Fructose-Rich Beverages and the Risk of Gout in Women. Retrieved May 5, 2015, from http://www.ncbi.nlm.nih.gov/pmc/articles/PMC3058904/

[166] Bazzano, L. (2008, April 4). Intake of Fruit, Vegetables, and Fruit Juices and Risk of Diabetes in Women. Retrieved May 5, 2015, from http://care.diabetesjournals.org/content/31/7/1311.abstract?sid=78c93e1d-7ad7-463b-8e77-b27826ffe640

[167] Robey, I. (2012, August 1). Examining the relationship between diet-induced acidosis and cancer. Retrieved May 5, 2015, from http://www.ncbi.nlm.nih.gov/pmc/articles/PMC3571898/

[168] Higher dietary acid load increases risk of diabetes, study says. (n.d.). Retrieved May 5, 2015, from http://www.sciencedaily.com/releases/2013/11/131111185514.htm

[169] Drewnowski, A. (2000, December). Bitter taste, phytonutrients, and the consumer: A review1,2,3. Retrieved May 5, 2015, from http://ajcn.nutrition.org/content/72/6/1424.full

[170] Healthy and Unhealthy Fats: Eat Healthy Fats | POS Pilot Plant Corporation (n.d.). Retrieved May 6, 2015, from http://www.aneggadayisok.ca/managing-cholesterol/healthy-tips-for-managing-cholesterol/healthy-fats-vs-unhealthy-fats/

[171] Estruch, R. (2013, April 4). Primary prevention of cardiovascular disease with a Mediterranean diet. Retrieved May 6, 2015, from http://www.ncbi.nlm.nih.gov/pubmed/23432189

[172] Beltrán, G. (2004, June 2). Influence of harvest date and crop yield on the fatty acid composition of virgin olive oils from cv. Picual. Retrieved May 6, 2015, from http://www.ncbi.nlm.nih.gov/pubmed/15161211

[173] Frankel, E. (2011, April 1). Evaluation of Extra-Virgin Olive Oil Sold in California. Retrieved May 6, 2015, from http://olivecenter.ucdavis.edu/research/files/report041211finalreduced.pdf

[174] Eat Wild - Super Natural. (n.d.). Retrieved May 6, 2015, from http://www.eatwild.com/articles/superhealthy.html

[175] FDA Ban PHO 2018. (n.d.). Retrieved September 17, 2015, from http://blogs.fda.gov/fdavoice/index.php/2015/06/protecting-consumers-from-trans-fat/

[176] Trans Fats | American Heart Association. (n.d.). Retrieved May 6, 2015, from http://www.heart.org/HEARTORG/GettingHealthy/FatsAndOils/Fats101/Trans-Fats_UCM_301120_Article.jsp

[177] Remig, V. (2010, April). Trans fats in America: A review of their use, consumption, health implications, and regulation. Retrieved May 6, 2015, from http://www.ncbi.nlm.nih.gov/pubmed/20338284

[178] Foods highest in Total trans fatty acids. (n.d.). Retrieved May 6, 2015, from http://nutritiondata.self.com/foods-000071000000000000000.html

[179] Stender, S. (2006, May). A trans world journey. Retrieved May 6, 2015, from http://www.sciencedirect.com/science/article/pii/S1567568806000377

[180] Countries Compared by Health Obesity. International Statistics OECD. (n.d.). Retrieved May 6, 2015, from http://www.nationmaster.com/country-info/stats/Health/Obesity

[181] Kavanagh, K. (2007, July 1). Trans fat diet induces abdominal obesity and changes in insulin sensitivity in monkeys. Retrieved May 6, 2015, from http://www.ncbi.nlm.nih.gov/pubmed/17636085

[182] Luevano-Contreras, C., & Chapman-Novakofski, K. (2010, December 13). Dietary Advanced Glycation End Products and Aging. Retrieved May 6, 2015, from http://www.ncbi.nlm.nih.gov/pmc/articles/PMC3257625/?tool=pubmed

[183] Nutrition Facts and Analysis for Syrups, corn, high-fructose. (n.d.). Retrieved May 6, 2015, from http://nutritiondata.self.com/facts/sweets/5600/2

[184] Vos, M., Kimmons, J., Gillespie, C., Welsh, J., & Blanck, H. (2008, July 9). Dietary Fructose Consumption Among US Children and Adults: The Third National Health and Nutrition Examination Survey. Retrieved May 6, 2015, from http://www.ncbi.nlm.nih.gov/pmc/articles/PMC2525476/

[185] Bray, G. (2007, October). How bad is fructose?1,2. Retrieved May 6, 2015, from http://ajcn.nutrition.org/content/86/4/895.full

[186] Warren Buffett's secret to staying young: "I eat like a six-year-old.". (2015, February 25). Retrieved May 6, 2015, from http://fortune.com/2015/02/25/warren-buffett-diet-coke/

[187] 104-year-old woman shares her secret: 3 cans of Dr. Pepper a day. (2015, March 19). Retrieved May 6, 2015, from http://fox2now.com/2015/03/19/104-year-old-woman-shares-her-secret-3-cans-of-dr-pepper-a-day/

[188] Ludwig, D. (2001, February 17). Relation between consumption of sugar-sweetened drinks and childhood obesity: A prospective, observational analysis. Retrieved May 6, 2015, from http://www.ncbi.nlm.nih.gov/pubmed/11229668

[189] Choi, H. (2010, November 24). Fructose-rich beverages and risk of gout in women. Retrieved May 6, 2015, from http://www.ncbi.nlm.nih.gov/pubmed/21068145

[190] Sparvero, L., Asafu-Adjei, D. (2009, March 17). RAGE (Receptor for Advanced Glycation Endproducts), RAGE Ligands, and their role in Cancer and Inflammation. Retrieved May 6, 2015, from http://www.ncbi.nlm.nih.gov/pmc/articles/PMC2666642/

[191] Brant, A. (2007, April 1). Baker's asthma. Retrieved May 6, 2015, from http://www.ncbi.nlm.nih.gov/pubmed/17351468

[192] Shewry, P. (2009, February 13). Wheat. Retrieved May 6, 2015, from http://jxb.oxfordjournals.org/content/60/6/1537.full

[193] Van de Wouw, M. (2010, April 1). Genetic diversity trends in twentieth century crop cultivars: A meta analysis. Retrieved May 6, 2015, from http://www.ncbi.nlm.nih.gov/pubmed/20054521/

[194] Broeck, H., Jong, H. (2010, July 28). Presence of celiac disease epitopes in modern and old hexaploid wheat varieties: Wheat breeding may have contributed to increased prevalence of celiac disease. Retrieved May 6, 2015, from http://www.ncbi.nlm.nih.gov/pmc/articles/PMC2963738/

[195] Olmstead, A., & Rhode, P. (2010, December 27). Adapting North American wheat production to climatic challenges, 1839–2009. Retrieved May 6, 2015, from http://www.ncbi.nlm.nih.gov/pmc/articles/PMC3021086/

[196] World Wheat Production, World Maize Production, World Rice Production. (n.d.). Retrieved May 6, 2015, from http://www.nue.okstate.edu/Crop_Information/World_Wheat_Production.htm

[197] Rubio-Tapia, A. (2009, July 1). Increased prevalence and mortality in undiagnosed celiac disease. Retrieved May 6, 2015, from http://www.ncbi.nlm.nih.gov/pubmed/19362553/

[198] Lohi, S. (2007, November 1). Increasing prevalence of coeliac disease over time. Retrieved May 6, 2015, from http://www.ncbi.nlm.nih.gov/pubmed/17944736/

[199] Kappler, M., Krauss-Etschmann, S., Diehl, V., Zeilhofer, H., & Koletzko, S. (2006, January 28). Detection of secretory IgA antibodies against gliadin and human tissue transglutaminase in stool to screen for coeliac disease in children: Validation study. Retrieved May 6, 2015, from http://www.ncbi.nlm.nih.gov/pmc/articles/PMC1352053/

[200] Daniëlle, A. (2010, May 5). Diagnostic Testing for Celiac Disease Among Patients With Abdominal Symptoms. Retrieved May 6, 2015, from http://jama.jamanetwork.com/article.aspx?articleid=185775

[201] Bizzaro, N. (2012, June 1). Cutting-edge issues in celiac disease and in gluten intolerance. Retrieved May 6, 2015, from http://www.ncbi.nlm.nih.gov/pubmed/21181303

[202] Fasano, A. (2003, February 10). Prevalence of celiac disease in at-risk and not-at-risk groups in the United States: A large multicenter study. Retrieved May 6, 2015, from http://www.ncbi.nlm.nih.gov/pubmed/12578508

[203] Anderson, J. (n.d.). How Many People Have Gluten Sensitivity. Retrieved May 6, 2015, from http://celiacdisease.about.com/od/glutenintolerance/a/How-Many-People-Have-Gluten-Sensitivity.htm

[204] Katcher, H. (2008). The effects of a whole grain–enriched hypocaloric diet on cardiovascular disease risk factors in men and women with metabolic syndrome1,2,3. Retrieved May 6, 2015, from http://ajcn.nutrition.org/content/87/1/79.abstract?sid=6a2dfac6-858a-466f-8435-eb1f1ecc3127

[205] Masters, R., Liese, A., Haffner, S., Wagenknecht, L., & Hanley, A. (2010, March 1). Whole and Refined Grain Intakes Are Related to Inflammatory Protein Concentrations in Human Plasma. Retrieved May 6, 2015, from http://www.ncbi.nlm.nih.gov/pmc/articles/PMC2821887/

[206] Teitelbaum, J. (2011). Iodine Deficiency - An Old Epidemic Is Back. Retrieved May 15, 2015, from http://www.psychologytoday.com/blog/complementary-medicine/201108/iodine-deficiency-old-epidemic-is-back

[207] Lisotto, C., Mainardi, F., Maggioni, F., & Zanchin, G. (2013, February 21). The comorbidity between migraine and hypothyroidism. Retrieved May 15, 2015, from http://www.ncbi.nlm.nih.gov/pmc/articles/PMC3620300/

[208] Messina, M. (2006). Effects of soy protein and soybean isoflavones on thyroid function in healthy adults and hypothyroid patients: A review of the relevant literature. Retrieved May 15, 2015, from http://www.ncbi.nlm.nih.gov/pubmed/16571087

[209] FDA. (n.d.). Health Claim Notification for Whole Grain Foods. Retrieved May 6, 2015, from http://www.fda.gov/Food/IngredientsPackagingLabeling/LabelingNutrition/ucm073639.htm

[210] Mozaffarian, R. (2013, January 4). Identifying whole grain foods: A comparison of different approaches for selecting more healthful whole grain products. Retrieved May 6, 2015, from http://www.ncbi.nlm.nih.gov/pubmed/23286205

[211] Menéndez-Buxadera, A. (2007, November 12). Multi-trait and random regression approaches for addressing the wide range of weaning ages in Asturiana de los Valles beef cattle for genetic parameter estimation. Retrieved May 6, 2015, from http://www.ncbi.nlm.nih.gov/pubmed/17998432

[212] What is Lactose Intolerance? (n.d.). Retrieved May 6, 2015, from http://www.pcrm.org/search/?cid=254

[213] Tishkoff, S. (2006, December 10). Convergent adaptation of human lactase persistence in Africa and Europe. Retrieved May 6, 2015, from http://www.ncbi.nlm.nih.gov/pmc/articles/PMC2672153/

[214] Crittenden, R. (2005, December 1). Cow's milk allergy: A complex disorder. Retrieved May 6, 2015, from http://www.ncbi.nlm.nih.gov/pubmed/16373958

[215] Fortt, R. (1997, September 1). The identification of 'casein' in human breast cancer. Retrieved May 6, 2015, from http://www.ncbi.nlm.nih.gov/pubmed/385473

[216] Hebert, J. (1998, November 4). Nutritional and socioeconomic factors in relation to prostate cancer mortality: A cross-national study. Retrieved May 6, 2015, from http://www.ncbi.nlm.nih.gov/pubmed/9811313

[217] Milk Consumption and Prostate Cancer. (n.d.). Retrieved May 6, 2015, from http://www.pcrm.org/health/health-topics/milk-consumption-and-prostate-cancer

[218] Hirayama, T. (1997, November 1). Epidemiology of prostate cancer with special reference to the role of diet. Retrieved May 6, 2015, from http://www.ncbi.nlm.nih.gov/pubmed/537622

Citations

[219] Ratner, D. (1983, September 1). Milk protein-free diet for nonseasonal asthma and migraine in lactase-deficient patients. Retrieved May 6, 2015, from http://www.ncbi.nlm.nih.gov/pubmed/6643018

[220] Berkey, C. (2005, June 1). Milk, Dairy Fat, Dietary Calcium, and Weight Gain. Retrieved May 6, 2015, from http://archpedi.jamanetwork.com/article.aspx?articleid=486041

[221] Rist, P. (2015, August 15). Dietary patterns according to headache and migraine status: A cross-sectional study. Retrieved September 17, 2015, from http://www.ncbi.nlm.nih.gov/pubmed/25424709

[222] Cordain, L. (2002, December 1). Acne vulgaris: A disease of Western civilization. Retrieved May 6, 2015, from http://www.ncbi.nlm.nih.gov/pubmed/12472346?dopt=AbstractPlus

[223] Adebamowo, C. (2008, May). Milk consumption and acne in teenaged boys. Retrieved May 6, 2015, from http://www.jaad.org/article/S0190-9622(07)02402-4/

[224] Ferdowsian, H. (2010, March 1). Does diet really affect acne? Retrieved May 6, 2015, from http://www.ncbi.nlm.nih.gov/pubmed/20361171

[225] Unger, A. (1952, September 1). Migraine is an allergic disease. Retrieved May 5, 2015, from http://www.sciencedirect.com/science/article/pii/0021870752900075

[226] Mattes, R. (2009). Nonnutritive sweetener consumption in humans: Effects on appetite and food intake and their putative mechanisms. Retrieved May 6, 2015, from http://www.ncbi.nlm.nih.gov/pubmed/19056571/

[227] HSC NEWS - New analysis suggests 'diet soda paradox' – less sugar, more weight. (n.d.). Retrieved May 6, 2015, from http://www.uthscsa.edu/hscnews/singleformat2.asp?newID=1539

[228] Rogers, P. (1988). Uncoupling sweet taste and calories: Comparison of the effects of glucose and three intense sweeteners on hunger and food intake. Retrieved May 7, 2015, from http://www.ncbi.nlm.nih.gov/pubmed/3200909

[229] Fagherazzi, G. (2013, January 30). Consumption of artificially and sugar-sweetened beverages and incident type 2 diabetes in the Etude Epidémiologique... Retrieved May 7, 2015, from http://ajcn.nutrition.org/content/early/2013/01/30/ajcn.112.050997

[230] Swithers, S. (2008, February 1). Result FiltersA role for sweet taste: Calorie predictive relations in energy regulation by rats. Retrieved May 7, 2015, from http://www.ncbi.nlm.nih.gov/pubmed/18298259

[231] BRAIN SEROTONIN CHANGES IN PHENYLALANINE-FED RATS. (2006, October 4). Retrieved May 7, 2015, from http://onlinelibrary.wiley.com/doi/10.1111/j.1471-4159.1969.tb08990.x/abstract

[232] FDA Docket # 02P-0317. (n.d.). Retrieved May 7, 2015, from http://www.fda.gov/ohrms/dockets/dailys/03/Jan03/012203/02P-0317_emc-000196.txt

[233] Medical Management Guidelines for Formaldehyde. (n.d.). Retrieved May 7, 2015, from http://www.atsdr.cdc.gov/mmg/mmg.asp?id=216&tid=39

[234] Dockets, FDA. (2004, July 8). Retrieved May 7, 2015, from http://www.fda.gov/ohrms/dockets/dailys/04/july04/071204/02P-0317-emc00346.txt

[235] FDA Docket # 02P-0317 Recall Aspartame. (2003, January 12). Retrieved May 7, 2015, from http://www.fda.gov/ohrms/dockets/dailys/03/jan03/012203/02p-0317_emc-000199.txt

[236] Aspartame | C14H18N2O5 - PubChem. (n.d.). Retrieved May 7, 2015, from http://pubchem.ncbi.nlm.nih.gov/compound/aspartame#section=Metabolism-Metabolites

[237] Stegink, L. (1981, February 1). Blood methanol concentrations in normal adult subjects administered abuse doses of aspartame. Retrieved May 7, 2015, from http://www.ncbi.nlm.nih.gov/pubmed/7230276

[238] Olney, J. (1980). Brain damage in mice from voluntary ingestion of glutamate and aspartate. Retrieved May 7, 2015, from http://www.ncbi.nlm.nih.gov/pubmed/7290308

[239] Deshpande, L. (2007, August 1). Activation of a novel injury-induced calcium-permeable channel that plays a key role in causing extended neuronal depolarization and initiating neuronal death in excitotoxic neuronal injury. Retrieved May 7, 2015, from http://www.ncbi.nlm.nih.gov/pubmed/17483292

[240] Olney, J. (1996, November 1). Increasing brain tumor rates: Is there a link to aspartame? Retrieved May 7, 2015, from http://www.ncbi.nlm.nih.gov/pubmed/8939194

[241] Warner, M. (2006, February 11). The Lowdown on Sweet? Retrieved May 7, 2015, from http://www.nytimes.com/2006/02/12/business/yourmoney/12sweet.html?ei=5090&en=f5f173a4cc33d534&ex=1297400400&partner=rssuserland&emc=rss&pagewanted=all&_r=0

[242] Gold, M. (2002, January 12). Docket # 02P-0317 Recall Aspartame as a Neurotoxic Drug: File #7: Aspartame History. Retrieved May 7, 2015, from http://www.fda.gov/ohrms/dockets/dailys/03/Jan03/012203/02P-0317_emc-000202.txt

[243] Aspartame Fraud. (n.d.). Retrieved May 7, 2015, from http://www.mercola.com/article/aspartame/fraud.htm

[244] Tangvoranuntakul, P. (2003, October 14). Human uptake and incorporation of an immunogenic nonhuman dietary sialic acid. Retrieved May 7, 2015, from http://www.ncbi.nlm.nih.gov/pubmed/14523234

[245] How Eating Red Meat Can Spur Cancer Progression. (n.d.). Retrieved May 7, 2015, from http://ucsdnews.ucsd.edu/archive/newsrel/health/11-08RedMeatCancer.asp

[246] Lanou, A., & Svenson, B. (2011). Reduced cancer risk in vegetarians: An analysis of recent reports. Retrieved September 10, 2015, from http://www.ncbi.nlm.nih.gov/pmc/articles/PMC3048091/

[247] Tuso, P., Ismail, M., Ha, B., & Bartolotto, C. (2013). Nutritional Update for Physicians: Plant-Based Diets. Retrieved September 10, 2015, from http://www.ncbi.nlm.nih.gov/pmc/articles/PMC3662288/

[248] Varki, A. (n.d.). Uniquely human evolution of sialic acid genetics and biology, UCSD. Retrieved May 7, 2015, from http://cmm.ucsd.edu/lab_pages/varki/varkilab/Publications/B143.pdf

[249] McDougall, J. (2002, February). Effects of a very low-fat, vegan diet in subjects with rheumatoid arthritis. Retrieved May 7, 2015, from http://www.ncbi.nlm.nih.gov/pubmed/11890437

[250] Varki, A. (n.d.). Evolutionary perspectives on the origins of disease. Retrieved May 7, 2015, from http://cmm.ucsd.edu/varki/varkilab/Publications/B137.pdf

[251] Hodgson, J. (2007, February). Increased Lean Red Meat Intake Does Not Elevate Markers of Oxidative Stress and Inflammation in Humans. Retrieved May 7, 2015, from http://jn.nutrition.org/content/137/2/363.full

[252] University of Maryland Medical Center. (n.d.). Omega-6 fatty acids. Retrieved May 7, 2015, from http://umm.edu/health/medical/altmed/supplement/omega6-fatty-acids

[253] Daley, C., Abbott, A., Doyle, P., Nader, G., & Larson, S. (2010, March 10). A review of fatty acid profiles and antioxidant content in grass-fed and grain-fed beef. Retrieved May 7, 2015, from http://www.ncbi.nlm.nih.gov/pmc/articles/PMC2846864/

[254] Health Benefits of Grass-Fed Products. (n.d.). Retrieved May 7, 2015, from http://www.eatwild.com/healthbenefits.htm

[255] Harel, Z. (2002, August). Supplementation with omega-3 polyunsaturated fatty acids in the management of recurrent migraines in adolescents. Retrieved May 7, 2015, from http://www.ncbi.nlm.nih.gov/pubmed/12127385

[256] Maroon, J. (2006, April 1). Omega-3 fatty acids (fish oil) as an anti-inflammatory: An alternative to nonsteroidal anti-inflammatory drugs for discogenic pain. Retrieved May 7, 2015, from http://www.ncbi.nlm.nih.gov/pubmed/16531187

[257] Non-steroidal anti-inflammatory drugs (NSAIDs) Oregon State University. (n.d.). Retrieved May 7, 2015, from http://www.omapure.com/Can_Help/nsaid.html

[258] Peng, Y., Shi, H., Qi, X., Xiao, C., Zhong, H., Ma, R., & Su, B. (2010, January 20). The ADH1B Arg47His polymorphism in East Asian populations and expansion of rice domestication in history. Retrieved May 7, 2015, from http://www.ncbi.nlm.nih.gov/pmc/articles/PMC2823730/

[259] Maxwell, C., Spangenberg, R., Hoek, J., Silberstein, S., & Oshinsky, M. (2010, December 31). Acetate Causes Alcohol Hangover Headache in Rats. Retrieved May 7, 2015, from http://www.ncbi.nlm.nih.gov/pmc/articles/PMC3013144/

[260] Acetaldehyde. (n.d.). Retrieved May 8, 2015, from http://en.wikipedia.org/wiki/Acetaldehyde

[261] ACETALDEHYDE | Scientific Committee on Cosmetic Products and Non-food. (2004, May 25). Retrieved May 8, 2015, from http://ec.europa.eu/health/ph_risk/committees/sccp/documents/out275_en.pdf

[262] Jung, J. (2014, April). Hypertension associated with alcohol consumption based on the facial flushing reaction to drinking. Retrieved May 8, 2015, from http://www.ncbi.nlm.nih.gov/pubmed/24256516

[263] Waldschmidt, T., Cook, R., & Kovacs, E. (2009, March 1). Alcohol and Inflammation & Immune Responses: Summary of the 2006 Alcohol and Immunology Research Interest Group (AIRIG) meeting. Retrieved May 8, 2015, from http://www.ncbi.nlm.nih.gov/pmc/articles/PMC2377009/

[264] Wang, H., Zakhari, S., & Jung, M. (2010, March 21). Alcohol, inflammation, and gut-liver-brain interactions in tissue damage and disease development. Retrieved May 8, 2015, from http://www.ncbi.nlm.nih.gov/pmc/articles/PMC2842521/

[265] Swift, R. (1998). Alcohol hangover: Mechanisms and mediators. Retrieved May 8, 2015, from http://www.ncbi.nlm.nih.gov/pubmed/15706734

[266] Volpato, S. (2004, February 10). Relationship of alcohol intake with inflammatory markers and plasminogen activator inhibitor-1 in well-functioning older adults: The Health, Aging, and Body Composition study. Retrieved May 8, 2015, from http://www.ncbi.nlm.nih.gov/pubmed/14769682

[267] Lu, B. (2010, December 1). Alcohol consumption and markers of inflammation in women with preclinical rheumatoid arthritis. Retrieved May 8, 2015, from http://www.ncbi.nlm.nih.gov/pubmed/20827783

[268] This is why alcohol doesn't come with nutrition facts. (2015, March 14). Retrieved May 8, 2015, from http://www.vox.com/2014/11/12/7195573/alcohol-nutrition

[269] 'No trouble brewing,' beer industry insists. (n.d.). Retrieved May 8, 2015, from http://www.chinadaily.com.cn/english/doc/2005-07/14/content_460109.htm

[270] Panconesi, A. (2011, June). Alcohol and migraine: What should we tell patients? Retrieved May 8, 2015, from http://www.ncbi.nlm.nih.gov/pubmed/21336550

[271] Simpson, N. (2007, December 1). Sleep and inflammation. Retrieved May 8, 2015, from http://www.ncbi.nlm.nih.gov/pubmed/18240557

[272] Tsai, G. (1998, June 1). Increased glutamatergic neurotransmission and oxidative stress after alcohol withdrawal. Retrieved May 8, 2015, from http://www.ncbi.nlm.nih.gov/pubmed/9619143

[273] FDA. (2009). Acetaminophen Overdose and Liver Injury — Background and Options for Reducing Injury. Retrieved May 8, 2015, from http://www.fda.gov/downloads/AdvisoryCommittees/CommitteesMeetingMaterials/Drugs/DrugSafetyandRiskManagementAdvisoryCommittee/UCM164897.pdf

[274] UC Health - UC San Diego, Acute Liver Failure from Acetaminophen Overdose. (n.d.). Retrieved May 8, 2015, from http://health.ucsd.edu/specialties/gastro/areas-expertise/liver-center/patient-resources/Pages/acetaminophen.aspx

[275] Why Coconut Water Is The Best Sports Drink. (n.d.). Retrieved May 8, 2015, from http://articles.mercola.com/sites/articles/archive/2011/11/27/coconut-water-ultimate-rehydrator.aspx

[276] Gibson, A., Woodside, J. (2012, September 12). Alcohol increases homocysteine and reduces B vitamin concentration in healthy male volunteers—a randomized, crossover intervention study. Retrieved May 8, 2015, from http://www.ncbi.nlm.nih.gov/pmc/articles/PMC2572692/

[277] National Institute on Alcohol Abuse and Alcoholism (NIAAA). (n.d.). Retrieved May 8, 2015, from http://www.niaaa.nih.gov/

[278] Khan, M. (1973, December). Alcohol-induced hangover. A double-blind comparison of pyritinol and placebo in preventing hangover symptoms. Retrieved May 8, 2015, from http://www.ncbi.nlm.nih.gov/pubmed/4588294

[279] Warner, J. (n.d.). Low Vitamin B6 Linked to Inflammation. Retrieved May 8, 2015, from http://www.webmd.com/heart/news/20120619/low-vitamin-b6-linked-to-inflammation

[280] McDowell, L. (2007, January 31). Vitamins and minerals functioning as antioxidants with supplementation considerations | University of Florida. Retrieved May 8, 2015, from http://dairy.ifas.ufl.edu/rns/2007/McDowell.pdf

[281] Alleyne, T. (2005). The control of hypertension by use of coconut water and mauby: Two tropical food drinks. Retrieved May 8, 2015, from http://www.ncbi.nlm.nih.gov/pubmed/15892382

[282] Pittler, M., Verster, J., & Ernst, E. (2005, December 24). Interventions for preventing or treating alcohol hangover: Systematic review of randomised controlled trials. Retrieved May 8, 2015, from http://www.ncbi.nlm.nih.gov/pmc/articles/PMC1322250/

[283] Ohtsuka, Y. (1997, December 1). Reducing cell membrane n-6 fatty acids attenuate mucosal damage in food-sensitive enteropathy in mice. Retrieved May 8, 2015, from http://www.ncbi.nlm.nih.gov/pubmed/9396566

[284] Vojdani, A. (2013). Cross-Reaction between Gliadin and Different Food and Tissue Antigens. Retrieved May 8, 2015, from http://www.scirp.org/Journal/PaperInformation.aspx?paperID=26626#.VUzBMhf6m1k

[285] Cabrera-Chávez, F. (2008, January 15). Transglutaminase treatment of wheat and maize prolamins of bread increases the serum IgA reactivity of celiac disease patients. Retrieved May 8, 2015, from http://www.ncbi.nlm.nih.gov/pubmed/18193828

[286] Cabrera-Chávez, F. (2012, March 1). Maize prolamins resistant to peptic-tryptic digestion maintain immune-recognition by IgA from some celiac disease patients. Retrieved May 8, 2015, from http://www.ncbi.nlm.nih.gov/pubmed/22298027

[287] Bray, G. (2004, October 1). Consumption of high-fructose corn syrup in beverages may play a role in the epidemic of obesity. Retrieved May 8, 2015, from http://www.ncbi.nlm.nih.gov/pubmed/15051594

[288] Corn Allergen List. (n.d.). Retrieved May 8, 2015, from http://www.cornallergens.com/list/corn-allergen-list.php

[289] Foods High in Glutamic acid(per 100 g edible portion). (n.d.). Retrieved May 8, 2015, from http://wholefoodcatalog.info/nutrient/glutamic_acid/foods/high/

[290] Asthma and Allergy Foundation of America. (n.d.). Retrieved May 8, 2015, from http://www.aafa.org

[291] Cordle, C. (2004, May 1). Soy protein allergy: Incidence and relative severity. Retrieved May 8, 2015, from http://www.ncbi.nlm.nih.gov/pubmed/15113974

[292] Soy Protein Intolerance Clinical Presentation. (n.d.). Retrieved May 8, 2015, from http://emedicine.medscape.com/article/932026-clinical

[293] Migraine DC Forum. (n.d.). Retrieved May 11, 2014, from http://www.migrainepage.com/dcforum/discussion/14166.html

[294] HOW IT IS MADE | Prosciutto di Parma. (n.d.). Retrieved May 11, 2015, from http://www.prosciuttodiparma.com/en_UK/prosciutto/how

[295] Scientific Opinion on risk based control of biogenic amine formation in fermented foods | European Food Safety Authority. (2011). Retrieved May 11, 2015, from http://www.efsa.europa.eu/en/search/doc/2393.pdf

[296] Ladero, V. (2010). Toxicological Effects of Dietary Biogenic Amines. Retrieved May 11, 2015, from http://www.ingentaconnect.com/content/ben/cnf/2010/00000006/00000002/art00004

[297] Wimbiscus, M. (2010, December). MAO inhibitors: Risks, benefits, and lore. Retrieved May 11, 2015, from http://www.ncbi.nlm.nih.gov/pubmed/21147941

[298] Jansen, S. (2003). Intolerance to dietary biogenic amines: A review. Retrieved May 11, 2015, from http://www.ncbi.nlm.nih.gov/pubmed/14533654

[299] Millichap, J. (2003). The diet factor in pediatric and adolescent migraine. Retrieved May 11, 2015, from http://www.ncbi.nlm.nih.gov/pubmed/12657413

[300] Ladero, V. (2010). Toxicological Effects of Dietary Biogenic Amines. Retrieved May 11, 2015, from http://www.ingentaconnect.com/content/ben/cnf/2010/00000006/00000002/art00004

[301] Berlin, I. (2001, March 1). Monoamine oxidases and tobacco smoking. Retrieved May 11, 2015, from http://www.ncbi.nlm.nih.gov/pubmed/11343627

[302] Moret, S. (2005, February 1). A survey on free biogenic amine content of fresh and preserved vegetables. Retrieved May 11, 2015, from http://www.sciencedirect.com/science/article/pii/S0308814604002079

[303] Shalaby, A. (1996). Significance of biogenic amines to food safety and human health. Retrieved May 11, 2015, from http://www.sciencedirect.com/science/article/pii/S096399699600066X

[304] D'Andrea, G. (2004, May 25). Elevated levels of circulating trace amines in primary headaches. Retrieved May 5, 2015, from http://www.ncbi.nlm.nih.gov/pubmed/15159465

[305] Vieira, S. (2007). Profile and levels of bioactive amines in orange juice and orange soft drink. Retrieved May 11, 2015, from http://www.sciencedirect.com/science/article/pii/S0308814605009520

[306] Shalaby, A. (1996). Significance of biogenic amines to food safety and human health. Retrieved May 11, 2015, from http://www.sciencedirect.com/science/article/pii/S096399699600066X

[307] Walker, S. (1996, October 1). Tyramine content of previously restricted foods in monoamine oxidase inhibitor diets. Retrieved May 11, 2015, from http://www.ncbi.nlm.nih.gov/pubmed/8889911

[308] Adão, R. (2005). Bioactive amines and carbohydrate changes during ripening of `Prata' banana (Musa acuminata × M. balbisiana). Retrieved May 11, 2015, from http://www.sciencedirect.com/science/article/pii/S030881460400384X

[309] Young, S. (2007, November 1). How to increase serotonin in the human brain without drugs. Retrieved May 11, 2015, from http://www.ncbi.nlm.nih.gov/pmc/articles/PMC2077351/

[310] Moret, S. (2005, February 1). A survey on free biogenic amine content of fresh and preserved vegetables. Retrieved May 11, 2015, from http://www.sciencedirect.com/science/article/pii/S0308814604002079

[311] Shalaby, A. (1996). Significance of biogenic amines to food safety and human health. Retrieved May 11, 2015, from http://www.sciencedirect.com/science/article/pii/S096399699600066X

[312] Veciana-Nogues, M. (1996, November 11). Changes in Biogenic Amines during the Manufacture and Storage of Semipreserved Anchovies. Retrieved May 11, 2015, from http://www.ingentaconnect.com/content/iafp/jfp/1996/00000059/00000011/art00013

[313] Jae-Hyung, M. (2002, March 7). Biogenic amines in Jeotkals, Korean salted and fermented fish products. Retrieved May 11, 2015, from http://www.sciencedirect.com/science/article/pii/S0308814602001504

[314] Scientific Opinion on risk based control of biogenic amine formation in fermented foods | European Food Safety Authority. (2011). Retrieved May 11, 2015, from http://www.efsa.europa.eu/en/search/doc/2393.pdf

[315] Panconesi, A. (2008, January 30). Alcohol and migraine: Trigger factor, consumption, mechanisms. A review. Retrieved May 11, 2015, from http://www.ncbi.nlm.nih.gov/pmc/articles/PMC3476173/

[316] Shalaby, A. (1996). Significance of biogenic amines to food safety and human health. Retrieved May 11, 2015, from http://www.sciencedirect.com/science/article/pii/S096399699600066X

[317] Walker, S. (1996, October 1). Tyramine content of previously restricted foods in monoamine oxidase inhibitor diets. Retrieved May 11, 2015, from http://www.ncbi.nlm.nih.gov/pubmed/8889911

[318] Shalaby, A. (1996). Significance of biogenic amines to food safety and human health. Retrieved May 11, 2015, from http://www.sciencedirect.com/science/article/pii/S096399699600066X

[319] Walker, S. (1996, October 1). Tyramine content of previously restricted foods in monoamine oxidase inhibitor diets. Retrieved May 11, 2015, from http://www.ncbi.nlm.nih.gov/pubmed/8889911

[320] Ladero, V. (2010). Toxicological Effects of Dietary Biogenic Amines. Retrieved May 11, 2015, from http://www.ingentaconnect.com/content/ben/cnf/2010/00000006/00000002/art00004

[321] Walker, S. (1996, October 1). Tyramine content of previously restricted foods in monoamine oxidase inhibitor diets. Retrieved May 11, 2015, from http://www.ncbi.nlm.nih.gov/pubmed/8889911

[322] Scientific Opinion on risk based control of biogenic amine formation in fermented foods | European Food Safety Authority. (2011). Retrieved May 11, 2015, from http://www.efsa.europa.eu/en/search/doc/2393.pdf

[323] Ladero, V. (2010). Toxicological Effects of Dietary Biogenic Amines. Retrieved May 11, 2015, from http://www.ingentaconnect.com/content/ben/cnf/2010/00000006/00000002/art00004

[324] Ladero, V. (2010). Toxicological Effects of Dietary Biogenic Amines. Retrieved May 11, 2015, from http://www.ingentaconnect.com/content/ben/cnf/2010/00000006/00000002/art00004

[325] García-García, P. (2001, March 1). Biogenic amines in packed table olives and pickles. Retrieved May 11, 2015, from http://www.ncbi.nlm.nih.gov/pubmed/11252482

[326] Ekici, K. (2004). Histamine Contents of Some Commercial Vegetable Pickles. Retrieved May 11, 2015, from http://www.pjbs.org/pjnonline/fin201.pdf

[327] Ren, J. (2012, April 12). Pickled food and risk of gastric cancer--a systematic review and meta-analysis of English and Chinese literature. Retrieved May 11, 2015, from http://www.ncbi.nlm.nih.gov/pubmed/22499775

[328] Shalaby, A. (1996). Significance of biogenic amines to food safety and human health. Retrieved May 11, 2015, from http://www.sciencedirect.com/science/article/pii/S096399699600066X

[329] Yung-Hsiang, T. (2007). Histamine formation by histamine-forming bacteria in douchi, a Chinese traditional fermented soybean product. Retrieved May 11, 2015, from http://www.sciencedirect.com/science/article/pii/S0308814606008259

[330] Freed, D. (1999, April 17). Do dietary lectins cause disease? : The evidence is suggestive—and raises interesting possibilities for treatment . Retrieved May 11,

2015, from http://www.ncbi.nlm.nih.gov/pmc/articles/PMC1115436/#!po=8.33333

[331] Cummings, R. (2009). Antibodies and Lectins in Glycan Analysis. Retrieved May 11, 2015, from http://www.ncbi.nlm.nih.gov/books/NBK1919/

[332] Department of Animal Science - Plants Poisonous to Livestock. (n.d.). Retrieved May 11, 2015, from http://www.ansci.cornell.edu/plants/toxicagents/lectins.html

[333] Watzl, B. (2001, April). Dietary wheat germ agglutinin modulates ovalbumin-induced immune responses in Brown Norway rats. Retrieved May 11, 2015, from http://www.ncbi.nlm.nih.gov/pubmed/11348563

[334] Monte, L. (2014, March 1). Lectin of Abelmoschus esculentus (okra) promotes selective antitumor effects in human breast cancer cells. Retrieved May 11, 2015, from http://www.ncbi.nlm.nih.gov/pubmed/24129958

[335] Maher, P. (1996, October 15). The role of monoamine metabolism in oxidative glutamate toxicity. Retrieved May 11, 2015, from http://www.ncbi.nlm.nih.gov/pubmed/8815918

[336] Maintz, L. (2008, May 22). Effects of histamine and diamine oxidase activities on pregnancy: A critical review. Retrieved May 11, 2015, from http://www.ncbi.nlm.nih.gov/pubmed/18499706?dopt=AbstractPlus

[337] Silberstein, S. (1997, February). Migraine and pregnancy. Retrieved May 11, 2015, from http://www.ncbi.nlm.nih.gov/pubmed/9058407

[338] Maintz, L. (2008, May 22). Effects of histamine and diamine oxidase activities on pregnancy: A critical review. Retrieved May 11, 2015, from http://www.ncbi.nlm.nih.gov/pubmed/18499706

[339] García-Martín, E. (2015, January 22). Diamine oxidase rs10156191 and rs2052129 variants are associated with the risk for migraine. Retrieved May 11, 2015, from http://www.ncbi.nlm.nih.gov/pubmed/25612138

[340] Moser, J. (2013, September 25). Enzyme Supplementation Useful and Safe in Treating Episodic Migraine: Presented at WCN. Retrieved May 11, 2015, from http://www.firstwordpharma.com/node/1141756?tsid.#axzz2pvl68jEG

[341] Testing if Your DAO Level is Low. (n.d.). Retrieved May 11, 2015, from http://www.thedailyheadache.com/tag/diamine-oxidase

[342] Glycemic index and glycemic load for 100 foods - Harvard Health. (n.d.). Retrieved May 8, 2015, from http://www.health.harvard.edu/newsweek/Glycemic_index_and_glycemic_load_for_100_foods.htm

Citations

[343] Babu, P. (2009). Brown Rice-Beyond the Color Reviving a Lost Health Food - A Review. Retrieved May 8, 2015, from http://www.idosi.org/aeja/2(2)09/4.pdf?origin=publication_detail

[344] Sun, Q., Spiegelman, D., Dam, R., Holmes, M., Malik, V., Willett, W., & Hu, F. (2010, June 14). White Rice, Brown Rice, and Risk of Type 2 Diabetes in US Men and Women. Retrieved May 8, 2015, from http://www.ncbi.nlm.nih.gov/pmc/articles/PMC3024208/

[345] Hu, E., Pan, A., Malik, V., & Sun, Q. (2012, March 15). White rice consumption and risk of type 2 diabetes: Meta-analysis and systematic review. Retrieved May 8, 2015, from http://www.ncbi.nlm.nih.gov/pmc/articles/PMC3307808/

[346] Hoshi, A. (1995). Risk factors for mortality and mortality rate of sumo wrestlers. Retrieved May 13, 2015, from http://www.ncbi.nlm.nih.gov/pubmed/7474495

[347] Suvarna, B. (2008). Rice, the Allergen. Retrieved May 8, 2015, from http://www.nepjol.info/index.php/NJST/article/viewFile/3187/2772

[348] Riccardi, G. (2008). Role of glycemic index and glycemic load in the healthy state, in prediabetes, and in diabetes. Retrieved May 8, 2015, from http://ajcn.nutrition.org/content/87/1/269S.full

[349] Liu, S. (2003, November 1). Relation between changes in intakes of dietary fiber and grain products and changes in weight and development of obesity among middle-aged women. Retrieved May 8, 2015, from http://ajcn.nutrition.org/content/78/5/920.short

[350] Nutrition Facts Analysis for Rice, white, long-grain, regular, cooked. (n.d.). Retrieved May 8, 2015, from http://nutritiondata.self.com/facts/cereal-grains-and-pasta/5712/2

[351] Simopoulos, A. (2002, October). The importance of the ratio of omega-6/omega-3 essential fatty acids. Retrieved May 8, 2015, from http://www.ncbi.nlm.nih.gov/pubmed/12442909

[352] Dockets, FDA. (2004, July 8). Retrieved May 7, 2015, from http://www.fda.gov/ohrms/dockets/dailys/04/july04/071204/02P-0317-emc00346.txt

[353] Phenylalanine, Uses and Risk WebMD. (n.d.). Retrieved November 13, 2015, from http://www.webmd.com/vitamins-supplements/ingredientmono-653-phenylalanine.aspx?activeingredientid=653&activeingredientname=phenylalanine

[354] Nutrition facts, calories in food, labels, nutritional information and analysis – NutritionData.com . (n.d.). Retrieved May 5, 2015, from http://nutritiondata.self.com

[355] Nutrition facts, calories in food, labels, nutritional information and analysis – NutritionData.com . (n.d.). Retrieved May 5, 2015, from http://nutritiondata.self.com

[356] USDA. (n.d.). Meat and Poultry Labeling Terms. Retrieved May 8, 2015, from http://www.fsis.usda.gov/wps/portal/fsis/topics/food-safety-education/get-answers/food-safety-fact-sheets/food-labeling/meat-and-poultry-labeling-terms/meat-and-poultry-labeling-terms

[357] Meet Real Free-Range Eggs. (n.d.). Retrieved May 8, 2015, from http://www.motherearthnews.com/real-food/tests-reveal-healthier-eggs.aspx?PageId=1#axzz2yJQ2tFbO

[358] Karsten, H. (2010, March 1). Vitamins A, E and fatty acid composition of the eggs of caged hens and pastured hens. Retrieved May 8, 2015, from http://journals.cambridge.org/action/displayAbstract?fromPage=online&aid=7219036

[359] Hu, F. (1999, April 21). A Prospective Study of Egg Consumption and Risk of Cardiovascular Disease in Men and Women. Retrieved May 8, 2015, from http://jama.jamanetwork.com/article.aspx?articleid=189529

[360] Trichopoulou, A. (2006, June 1). Diet and physical activity in relation to overall mortality amongst adult diabetics in a general population cohort. Retrieved May 8, 2015, from http://www.ncbi.nlm.nih.gov/pubmed/16704559

[361] Katz, D. (2011, November 15). Cocoa and chocolate in human health and disease. Retrieved May 8, 2015, from http://www.ncbi.nlm.nih.gov/pubmed/21470061

[362] De Araujo, Q. (2013, August 24). Cacao and Human Health: From Head to Foot - A Review. Retrieved May 8, 2015, from http://www.ncbi.nlm.nih.gov/pubmed/24915376

[363] Bergman, J. (2001, December 1). Psychomotor stimulant effects of beta-phenylethylamine in monkeys treated with MAO-B inhibitors. Retrieved May 8, 2015, from http://www.ncbi.nlm.nih.gov/pubmed/11797065

[364] Cornell University Department of Animal Science - Plants Poisonous to Livestock. (n.d.). Retrieved May 8, 2015, from http://www.ansci.cornell.edu/plants/toxicagents/tannin.html

[365] Pizza, V. (2013, April 30). Food Intolerance in Migraine, Neurosciences Department, Second University of Naples. Retrieved May 8, 2015, from http://pharmacologyonline.silae.it/files/archives/2013/vol1/PhOL_2013_1_A004_024_Pizza.pdf

[366] Chung, K. (1999, August). Tannins and human health: A review. Retrieved May 11, 2015, from http://www.ncbi.nlm.nih.gov/pubmed/9759559

[367] Seeram, N. (2008, February 13). Berry fruits: Compositional elements, biochemical activities, and the impact of their intake on human health, performance, and disease. Retrieved May 11, 2015, from http://www.ncbi.nlm.nih.gov/pubmed/18211023

[368] Rossi, L. (2008, December). Benefits from dietary polyphenols for brain aging and Alzheimer's disease. Retrieved May 11, 2015, from http://www.ncbi.nlm.nih.gov/pubmed/18415677

[369] Barone, J. (1996). Caffeine consumption. Retrieved May 11, 2015, from http://www.ncbi.nlm.nih.gov/pubmed/8603790

[370] Moffett, A. (1974, April). Effect of chocolate in migraine: A double-blind study. Retrieved May 11, 2015, from http://www.ncbi.nlm.nih.gov/pubmed/4838915

[371] Salfield, S. (1987, May). Controlled study of exclusion of dietary vasoactive amines in migraine. Retrieved May 11, 2015, from http://www.ncbi.nlm.nih.gov/pubmed/3038036

[372] Marcus, D. (1997, December 1). A double-blind provocative study of chocolate as a trigger of headache. Retrieved May 11, 2015, from http://www.ncbi.nlm.nih.gov/pubmed/9453274

[373] Waterhouse, A. (n.d.). Sulfites | Waterhouse Labs, UC Davis. Retrieved May 11, 2015, from http://waterhouse.ucdavis.edu/whats-in-wine/sulfites-in-wine

[374] AP News. (1986, July 8). FDA Bans Sulfites on Fresh Fruits, Vegetables. Retrieved May 11, 2015, from http://www.apnewsarchive.com/1986/FDA-Bans-Sulfites-on-Fresh-Fruits-Vegetables/id-2f37f730b64242079996cbcd6df60b8e

[375] Lester, M. (1995, June 1). Sulfite sensitivity: Significance in human health. Retrieved May 11, 2015, from http://www.ncbi.nlm.nih.gov/pubmed/8586770

[376] Taylor, S. (2001, September 1). Food Allergies and Other Food Sensitivities - IFT.org. Retrieved May 11, 2015, from http://www.ift.org/knowledge-center/read-ift-publications/science-reports/scientific-status-summaries/food-allergies-and-other-food-sensitivities.aspx

[377] Do you need to buy sulfite-free to avoid red wine headaches. (n.d.). Retrieved May 11, 2014, from http://www.examiner.com/article/do-you-need-to-buy-sulfite-free-to-avoid-red-wine-headaches

[378] Sulfites | University of Nebraska-Lincoln. (n.d.). Retrieved May 11, 2015, from http://farrp.unl.edu/sulfites-usa

[379] Sulfites: Separating Fact from Fiction | University of Florida. (n.d.). Retrieved May 11, 2015, from http://edis.ifas.ufl.edu/fy731

[380] Nitrate in vegetables - Scientific Opinion of the Panel on Contaminants in the Food chain | European Food Safety Authority. (2008, June 5). Retrieved May 11, 2015, from http://www.efsa.europa.eu/en/efsajournal/pub/689.htm

[381] De Mey, E. (2014, February). The occurrence of N-nitrosamines, residual nitrite and biogenic amines in commercial dry fermented sausages and evaluation of their occasional relation. Retrieved May 11, 2015, from http://www.ncbi.nlm.nih.gov/pubmed/24200576

[382] Nabrzyski, M. (1994). The content of nitrates and nitrites in fruits, vegetables and other foodstuffs. Retrieved May 11, 2015, from http://www.ncbi.nlm.nih.gov/pubmed/7777773

[383] Monte, S. (2012). Brain Insulin Resistance and Deficiency as Therapeutic Targets in Alzheimer's Disease. Retrieved May 12, 2015, from http://www.ncbi.nlm.nih.gov/pmc/articles/PMC3349985/?report=classic

[384] Scanlan, R. (2000). Nitrosamines and Cancer. Retrieved May 12, 2015, from http://lpi.oregonstate.edu/research-newsletter

[385] Dykhuizen, R., Frazer, R., Duncan, C., Smith, C., Golden, M., Benjamin, N., & Leifert, C. (1996, June 1). Antimicrobial effect of acidified nitrite on gut pathogens: Importance of dietary nitrate in host defense. Retrieved May 12, 2015, from http://www.ncbi.nlm.nih.gov/pmc/articles/PMC163343/

[386] Qin, J., Yang, L., Chen, B., Wang, X., Li, F., Liao, P., & He, L. (2008, December 7). Interaction of methylenetetrahydrofolate reductase C677T, cytochrome P4502E1 polymorphism and environment factors in esophageal cancer in Kazakh population. Retrieved May 12, 2015, from http://www.ncbi.nlm.nih.gov/pmc/articles/PMC2773864/

[387] DeLaMonte, S. (2011, April 6). Alzheimer's: Diabetes of the Brain? By Dr. Suzanne DeLaMonte Alpert Medical School, Brown University Neuropathologist, Rhode Island Hospital.

[388] How Male and Female Brains Differ | WebMD. (n.d.). Retrieved May 12, 2015, from http://www.webmd.com/balance/features/how-male-female-brains-differ?page=2

[389] Paterson, R., Uchino, K., Emsley, H., & Pullicino, P. (2013, May 18). Recurrent Stereotyped Episodes in Cerebral Amyloid Angiopathy: Response to Migraine Prophylaxis in Two Patients. Retrieved May 12, 2015, from http://www.ncbi.nlm.nih.gov/pmc/articles/PMC3670647/?report=classic

[390] Kruuse, C. (2003). Migraine can be induced by sildenafil without changes in middle cerebral artery diameter. Retrieved May 11, 2015, from http://www.ncbi.nlm.nih.gov/pubmed/12477710

[391] Brown, G. (2003, June 1). Inflammatory neurodegeneration mediated by nitric oxide, glutamate, and mitochondria. Retrieved May 11, 2015, from http://www.ncbi.nlm.nih.gov/pubmed/12845153

[392] Reid, I. (1994). Role of nitric oxide in the regulation of renin and vasopressin secretion. Retrieved May 14, 2015, from http://www.ncbi.nlm.nih.gov/pubmed/7534728

[393] Schüller, H. (1992, May 1). Nitrosamine-induced Lung Carcinogenesis and Ca2/Calmodulin Antagonists1. Retrieved May 14, 2015, from http://www.ncbi.nlm.nih.gov/pubmed/1314135

[394] Bigal, M. (2008, October 1). Memantine in the preventive treatment of refractory migraine. Retrieved May 12, 2015, from http://www.ncbi.nlm.nih.gov/pubmed/19031499

[395] Byrd, A. (2008). Migraine Headache: A Precursor to Alzheimer's Disease? Retrieved May 12, 2015, from https://ispub.com/IJH/8/2/11263

[396] Reger, M. (2004, March 1). Effects of beta-hydroxybutyrate on cognition in memory-impaired adults. Retrieved May 12, 2015, from http://www.ncbi.nlm.nih.gov/pubmed/15123336

[397] Health Weather Maps. (n.d.). Retrieved May 14, 2015, from http://www.accuweather.com/en/us/national/health-maps

[398] Taylor, J. (2013, October 7). Avoiding Migraines Resulting from Changes in Barometric Pressure. Retrieved May 15, 2015, from http://blog.securevideo.com/2013/10/07/avoiding-migraines-resulting-from-changes-in-barometric-pressure/

[399] Kelly, P. (2007). Directly measured cabin pressure conditions during Boeing 747-400 commercial aircraft flights. Retrieved May 15, 2015, from http://www.ncbi.nlm.nih.gov/pubmed/17587417

[400] US City Barometric Pressure Records. (n.d.). Retrieved May 15, 2015, from http://www.wunderground.com/resources/pressure_records.asp?MR=1

[401] Kimoto, K. (2011). Influence of barometric pressure in patients with migraine headache. Retrieved May 15, 2015, from http://www.ncbi.nlm.nih.gov/pubmed/21921370

[402] People With Joint Pain Can Really Forecast Thunderstorms. (2008). Retrieved May 14, 2015, from http://www.sciencedaily.com/releases/2008/05/080530174619.htm

[403] Brenner, B., Cheng, D., Clark, S., & Camargo, C. (2011). Positive Association between Altitude and Suicide in 2584 US Counties. Retrieved May 15, 2015, from http://www.ncbi.nlm.nih.gov/pmc/articles/PMC3114154/

[404] Ray, K. (2011). Hypobaric hypoxia modulates brain biogenic amines and disturbs sleep architecture. Retrieved May 15, 2015, from http://www.ncbi.nlm.nih.gov/pubmed/21075155

[405] Leibeluft, E. (1998). Why Are So Many Women Depressed? | Scientific American. Retrieved May 15, 2015, from http://www.cmu.edu/CSR/case_studies/depressed_women.html

[406] Study Finds Utah Leads Nation in Antidepressant Use. (2002, February 20). Retrieved May 15, 2015, from http://articles.latimes.com/2002/feb/20/news/mn-28924

[407] There's a Suicide Epidemic in Utah - And One Neuroscientist Thinks He Knows Why. (2014, November 17). Retrieved May 15, 2015, from http://mic.com/articles/104096/there-s-a-suicide-epidemic-in-utah-and-one-neuroscientist-thinks-he-knows-why

[408] Sun, L. (2014). Potential biomarkers predicting risk of pulmonary hypertension in congenital heart disease: The role of homocysteine and hydrogen sulfide. Retrieved May 15, 2015, from http://www.ncbi.nlm.nih.gov/pubmed/24571884

[409] Association between C677T polymorphism of MTHFR gene and development of high altitude pulmonary hypertension (HAPH). (W/Citations). (n.d.). Retrieved May 15, 2015, from http://www.ers-education.org/Media/Media.aspx?idMedia=8675

[410] Yudkin, D. (2015). Without Friends or Family, even Extraordinary Experiences are Disappointing. Retrieved May 15, 2015, from http://www.scientificamerican.com/article/without-friends-or-family-even-extraordinary-experiences-are-disappointing/?WT.mc_id=SA_Facebook

[411] Migraine sensitivity to smells symptoms. (n.d.). Retrieved May 15, 2015, from http://migraine.com/migraine-symptoms/sensitivity-to-smells/

[412] Lima, A. (2011). Odors as triggering and worsening factors for migraine in men. Retrieved May 15, 2015, from http://www.ncbi.nlm.nih.gov/pubmed/21625759

[413] Not So Sexy, Hidden Chemicals in Perfume and Cologne | EWG. (2010). Retrieved May 15, 2015, from http://www.ewg.org/research/not-so-sexy

[414] Trasande, L. (2015, March 5). Estimating Burden and Disease Costs of Exposure to Endocrine-Disrupting Chemicals in the European Union. Retrieved May 15, 2015, from http://press.endocrine.org/doi/10.1210/jc.2014-4324

[415] Tony Robbins - 30 years of stuttering, cured in 7 minutes! (n.d.). Retrieved May 15, 2015, from https://youtu.be/3eOJaprDCDA

[416] Newhouse, P. (1988). Intravenous nicotine in Alzheimer's disease: A pilot study. Retrieved May 11, 2015, from http://www.ncbi.nlm.nih.gov/pubmed/3137593

Citations

[417] McClernon, F. (2006, November). Transdermal nicotine attenuates depression symptoms in nonsmokers: A double-blind, placebo-controlled trial. Retrieved May 11, 2015, from http://www.ncbi.nlm.nih.gov/pubmed/16977477

[418] Nicotine Stimulates New Blood Vessel Formation; Also Promotes Tumor Growth And Atherosclerosis. (2001, July 31). Retrieved May 11, 2015, from http://www.sciencedaily.com/releases/2001/07/010730075130.htm

[419] CDC. (n.d.). Facts About Cyanide. Retrieved May 11, 2015, from http://www.bt.cdc.gov/agent/cyanide/basics/facts.asp

[420] López-Mesonero, L., Márquez, S., Parra, P., Gámez-Leyva, G., Muñoz, P., & Pascual, J. (2009). Smoking as a precipitating factor for migraine: a survey in medical students. *The Journal of Headache and Pain*, *10*(2), 101.

[421] Jéquier, E. (2002, September 1). Pathways to obesity. Retrieved May 11, 2015, from http://www.ncbi.nlm.nih.gov/pubmed/12174324

[422] Veldhorst, M. (2010, June 22). Presence or absence of carbohydrates and the proportion of fat in a high-protein diet affect appetite... Retrieved May 12, 2015, from http://www.ncbi.nlm.nih.gov/pubmed/20565999

[423] Johnston, C. (2002, February). Postprandial thermogenesis is increased 100% on a high-protein, low-fat diet versus a high-carbohydrate, low-fat diet in healthy, young women. Retrieved May 12, 2015, from http://www.ncbi.nlm.nih.gov/pubmed/11838888

[424] Weigle, D. (2005, July 1). A high-protein diet induces sustained reductions in appetite, ad libitum caloric intake, and body weight despite compensatory changes in diurnal plasma leptin and ghrelin concentrations. Retrieved May 12, 2015, from http://ajcn.nutrition.org/content/82/1/41.abstract

[425] Glycemic index and glycemic load for 100 foods - Harvard Health. (n.d.). Retrieved May 8, 2015, from http://www.health.harvard.edu/newsweek/Glycemic_index_and_glycemic_load_for_100_foods.htm

[426] National Toxicology Program 13th Report on Carcinogens. (n.d.). Retrieved May 12, 2015, from http://ntp.niehs.nih.gov/pubhealth/roc/roc13/index.html

[427] Dabelea, D. (2014, May 17). Prevalence of Type 1 and Type 2 Diabetes, 2001 to 2009 | JAMA. Retrieved May 12, 2015, from http://jama.jamanetwork.com/article.aspx?articleid=1866098

[428] Festa, A. (2000, February 2). Chronic Subclinical Inflammation as Part of the Insulin Resistance Syndrome | AHA. Retrieved May 12, 2015, from http://circ.ahajournals.org/content/102/1/42.full

[429] Harris, G. (2005, March 1). F.D.A. Official Admits 'Lapses' on Vioxx. Retrieved May 12, 2015, from http://www.nytimes.com/2005/03/02/politics/02fda.html

[430] Psaty, B. (2008, April 16). Reporting Mortality Findings in Trials of Rofecoxib for Alzheimer Disease or Cognitive Impairment. Retrieved May 12, 2015, from http://jama.jamanetwork.com/article.aspx?articleid=181772

[431] Despite Warnings, Drug Giant Took Long Path to Vioxx Recall. (2004, November 13). Retrieved May 12, 2015, from http://www.nytimes.com/2004/11/14/business/14merck.html?pagewanted=3&_r=2&

[432] Bird, N. (2009). Ice cream headache--site, duration, and relationship to migraine. Retrieved May 12, 2015, from http://www.ncbi.nlm.nih.gov/pubmed/1555929

[433] Fuh, J. (2003, December 1). Ice-cream headache--a large survey of 8359 adolescents. Retrieved May 12, 2015, from http://www.ncbi.nlm.nih.gov/pubmed/14984231

[434] Kirthi, V. (2013, April 30). Aspirin with or without an antiemetic for acute migraine headaches in adults. Retrieved May 6, 2015, from http://www.ncbi.nlm.nih.gov/pubmed/23633350

[435] Shapiro, R. (n.d.). Caffeine and Migraine | ACHE. Retrieved May 12, 2015, from http://www.achenet.org/resources/caffeine_and_migraine/

[436] Solinas, M. (2002, August 1). Caffeine induces dopamine and glutamate release in the shell of the nucleus accumbens. Retrieved May 12, 2015, from http://www.ncbi.nlm.nih.gov/pubmed/12151508

[437] Gomes, C. (2011, May 1). Adenosine receptors and brain diseases: Neuroprotection and neurodegeneration. Retrieved May 12, 2015, from http://www.ncbi.nlm.nih.gov/pubmed/21145878

[438] Tauler, P. (2013, July 1). Effects of caffeine on the inflammatory response induced by a 15-km run competition. Retrieved May 12, 2015, from http://www.ncbi.nlm.nih.gov/pubmed/23299767

[439] Lovallo, W. (2006, May 2). Cortisol responses to mental stress, exercise, and meals following caffeine intake in men and women. Retrieved May 12, 2015, from http://www.ncbi.nlm.nih.gov/pubmed/16631247

[440] Biaggioni, I. (2002, February 1). Caffeine: A Cause of Insulin Resistance? Retrieved May 12, 2015, from http://care.diabetesjournals.org/content/25/2/399.full

[441] Van Dam, R. (n.d.). Coffee, Caffeine, and Risk of Type 2 Diabetes: American Diabetes Association. Retrieved November 16, 2015, from http://care.diabetesjournals.org/content/29/2/398.full

Citations

[442] Soliman, K. (2002, December 4). Incidence, level, and behavior of aflatoxins during coffee bean roasting and decaffeination. Retrieved May 12, 2015, from http://www.ncbi.nlm.nih.gov/pubmed/12452679

[443] Batista, L. (2009, September 1). Ochratoxin A in coffee beans (Coffea arabica L.) processed by dry and wet methods. Retrieved May 12, 2015, from http://www.sciencedirect.com/science/article/pii/S0956713508002818

[444] Van der Stegen. (2001). Effect of roasting conditions on reduction of ochratoxin a in coffee. Retrieved May 12, 2015, from http://www.ncbi.nlm.nih.gov/pubmed/11600012

[445] Stegen, V. (1997). Screening of European coffee final products for occurrence of ochratoxin A (OTA). Retrieved May 12, 2015, from http://www.ncbi.nlm.nih.gov/pubmed/9135718

[446] Hope, J., & Hope, B. (2011, December 29). A Review of the Diagnosis and Treatment of Ochratoxin A Inhalational Exposure Associated with Human Illness and Kidney Disease including Focal Segmental Glomerulosclerosis. Retrieved May 12, 2015, from http://www.ncbi.nlm.nih.gov/pmc/articles/PMC3255309/

[447] Juliano, L. (2004, September 21). A critical review of caffeine withdrawal: Empirical validation of symptoms and signs, incidence, severity, and associated features. Retrieved May 12, 2015, from http://www.ncbi.nlm.nih.gov/pubmed/15448977

[448] Noseda, R., Kainz, V., Jakubowski, M., Gooley, J., Saper, C., Digre, K., & Burstein, R. (2010, August 1). A neural mechanism for exacerbation of headache by light. Retrieved May 15, 2015, from http://www.ncbi.nlm.nih.gov/pmc/articles/PMC2818758/

[449] Delezie, J. (2011). Interactions between metabolism and circadian clocks: Reciprocal disturbances. Retrieved May 15, 2015, from http://www.ncbi.nlm.nih.gov/pubmed/22211891

[450] Macular Degeneration: MedlinePlus. (n.d.). Retrieved May 15, 2015, from http://www.nlm.nih.gov/medlineplus/maculardegeneration.html

[451] Scientists discover drug that could combat migraines. (2013). Retrieved May 15, 2015, from http://www.medicalnewstoday.com/articles/265330.php

[452] Blue-blocking Glasses To Improve Sleep And ADHD Symptoms Developed. (2007). Retrieved May 15, 2015, from http://www.sciencedaily.com/releases/2007/11/071112143308.htm

[453] Sasseville, A. (2006). Blue blocker glasses impede the capacity of bright light to suppress melatonin production. Retrieved May 15, 2015, from http://www.ncbi.nlm.nih.gov/pubmed/16842544

[454] Calhoun, A. (2007, September 1). Behavioral sleep modification may revert transformed migraine to episodic migraine. Retrieved May 13, 2015, from http://www.ncbi.nlm.nih.gov/pubmed/17883522

[455] Chronic Migraine | Migraine Trust. (n.d.). Retrieved May 13, 2015, from http://www.migrainetrust.org/chronic-migraine

[456] Bettendorff, L. (1996). Paradoxical sleep deprivation increases the content of glutamate and glutamine in rat cerebral cortex. Retrieved May 13, 2015, from http://www.ncbi.nlm.nih.gov/pubmed/8650466

[457] Novati, A. (2012, February 1). Chronic partial sleep deprivation reduces brain sensitivity to glutamate N-methyl-D-aspartate receptor-mediated neurotoxicity. Retrieved May 13, 2015, from http://www.ncbi.nlm.nih.gov/pubmed/21672070

[458] Feature, D. (n.d.). Do Your Sleep Habits Trigger Migraines? Retrieved May 13, 2015, from http://www.webmd.com/migraines-headaches/features/do-your-sleep-habits-trigger-migraines

[459] Feature, D. (n.d.). Do Your Sleep Habits Trigger Migraines? Retrieved May 13, 2015, from http://www.webmd.com/migraines-headaches/features/do-your-sleep-habits-trigger-migraines

[460] Kodama, T. (1998, January 5). Enhanced glutamate release during REM sleep in the rostromedial medulla as measured by in vivo microdialysis. Retrieved May 13, 2015, from http://www.ncbi.nlm.nih.gov/pubmed/9497097

[461] Napping may not be such a no-no - Harvard Health. (2014, November 19). Retrieved May 13, 2015, from http://www.health.harvard.edu/newsletters/Harvard_Health_Letter/2009/November/napping-may-not-be-such-a-no-no

[462] Calhoun, A. (2007, September 1). Behavioral sleep modification may revert transformed migraine to episodic migraine. Retrieved May 13, 2015, from http://www.ncbi.nlm.nih.gov/pubmed/17883522

[463] Migraines no longer a concern for Percy Harvin. (2013, March 13). Retrieved May 13, 2015, from http://profootballtalk.nbcsports.com/2013/03/13/migraines-no-longer-a-concern-for-percy-harvin/

[464] Sleepless Nights May Put The Aging Brain At Risk Of Dementia. (2012, August 27). Retrieved May 13, 2015, from http://www.npr.org/sections/health-shots/2012/08/27/159983037/sleepless-nights-may-put-the-aging-brain-at-risk-of-dementia

[465] Sleep, Learning, and Memory | Harvard. (n.d.). Retrieved May 13, 2015, from http://healthysleep.med.harvard.edu/healthy/matters/benefits-of-sleep/learning-memory

Citations

[466] Sleep and Disease Risk. (n.d.). Retrieved May 13, 2015, from http://healthysleep.med.harvard.edu/healthy/matters/consequences/sleep-and-disease-risk

[467] Poor Sleep Linked to Firefighter Deaths | Time. (2014, November 14). Retrieved May 13, 2015, from http://time.com/3584980/sleep-problems-firefighters-death-insomnia-shift-work-sleep-apnea/

[468] Sleep: The Ultimate Brainwasher? (2013, October 17). Retrieved May 13, 2015, from http://news.sciencemag.org/brain-behavior/2013/10/sleep-ultimate-brainwasher

[469] Acknowledging Preindustrial Patterns of Sleep May Revolutionize Approach to Sleep Dysfunction. (n.d.). Retrieved May 13, 2015, from http://www.psychiatrictimes.com/sleep-disorders/acknowledging-preindustrial-patterns-sleep-may-revolutionize-approach-sleep-dysfunction

[470] Wehr, T. (1992, June 1). In short photoperiods, human sleep is biphasic. Retrieved May 13, 2015, from http://www.ncbi.nlm.nih.gov/pubmed/10607034

[471] Absurd New Ways Splenda is Deceiving You. (n.d.). Retrieved May 11, 2015, from http://articles.mercola.com/sites/articles/archive/2011/06/20/absurd-new-ways-splenda-is-deceiving-you.aspx

[472] Walton, R. (n.d.). Aspartame Studies: Correlation of Funding and Outcome | Northeastern Ohio Universities College of Medicine. Retrieved May 11, 2015, from http://www.worldstar.com/~trufax/online/aspartame.html

[473] Patel, R. (2006, September 1). Popular sweetner sucralose as a migraine trigger. Retrieved May 11, 2015, from http://www.ncbi.nlm.nih.gov/pubmed/16942478

[474] Teixido, M. (2013, May 3). Migraine safe foods listed by category. Retrieved May 11, 2015, from http://www.migrainedisorders.org/migraine-safe-foods-by-category/

[475] Hand, B. (n.d.). Common Foods that Can Trigger Migraines. Retrieved May 11, 2015, from http://www.sparkpeople.com/resource/nutrition_articles.asp?id=1840&page=2

[476] Migraine Diaries. (n.d.). Retrieved May 15, 2015, from http://diary.migrainetrust.org/assets/x/50044

[477] The Big-8: UNIVERSITY OF NEBRASKA. (n.d.). Retrieved September 11, 2015, from https://farrp.unl.edu/informallbig8

[478] Alpay, K. (2010, January 3). Diet restriction in migraine, based on IgG against foods: A clinical double-blind, randomised, cross-over trial. Retrieved May 8, 2015, from http://www.ncbi.nlm.nih.gov/pmc/articles/PMC2899772/pdf/10.1177_0333102410361404.pdf

[479] A Natural Approach to Migraines. (n.d.). Retrieved May 11, 2015, from http://www.pcrm.org/health/health-topics/a-natural-approach-to-migraines

[480] Spigt, M. (2005, September). Increasing the daily water intake for the prophylactic treatment of headache: A pilot trial. Retrieved May 12, 2015, from http://www.ncbi.nlm.nih.gov/pubmed/16128874

[481] Spigt, M. (2011, October 6). A randomized trial on the effects of regular water intake in patients with recurrent headaches. Retrieved May 12, 2015, from http://fampra.oxfordjournals.org/content/early/2011/11/22/fampra.cmr112.full

[482] Spigt, M. (2011, October 6). A randomized trial on the effects of regular water intake in patients with recurrent headaches. Retrieved May 12, 2015, from http://fampra.oxfordjournals.org/content/early/2011/11/22/fampra.cmr112.full

[483] Blau, J. (2004). Water-deprivation headache: A new headache with two variants. Retrieved May 12, 2015, from http://www.ncbi.nlm.nih.gov/pubmed/14979888/

[484] King, T., Toney, G., Tian, P., & Javors, M. (2012, June 8). Dehydration increases sodium-dependent glutamate uptake by hypothalamic paraventricular nucleus synaptosomes. Retrieved May 12, 2015, from http://www.ncbi.nlm.nih.gov/pmc/articles/PMC3370430/

[485] King, T. (2011). Dehydration increases sodium-dependent glutamate uptake by hypothalamic paraventricular nucleus synaptosomes. Retrieved May 12, 2015, from http://www.ncbi.nlm.nih.gov/pubmed/22286787

[486] Brown, R. (2001, April 1). The physiology of brain histamine. Retrieved May 12, 2015, from http://www.ncbi.nlm.nih.gov/pubmed/11164999

[487] Mukamal, K. (2009, March 10). Weather and air pollution as triggers of severe headaches. Retrieved May 12, 2015, from http://www.ncbi.nlm.nih.gov/pubmed/19273827

[488] Dennis, E. (2010, February 8). Water consumption increases weight loss during a hypocaloric diet intervention in middle-aged and older adults. Retrieved May 12, 2015, from http://www.ncbi.nlm.nih.gov/pubmed/19661958

[489] Boschmann, M. (2003, December 1). Water-induced thermogenesis. Retrieved May 12, 2015, from http://www.ncbi.nlm.nih.gov/pubmed/14671205

[490] Popkin, B., D'Anci, K., & Rosenberg, I. (2011, August 1). Water, Hydration and Health. Retrieved May 12, 2015, from http://www.ncbi.nlm.nih.gov/pmc/articles/PMC2908954/

[491] BBC Human Mammal, Human Hunter - Attenborough - Life of Mammals - BBC. (n.d.). Retrieved May 12, 2015, from http://youtu.be/826HMLoiE_o

Citations

[492] Maughan, R. (1996). Restoration of fluid balance after exercise-induced dehydration: Effects of food and fluid intake. Retrieved May 12, 2015, from http://www.ncbi.nlm.nih.gov/pubmed/8781863

[493] Azoulay, A., Garzon, P., & Eisenberg, M. (2001, March 1). Comparison of the Mineral Content of Tap Water and Bottled Waters. Retrieved May 12, 2015, from http://www.ncbi.nlm.nih.gov/pmc/articles/PMC1495189/

[494] Davenward, S. (2013). Silicon-rich mineral water as a non-invasive test of the 'aluminum hypothesis' in Alzheimer's disease. Retrieved May 12, 2015, from http://www.ncbi.nlm.nih.gov/pubmed/22976072

[495] Heil, D. (2010, September 13). Acid-base balance and hydration status following consumption of mineral-based alkaline bottled water. Retrieved May 12, 2015, from http://www.ncbi.nlm.nih.gov/pmc/articles/PMC3161391/

[496] Murray, R. (1978, December). Blood pressure responses to extremes of sodium intake in normal man. Retrieved May 12, 2015, from http://www.ncbi.nlm.nih.gov/pubmed/733808

[497] Graudal, N. (2005, October). Commentary: Possible role of salt intake in the development of essential hypertension. Retrieved May 12, 2015, from http://ije.oxfordjournals.org/content/34/5/972.full

[498] It's Time to End the War on Salt. (2011, July 8). Retrieved May 12, 2015, from http://www.scientificamerican.com/article/its-time-to-end-the-war-on-salt/

[499] A Brief History of Salt | Time. (1982, March 15). Retrieved May 12, 2015, from http://content.time.com/time/magazine/article/0,9171,925341-1,00.html

[500] Shaking Up the Salt Myth. (2012, June 6). Retrieved May 12, 2015, from http://chriskresser.com/specialreports/salt

[501] Stanton, A. (2014, November 4). Dehydration and Salt Deficiency Trigger Migraines - Hormones Matter. Retrieved May 12, 2015, from http://www.hormonesmatter.com/dehydration-salt-deficiency-trigger-migraines/

[502] Hamzany, Y. (2013, February 20). Is human saliva an indicator of the adverse health effects of using mobile phones? Retrieved May 12, 2015, from http://www.ncbi.nlm.nih.gov/pubmed/22894683

[503] MATERIAL SAFETY DATA SHEET Plutonium-241 Radioactivity NIST. (n.d.). Retrieved May 12, 2015, from https://www-s.nist.gov/srmors/msds/4340B-MSDS.pdf?CFID=7582730&CFTOKEN=97ad62e77a70d17a-C6E59DE1-D8E0-C0FF-B13A83B0504AA561&jsessionid=f03024285115bd826f5d1f732b1c485e59b2

[504] Environmental Health and Medicine Education | CDC. (n.d.). Retrieved May 12, 2015, from http://www.atsdr.cdc.gov/csem/csem.asp?csem=7&po=8

[505] Iodized Salt - Salt Institute. (2013, July 13). Retrieved May 12, 2015, from http://www.saltinstitute.org/news-articles/iodized-salt/

[506] Addisons Disease. Symptoms and Information | Patient.co.uk. (n.d.). Retrieved May 12, 2015, from http://www.patient.co.uk/health/addisons-disease-leaflet

[507] Addison disease: MedlinePlus Medical Encyclopedia. (n.d.). Retrieved May 14, 2015, from http://www.nlm.nih.gov/medlineplus/ency/article/000378.htm

[508] Hustad, S. (2004). Phenotypic expression of the methylenetetrahydrofolate reductase 677C--T polymorphism and flavin cofactor availability in thyroid dysfunction. Retrieved May 14, 2015, from http://www.ncbi.nlm.nih.gov/pubmed/15447919

[509] Report on Absorption of magnesium sulfate (Epsom salts) across the skin University of Birmingham. (n.d.). Retrieved May 12, 2015, from http://www.mgwater.com/transdermal.shtml

[510] Alderman, M. (2012, April 5). Dietary Sodium Intake and Cardiovascular Mortality: Controversy Resolved? Retrieved May 12, 2015, from http://ajh.oxfordjournals.org/content/25/7/727.abstract

[511] Tappy, L. (2010). Metabolic effects of fructose and the worldwide increase in obesity. Retrieved May 6, 2015, from http://www.ncbi.nlm.nih.gov/pubmed/20086073

[512] Liu, R. (2003, September 1). Health benefits of fruit and vegetables are from additive and synergistic combinations of phytochemicals. Retrieved May 12, 2015, from http://www.ncbi.nlm.nih.gov/pubmed/12936943

[513] Van Duyn, M. (2000, December 1). Overview of the health benefits of fruit and vegetable consumption for the dietetics professional: Selected literature. Retrieved May 12, 2015, from http://www.ncbi.nlm.nih.gov/pubmed/11138444

[514] World's Fattest Countries | Forbes. (n.d.). Retrieved May 12, 2015, from http://www.forbes.com/2007/02/07/worlds-fattest-countries-forbeslife-cx_ls_0208worldfat.html

[515] Stanhope, K. (2009, May 1). Consuming fructose-sweetened, not glucose-sweetened, beverages increases visceral adiposity and lipids and decreases insulin sensitivity in overweight/obese humans. Retrieved May 12, 2015, from http://www.ncbi.nlm.nih.gov/pmc/articles/PMC2673878/

[516] Livesey, G. (2008, November 1). Fructose consumption and consequences for glycation, plasma triacylglycerol, and body weight: Meta-analyses and meta-regression models of intervention studies. Retrieved May 12, 2015, from http://www.ncbi.nlm.nih.gov/pubmed/18996880

[517] USDA. (n.d.). National Nutrient Database Foods List. Retrieved May 12, 2015, from http://ndb.nal.usda.gov/ndb/

[518] Livesey, G. (2009). Fructose ingestion: dose-dependent responses in health research. *The Journal of nutrition*, *139*(6), 1246S.

[519] Chudnovskiy, R. (2014, October 8). Consumption of clarified grapefruit juice ameliorates high-fat diet induced insulin resistance and weight gain in mice. Retrieved May 12, 2015, from http://www.ncbi.nlm.nih.gov/pubmed/25296035

[520] Paoli, A., Rubini, A., Volek, J., & Grimaldi, K. (2013, June 26). Beyond weight loss: A review of the therapeutic uses of very-low-carbohydrate (ketogenic) diets. Retrieved May 12, 2015, from http://www.ncbi.nlm.nih.gov/pmc/articles/PMC3826507/

[521] Stafstrom, C., & Rho, J. (2012, April 9). The Ketogenic Diet as a Treatment Paradigm for Diverse Neurological Disorders. Retrieved May 12, 2015, from http://www.ncbi.nlm.nih.gov/pmc/articles/PMC3321471/

[522] Medina, J. (2005, January 5). Lactate utilization by brain cells and its role in CNS development. Retrieved May 12, 2015, from http://www.ncbi.nlm.nih.gov/pubmed/15573408

[523] Manninen, A. (2004, December 31). Metabolic Effects of the Very-Low-Carbohydrate Diets: Misunderstood "Villains" of Human Metabolism. Retrieved May 12, 2015, from http://www.ncbi.nlm.nih.gov/pmc/articles/PMC2129159/

[524] Hyperglycemic Crises in Adult Patients With Diabetes | ADA. (2009). Retrieved May 12, 2015, from http://care.diabetesjournals.org/content/32/7/1335.full

[525] Paoli, A., Rubini, A., Volek, J., & Grimaldi, K. (2013, June 26). Beyond weight loss: A review of the therapeutic uses of very-low-carbohydrate (ketogenic) diets. Retrieved May 12, 2015, from http://www.ncbi.nlm.nih.gov/pmc/articles/PMC3826507/

[526] Paoli, A., Rubini, A., Volek, J., & Grimaldi, K. (2013, June 26). Beyond weight loss: A review of the therapeutic uses of very-low-carbohydrate (ketogenic) diets. Retrieved May 12, 2015, from http://www.ncbi.nlm.nih.gov/pmc/articles/PMC3826507/

[527] Lorenzo, C., Coppola, G., Sirianni, G., & Pierelli, F. (2013, February 21). Short term improvement of migraine headaches during ketogenic diet: A prospective observational study in a dietician clinical setting. Retrieved May 12, 2015, from http://www.ncbi.nlm.nih.gov/pmc/articles/PMC3620251/

[528] Nebeling, L. (1995, June 1). Implementing a ketogenic diet based on medium-chain triglyceride oil in pediatric patients with cancer. Retrieved May 12, 2015, from http://www.ncbi.nlm.nih.gov/pubmed/7759747

[529] Dhiman, T. (1999). Conjugated linoleic acid content of milk from cows fed different diets. Retrieved May 12, 2015, from http://www.ncbi.nlm.nih.gov/pubmed/10531600

[530] Hebeisen, D. (1993). Increased concentrations of omega-3 fatty acids in milk and platelet rich plasma of grass-fed cows. Retrieved May 12, 2015, from http://www.ncbi.nlm.nih.gov/pubmed/7905466

[531] Säemann, M. (2000, December 1). Anti-inflammatory effects of sodium butyrate on human monocytes: Potent inhibition of IL-12 and up-regulation of IL-10 production. Retrieved May 12, 2015, from http://www.ncbi.nlm.nih.gov/pubmed/11024006

[532] Hamer, H. (2008, January 15). Review article: The role of butyrate on colonic function. Retrieved May 12, 2015, from http://www.ncbi.nlm.nih.gov/pubmed/17973645

[533] Lührs, H. (2002, April 1). Butyrate inhibits NF-kappaB activation in lamina propria macrophages of patients with ulcerative colitis. Retrieved May 12, 2015, from http://www.ncbi.nlm.nih.gov/pubmed/11989838

[534] St-Onge, M. (2008). Weight-loss diet that includes consumption of medium-chain triacylglycerol oil leads to a greater rate of weight and fat mass loss than does olive oil. Retrieved May 12, 2015, from http://www.ncbi.nlm.nih.gov/pubmed/18326600

[535] Reger, M. (2004, March 1). Effects of beta-hydroxybutyrate on cognition in memory-impaired adults. Retrieved May 12, 2015, from http://www.ncbi.nlm.nih.gov/pubmed/15123336

[536] An Epic Debunking of The Saturated Fat Myth. (2013, May 29). Retrieved May 12, 2015, from http://authoritynutrition.com/it-aint-the-fat-people/

[537] Hite, A. (2010, October). In the face of contradictory evidence: Report of the Dietary Guidelines for Americans Committee. Retrieved May 12, 2015, from http://www.ncbi.nlm.nih.gov/pubmed/20888548

[538] Most Heart Attack Patients' Cholesterol Levels Did Not Indicate Cardiac Risk. (2009, January 13). Retrieved May 12, 2015, from http://www.sciencedaily.com/releases/2009/01/090112130653.htm

[539] Siri-Tarino, P., Sun, Q., Hu, F., & Krauss, R. (2010, January 13). Meta-analysis of prospective cohort studies evaluating the association of saturated fat with cardiovascular disease. Retrieved May 12, 2015, from http://www.ncbi.nlm.nih.gov/pmc/articles/PMC2824152/

[540] Most Heart Attack Patients' Cholesterol Levels Did Not Indicate Cardiac Risk. (2009, January 13). Retrieved May 12, 2015, from http://www.sciencedaily.com/releases/2009/01/090112130653.htm

[541] Sodero, A. (2012, February 17). Cholesterol loss during glutamate-mediated excitotoxicity. Retrieved May 12, 2015, from http://www.ncbi.nlm.nih.gov/pubmed/22343944

[542] Atif, F., Sayeed, I., Ishrat, T., & Stein, D. (2009, June 26). Progesterone with Vitamin D Affords Better Neuroprotection against Excitotoxicity in Cultured Cortical Neurons than Progesterone Alone. Retrieved May 12, 2015, from http://www.ncbi.nlm.nih.gov/pmc/articles/PMC2710287/

[543] Roberts, R. (2012). Relative intake of macronutrients impacts risk of mild cognitive impairment or dementia. Retrieved May 12, 2015, from http://www.ncbi.nlm.nih.gov/pubmed/22810099

[544] Paoli, A., Rubini, A., Volek, J., & Grimaldi, K. (2013, June 26). Beyond weight loss: A review of the therapeutic uses of very-low-carbohydrate (ketogenic) diets. Retrieved May 12, 2015, from http://www.ncbi.nlm.nih.gov/pmc/articles/PMC3826507/

[545] Lorenzo, C., Coppola, G., Sirianni, G., & Pierelli, F. (2013, February 21). Short term improvement of migraine headaches during ketogenic diet: A prospective observational study in a dietician clinical setting. Retrieved May 12, 2015, from http://www.ncbi.nlm.nih.gov/pmc/articles/PMC3620251/

[546] Paoli, A., Grimaldi, K., D'Agostino, D., Cenci, L., Moro, T., Bianco, A., & Palma, A. (2012, July 26). Ketogenic diet does not affect strength performance in elite artistic gymnasts. Retrieved May 12, 2015, from http://www.ncbi.nlm.nih.gov/pmc/articles/PMC3411406/

[547] FDA needs stronger rules to ensure the safety of dietary supplements - Harvard Health Blog. (2012, February 2). Retrieved May 13, 2015, from http://www.health.harvard.edu/blog/fda-needs-stronger-rules-to-ensure-the-safety-of-dietary-supplements-201202024182

[548] Newmaster, S., Grguric, M., Shanmughanandhan, D., Ramalingam, S., & Ragupathy, S. (2013, October 11). DNA barcoding detects contamination and substitution in North American herbal products. Retrieved May 13, 2015, from http://www.ncbi.nlm.nih.gov/pmc/articles/PMC3851815/

[549] What's in Those Supplements? | The New York Times. (2015, February 2). Retrieved May 13, 2015, from http://mobile.nytimes.com/blogs/well/2015/02/03/sidebar-whats-in-those-supplements/?ref=health&_r=1&referrer

[550] Many multivitamins don't have nutrients claimed in label. (2011, June 20). Retrieved May 13, 2015, from http://www.nbcnews.com/id/43429680/ns/health-diet_and_nutrition/t/many-multivitamins-dont-have-nutrients-claimed-label/#.VNuVzt51-GQ

[551] Maghbooli, M. (2014). Comparison between the efficacy of ginger and sumatriptan in the ablative treatment of the common migraine. Retrieved May 14, 2015, from http://www.ncbi.nlm.nih.gov/pubmed/23657930

[552] Mauskop, A. (1998). Role of magnesium in the pathogenesis and treatment of migraines. Retrieved May 13, 2015, from http://www.ncbi.nlm.nih.gov/pubmed/9523054

[553] Mauskop, A. (2012, March 18). Why all migraine patients should be treated with magnesium. Retrieved May 13, 2015, from http://www.ncbi.nlm.nih.gov/pubmed/22426836

[554] Barbagallo, M. (2003). Role of magnesium in insulin action, diabetes and cardio-metabolic syndrome X. Retrieved May 13, 2015, from http://www.ncbi.nlm.nih.gov/pubmed/12537988

[555] Bache, K., Slagsvold, T., & Stenmark, H. (2004, July 21). Defective downregulation of receptor tyrosine kinases in cancer. Retrieved May 13, 2015, from http://www.ncbi.nlm.nih.gov/pmc/articles/PMC514952/

[556] Davis, D. (2009). Declining Fruit and Vegetable Nutrient Composition: What Is the Evidence? Retrieved May 13, 2015, from http://hortsci.ashspublications.org/content/44/1/15.full

[557] Worthington, V. (2001). Nutritional quality of organic versus conventional fruits, vegetables, and grains. Retrieved May 13, 2015, from http://www.ncbi.nlm.nih.gov/pubmed/11327522

[558] Mayer, A. (1997). Historical changes in the mineral content of fruits and vegetables | British Food Journal. Retrieved May 13, 2015, from http://www.emeraldinsight.com/doi/abs/10.1108/00070709710181540

[559] Migraine headache | University of Maryland Medical Center. (n.d.). Retrieved May 13, 2015, from http://umm.edu/health/medical/altmed/condition/migraine-headache

[560] Peikert, A. (1996, June 1). Prophylaxis of migraine with oral magnesium: Results from a prospective, multi-center, placebo-controlled and double-blind randomized study. Retrieved May 13, 2015, from http://www.ncbi.nlm.nih.gov/pubmed/8792038

[561] Magnesium— Health Professional Fact Sheet. (n.d.). Retrieved May 13, 2015, from http://ods.od.nih.gov/factsheets/Magnesium-HealthProfessional/

[562] King, D. (2005, June 1). Dietary magnesium and C-reactive protein levels. Retrieved May 13, 2015, from http://www.ncbi.nlm.nih.gov/pubmed/15930481

[563] Pothmann, R. (2005, March 1). Migraine prevention in children and adolescents: Results of an open study with a special butterbur root extract. Retrieved May 13, 2015, from http://www.ncbi.nlm.nih.gov/pubmed/15836592

[564] Lipton, R. (2004, December 28). Petasites hybridus root (butterbur) is an effective preventive treatment for migraine. Retrieved May 13, 2015, from http://www.ncbi.nlm.nih.gov/pubmed/15623680

[565] Chang, Y. (2012, December 5). Coenzyme Q10 inhibits the release of glutamate in rat cerebrocortical nerve terminals by suppression of voltage-dependent calcium influx and mitogen-activated protein kinase signaling pathway. Retrieved May 13, 2015, from http://www.ncbi.nlm.nih.gov/pubmed/23167655

[566] Hershey, A. (2007, January 15). Coenzyme Q10 deficiency and response to supplementation in pediatric and adolescent migraine. Retrieved May 13, 2015, from http://www.ncbi.nlm.nih.gov/pubmed/17355497

[567] Sándor, P. (2005, February 22). Efficacy of coenzyme Q10 in migraine prophylaxis: A randomized controlled trial. Retrieved May 13, 2015, from http://www.ncbi.nlm.nih.gov/pubmed/15728298

[568] Rozen, T. (2002, March 1). Open label trial of coenzyme Q10 as a migraine preventive. Retrieved May 13, 2015, from http://www.ncbi.nlm.nih.gov/pubmed/11972582

[569] Ghirlanda, G. (1993). Evidence of plasma CoQ10-lowering effect by HMG-CoA reductase inhibitors: A double-blind, placebo-controlled study. Retrieved May 13, 2015, from http://www.ncbi.nlm.nih.gov/pubmed/8463436

[570] Parker, B., Gregory, S., Lorson, L., Polk, D., White, C., & Thompson, P. (2014, May 1). A Randomized Trial of Coenzyme Q10 in Patients with Statin Myopathy: Rationale and Study Design. Retrieved May 13, 2015, from http://www.ncbi.nlm.nih.gov/pmc/articles/PMC3671481/

[571] Tomlinson, S. (2005, May 1). Potential adverse effects of statins on muscle. Retrieved May 13, 2015, from http://www.ncbi.nlm.nih.gov/pubmed/15842193

[572] Pravst, I. (2010, April 1). Coenzyme Q10 contents in foods and fortification strategies. Retrieved May 13, 2015, from http://www.ncbi.nlm.nih.gov/pubmed/20301015

[573] What is vitamin B2? What is riboflavin? (2014). Retrieved May 13, 2015, from http://www.medicalnewstoday.com/articles/219561.php

[574] Boehnke, C. (2004, July 1). High-dose riboflavin treatment is efficacious in migraine prophylaxis: An open study in a tertiary care centre. Retrieved May 13, 2015, from http://www.ncbi.nlm.nih.gov/pubmed/15257686

[575] Maizels, M. (2004, September 22). A combination of riboflavin, magnesium, and feverfew for migraine prophylaxis: A randomized trial. Retrieved May 13, 2015, from http://www.ncbi.nlm.nih.gov/pubmed/15447697

[576] Dietary Reference Intakes for Thiamin, Riboflavin... | US National Library of Medicine. (1998). Retrieved May 13, 2015, from http://www.ncbi.nlm.nih.gov/books/NBK114322/

[577] "Natural" or Alternative Medications for Migraine Prevention | Medscape. (2006). Retrieved May 13, 2015, from http://www.medscape.com/viewarticle/533714_6

[578] Vitamin B12 (cobalamin) | University of Maryland Medical Center. (n.d.). Retrieved May 14, 2015, from https://umm.edu/health/medical/altmed/supplement/vitamin-b12-cobalamin

[579] Shaik, M. (2014). Do folate, vitamins B_6 and B_{12} play a role in the pathogenesis of migraine? The role of pharmacoepigenomics. Retrieved May 14, 2015, from http://europepmc.org/abstract/med/24040787

[580] Lea, R. (2009). The effects of vitamin supplementation and MTHFR (C677T) genotype on homocysteine-lowering and migraine disability. Retrieved May 14, 2015, from http://www.ncbi.nlm.nih.gov/pubmed/19384265

[581] French vegan couple whose baby died of vitamin deficiency after being fed solely on breast milk face jail for child neglect. (n.d.). Retrieved May 14, 2015, from http://www.dailymail.co.uk/news/article-1371172/French-vegan-couple-face-jail-child-neglect-baby-died-vitamin-deficiency.html

[582] Dagnelie, P. (1991). Vitamin B-12 from algae appears not to be bioavailable. Retrieved May 14, 2015, from http://www.ncbi.nlm.nih.gov/pubmed/2000824

[583] Dong, A. (1982). Serum vitamin B12 and blood cell values in vegetarians. Retrieved May 14, 2015, from http://www.ncbi.nlm.nih.gov/pubmed/6897159

[584] Oh, R. (2003, March 1). Vitamin B12 deficiency. Retrieved May 14, 2015, from http://www.ncbi.nlm.nih.gov/pubmed/12643357

[585] Tangney, C. (2011, September 27). Vitamin B12, cognition, and brain MRI measures: A cross-sectional examination. Retrieved May 14, 2015, from http://www.ncbi.nlm.nih.gov/pubmed/21947532

[586] Sethi, N. (2004). Neurological Manifestations Of Vitamin B-12 Deficiency | Saint Vincent's Hospital and Medical Center. Retrieved May 14, 2015, from https://ispub.com/IJNW/2/1/4476

[587] Wang, H. (2008, May 8). Vitamin B(12) and folate in relation to the development of Alzheimer's disease. Retrieved May 14, 2015, from http://www.ncbi.nlm.nih.gov/pubmed/11342684

[588] Tucker, K. (2000). Plasma vitamin B-12 concentrations relate to intake source in the Framingham Offspring study. Retrieved May 14, 2015, from http://www.ncbi.nlm.nih.gov/pubmed/10648266?dopt=Abstract

[589] Zhang, M., Han, W., Hu, S., & Xu, H. (2013, December 26). Methylcobalamin: A Potential Vitamin of Pain Killer. Retrieved May 14, 2015, from http://www.ncbi.nlm.nih.gov/pmc/articles/PMC3888748/

[590] Solomons, N. (2007). Food fortification with folic acid: Has the other shoe dropped? Retrieved May 14, 2015, from http://www.ncbi.nlm.nih.gov/pubmed/18038944

[591] Edwards, R. (2003). Chronic headaches in adults with spina bifida and associated hydrocephalus. Retrieved May 14, 2015, from http://www.ncbi.nlm.nih.gov/pubmed/14758561

[592] Powers, H. (n.d.). Folic acid under scrutiny. Retrieved May 14, 2015, from http://www.ncbi.nlm.nih.gov/pubmed/17697404

[593] Marinus, M. (n.d.). Folic Acid Metabolism | University of Massachusetts Medical School. Retrieved May 14, 2015, from http://users.umassmed.edu/martin.marinus/Mph200/FolicAcidMetabolism.pdf

[594] Bailey, S. (2009, September 8). The extremely slow and variable activity of dihydrofolate reductase in human liver and its implications for high folic acid intake. Retrieved May 14, 2015, from http://www.ncbi.nlm.nih.gov/pubmed/19706381

[595] Cario, H. (2011, February 11). Dihydrofolate reductase deficiency due to a homozygous DHFR mutation causes megaloblastic anemia and cerebral folate deficiency leading to severe neurologic disease. Retrieved May 14, 2015, from http://www.ncbi.nlm.nih.gov/pubmed/21310277

[596] Hirsch, S. (2009). Colon cancer in Chile before and after the start of the flour fortification program with folic acid. Retrieved May 14, 2015, from http://www.ncbi.nlm.nih.gov/pubmed/19190501

[597] Is your breakfast giving you cancer? (2010, March 29). Retrieved May 14, 2015, from http://www.nbcnews.com/id/35874922/ns/health-diet_and_nutrition/t/your-breakfast-giving-you-cancer/#.VVR2Qhf6m1l

[598] Vollset, S. (2013, March 23). Effects of folic acid supplementation on overall and site-specific cancer incidence during the randomised trials: Meta-analyses of data on 50,000 individuals. Retrieved May 14, 2015, from http://www.ncbi.nlm.nih.gov/pubmed/23352552

[599] Large amounts of folic acid shown to promote growth of breast cancer in rats. (2014, January 21). Retrieved May 14, 2015, from http://www.sciencedaily.com/releases/2014/01/140121183414.htm

[600] Food Labeling: Revision of the Nutrition and Supplement Facts Labels. (n.d.). Retrieved July 1, 2015, from https://www.federalregister.gov/articles/2014/03/03/2014-04387/food-labeling-revision-of-the-nutrition-and-supplement-facts-labels#h-78

[601] Smith, A. (2008, March 1). Is folic acid good for everyone? Retrieved May 14, 2015, from http://www.ncbi.nlm.nih.gov/pubmed/18326588

[602] Troen, A. (2006). Unmetabolized folic acid in plasma is associated with reduced natural killer cell cytotoxicity among postmenopausal women. Retrieved May 14, 2015, from http://www.ncbi.nlm.nih.gov/pubmed/16365081

[603] Kresser, C. (2012, March 9). The little known (but crucial) difference between folate and folic acid. Retrieved May 14, 2015, from http://chriskresser.com/folate-vs-folic-acid

[604] Folate | NIH. (n.d.). Retrieved May 14, 2015, from http://ods.od.nih.gov/factsheets/Folate-HealthProfessional/

[605] Boris, M. (2004). Association of MTHFR Gene Variants with Autism. Retrieved May 14, 2015, from http://www.jpands.org/vol9no4/boris.pdf

[606] Pizza, V., Agresta, A., Agresta, A., Lamaida, E., Lamaida, N., Infante, F., & Capasso, A. (2012, August 17). Migraine and Genetic Polymorphisms: An Overview. Retrieved May 14, 2015, from http://www.ncbi.nlm.nih.gov/pmc/articles/PMC3434423/

[607] Methylation Inhibited by Candida's Toxin - MTHFR.Net. (n.d.). Retrieved May 14, 2015, from http://mthfr.net/methylation-inhibited-by-candidas-toxin/2012/09/08/

[608] Maintz, L. (2008, May 22). Effects of histamine and diamine oxidase activities on pregnancy: A critical review. Retrieved May 14, 2015, from http://humupd.oxfordjournals.org/content/14/5/485.full.pdf

[609] Ziaee, A., Tehrani, N., Hosseinkhani, Z., Kazemifar, A., Javadi, A., & Karimzadeh, T. (2012). Effects of folic acid plus levothyroxine on serum homocysteine level in hypothyroidism. Retrieved May 14, 2015, from http://www.ncbi.nlm.nih.gov/pmc/articles/PMC3861905/

[610] Norman, A. (2008). From vitamin D to hormone D: Fundamentals of the vitamin D endocrine system essential for good health. Retrieved May 14, 2015, from http://www.ncbi.nlm.nih.gov/pubmed/18689389

[611] Vitamin D is Now the Most Popular Vitamin. (n.d.). Retrieved May 14, 2015, from http://www.orthomolecular.org/resources/omns/v09n01.shtml

[612] Atif, F., Sayeed, I., Ishrat, T., & Stein, D. (2009, June 26). Progesterone with Vitamin D Affords Better Neuroprotection against Excitotoxicity in Cultured

Cortical Neurons than Progesterone Alone. Retrieved May 14, 2015, from
http://www.ncbi.nlm.nih.gov/pmc/articles/PMC2710287/

[613] Norman, A. (2008). From vitamin D to hormone D: Fundamentals of the vitamin D endocrine system essential for good health. Retrieved May 14, 2015, from http://ajcn.nutrition.org/content/88/2/491S.long

[614] Vacek, J. (2012, February 1). Vitamin D deficiency and supplementation and relation to cardiovascular health. Retrieved May 14, 2015, from
http://www.ncbi.nlm.nih.gov/pubmed/22071212

[615] Low vitamin D levels linked to increased risks after noncardiac surgery. (2014, August 15). Retrieved May 14, 2015, from
http://www.sciencedaily.com/releases/2014/08/140815102033.htm

[616] Garland, C. (2009). Vitamin D for cancer prevention: Global perspective. Retrieved May 14, 2015, from http://www.ncbi.nlm.nih.gov/pubmed/19523595

[617] Lappe, J. (2007). Vitamin D and calcium supplementation reduces cancer risk: Results of a randomized trial. Retrieved May 14, 2015, from
http://www.ncbi.nlm.nih.gov/pubmed/17556697.

[618] Mohr, S. (2014, March). Meta-analysis of vitamin D sufficiency for improving survival of patients with breast cancer. Retrieved May 14, 2015, from
http://www.ncbi.nlm.nih.gov/pubmed/24596354

[619] Ginde, A., Liu, M., & Camargo, C. (2009, March 23). Demographic Differences and Trends of Vitamin D Insufficiency in the US Population, 1988–2004. Retrieved May 14, 2015, from http://www.ncbi.nlm.nih.gov/pmc/articles/PMC3447083/

[620] Harris, S. (2006). Vitamin D and African Americans. Retrieved May 14, 2015, from http://jn.nutrition.org/content/136/4/1126.full

[621] Reid, I. (1994). Role of nitric oxide in the regulation of renin and vasopressin secretion. Retrieved May 14, 2015, from
http://www.ncbi.nlm.nih.gov/pubmed/7534728

[622] Schüller, H. (1992, May 1). Nitrosamine-induced Lung Carcinogenesis and Ca2/Calmodulin Antagonists1. Retrieved May 14, 2015, from
http://www.ncbi.nlm.nih.gov/pubmed/1314135

[623] Causal link found between vitamin D, serotonin synthesis and autism in new study. (n.d.). Retrieved May 14, 2015, from
http://www.sciencedaily.com/releases/2014/02/140226110836.htm

[624] Anglin, R. (2013). Vitamin D deficiency and depression in adults: Systematic review and meta-analysis. Retrieved May 14, 2015, from
http://www.ncbi.nlm.nih.gov/pubmed/23377209

[625] Holick, M. (2006). High prevalence of vitamin D inadequacy and implications for health. Retrieved May 14, 2015, from http://www.ncbi.nlm.nih.gov/pubmed/16529140

[626] Bjelakovic, G. (2011). Vitamin D supplementation for prevention of mortality in adults. Retrieved May 14, 2015, from http://www.ncbi.nlm.nih.gov/m/pubmed/21735411/

[627] Vitamin D | NIH. (n.d.). Retrieved May 14, 2015, from http://ods.od.nih.gov/factsheets/VitaminD-HealthProfessional/#en11

[628] Warner, J. (n.d.). Too Little Vitamin D Puts Heart at Risk. Retrieved May 14, 2015, from http://www.webmd.com/heart-disease/news/20081201/too-little-vitamin-d-puts-heart-at-risk

[629] Indoor Tanning Is Not Safe | CDC. (2015, February 10). Retrieved May 14, 2015, from http://www.cdc.gov/cancer/skin/basic_info/indoor_tanning.htm

[630] Rhodes, L. (2003). Effect of eicosapentaenoic acid, an omega-3 polyunsaturated fatty acid, on UVR-related cancer risk in humans. An assessment of early genotoxic markers. Retrieved May 14, 2015, from http://www.ncbi.nlm.nih.gov/pubmed/12771037

[631] Diener, H. (2005). Efficacy and safety of 6.25 mg t.i.d. feverfew CO2-extract (MIG-99) in migraine prevention--a randomized, double-blind, multicentre, placebo-controlled study. Retrieved May 14, 2015, from http://www.ncbi.nlm.nih.gov/pubmed/16232154

[632] Feverfew. (n.d.). Retrieved May 14, 2014, from http://www.med.nyu.edu/content?ChunkIID=21713#ref14

[633] Murphy, J. (1988, July 23). Randomised double-blind placebo-controlled trial of feverfew in migraine prevention. Retrieved May 14, 2015, from http://www.ncbi.nlm.nih.gov/pubmed/2899663

[634] Lucas, L. (2011). Molecular mechanisms of inflammation. Anti-inflammatory benefits of virgin olive oil and the phenolic compound oleocanthal. Retrieved May 14, 2015, from http://www.ncbi.nlm.nih.gov/pubmed/21443487

[635] Bogani, P. (2007). Postprandial anti-inflammatory and antioxidant effects of extra virgin olive oil. Retrieved May 14, 2015, from http://www.ncbi.nlm.nih.gov/pubmed/16488419

[636] Ramsden, C. (2013, July 22). Targeted alteration of dietary n-3 and n-6 fatty acids for the treatment of chronic headaches: A randomized trial. Retrieved May 14, 2015, from http://www.ncbi.nlm.nih.gov/pubmed/23886520

[637] Marik, P. (2009). Omega-3 dietary supplements and the risk of cardiovascular events: A systematic review. Retrieved May 14, 2015, from http://www.ncbi.nlm.nih.gov/pubmed/19609891

[638] Burr, M. (2003). Lack of benefit of dietary advice to men with angina: Results of a controlled trial. Retrieved May 14, 2015, from http://www.ncbi.nlm.nih.gov/pubmed/12571649

[639] When it comes to fish oil, more is not better. (2010, October 25). Retrieved May 14, 2015, from http://chriskresser.com/when-it-comes-to-fish-oil-more-is-not-better

[640] Bunea, R. (2004). Evaluation of the effects of Neptune Krill Oil on the clinical course of hyperlipidemia. Retrieved May 14, 2015, from http://www.ncbi.nlm.nih.gov/pubmed/15656713

[641] Blasbalg, T. (2011). Changes in consumption of omega-3 and omega-6 fatty acids in the United States during the 20th century. Retrieved May 14, 2015, from http://www.ncbi.nlm.nih.gov/pubmed/21367944

[642] Hamel, E. (2007). Serotonin and migraine: Biology and clinical implications. Retrieved May 14, 2015, from http://www.ncbi.nlm.nih.gov/pubmed/17970989

[643] Titus, F. (1986). 5-Hydroxytryptophan versus methysergide in the prophylaxis of migraine. Randomized clinical trial. Retrieved May 14, 2015, from http://www.ncbi.nlm.nih.gov/pubmed/3536521

[644] 5-Hydroxytryptophan. (n.d.). Retrieved May 14, 2014, from http://www.med.nyu.edu/content?ChunkIID=21399

[645] Yoon, M. (2005). Evidence-based medicine in migraine prevention. Retrieved May 14, 2015, from http://www.ncbi.nlm.nih.gov/pubmed/15938666

[646] Ciranna, L. (2006). Serotonin as a Modulator of Glutamate- and GABA-Mediated Neurotransmission: Implications in Physiological Functions and in Pathology. Retrieved May 14, 2015, from http://www.ncbi.nlm.nih.gov/pmc/articles/PMC2430669/

[647] The Many Uses of 5-HTP. (2011). Retrieved May 14, 2015, from http://naturalmedicinejournal.com/journal/2011-10/many-uses-5-htp

[648] Peroutka, S. (2014, October 1). What turns on a migraine? A systematic review of migraine precipitating factors. Retrieved May 13, 2015, from http://www.ncbi.nlm.nih.gov/pubmed/25160711

[649] Dad's says on Facebook that he killed daughter to stop migraines. (2015, May 9). Retrieved May 13, 2015, from http://www.mirror.co.uk/news/world-news/father-reveals-killed-daughter-wife-5666661

[650] Robert Sapolsky discusses physiological effects of stress (Stanford University)). (n.d.). Retrieved May 13, 2015, from http://news.stanford.edu/news/2007/march7/sapolskysr-030707.html

[651] Stress A Major Health Problem in the US, Warns APA. (2007, October 24). Retrieved May 13, 2015, from http://www.apa.org/news/press/releases/2007/10/stress.aspx

[652] Baboon studies suggest strategies for coping with stress. (n.d.). Retrieved May 13, 2015, from http://news.stanford.edu/news/2001/february21/aaassapolsky-221.html

[653] Brandi, L. (1993, November 1). Insulin resistance of stress: Sites and mechanisms. Retrieved May 13, 2015, from http://www.ncbi.nlm.nih.gov/pubmed/8287639

[654] 35 School shooters/school related violence committed by those under the influence of psychiatric drugs | CCHR International. (n.d.). Retrieved May 13, 2015, from http://www.cchrint.org/school-shooters/

[655] Understanding our Bodies: Dopamine and Its Rewards. (2009). Retrieved May 13, 2015, from http://nutritionwonderland.com/2009/07/understanding-our-bodies-dopamine-rewards/

[656] BRAIN SEROTONIN CHANGES IN PHENYLALANINE-FED RATS. (2006, October 4). Retrieved May 7, 2015, from http://onlinelibrary.wiley.com/doi/10.1111/j.1471-4159.1969.tb08990.x/abstract

[657] Chen, H. (2013, January 9). Sweetened Drinks May Boost Depression, Coffee Reduce It. Retrieved May 7, 2015, from http://www.medscape.com/viewarticle/777356

[658] Causal link found between vitamin D, serotonin synthesis and autism in new study. (2014, February 26). Retrieved May 13, 2015, from http://www.sciencedaily.com/releases/2014/02/140226110836.htm

[659] Genuis, S. (2010, April 10). Keeping your sunny side up: How sunlight affects health and well-being. Retrieved May 13, 2015, from http://www.ncbi.nlm.nih.gov/pmc/articles/PMC1481673/

[660] Crockford, C., Wittig, R., Langergraber, K., Ziegler, T., Zuberbühler, K., & Deschner, T. (2013, March 22). Urinary oxytocin and social bonding in related and unrelated wild chimpanzees. Retrieved May 13, 2015, from http://www.ncbi.nlm.nih.gov/pmc/articles/PMC3574389/

[661] Oxytocin and social contact reduce anxiety: Hormone may be less effective at relieving stress for isolated animals. (2010, November 15). Retrieved May 13, 2015, from http://www.sciencedaily.com/releases/2010/11/101115160626.htm

Citations

[662] Nieman, D. (1993). Effects of high- vs moderate-intensity exercise on natural killer cell activity. Retrieved May 13, 2015, from http://www.ncbi.nlm.nih.gov/pubmed/8231757

[663] Leiber, D. (1986). Laughter and humor in critical care. Retrieved May 13, 2015, from http://www.ncbi.nlm.nih.gov/pubmed/3635471

[664] RSA Animate - Drive: The surprising truth about what motivates us. (n.d.). Retrieved May 13, 2015, from http://www.youtube.com/watch?v=u6XAPnuFjJc

[665] Brickman, P. (1978). Lottery winners and accident victims: Is happiness relative? Retrieved May 13, 2015, from http://www.ncbi.nlm.nih.gov/pubmed/690806

[666] Speciali, J. (2010, March 1). Migraine treatment and placebo effect. Retrieved May 13, 2015, from http://www.ncbi.nlm.nih.gov/pubmed/20187863

[667] Varkey, E. (2008, September 9). A study to evaluate the feasibility of an aerobic exercise program in patients with migraine. Retrieved May 13, 2015, from http://www.ncbi.nlm.nih.gov/pubmed/18783448

[668] Varkey, E., Cider, Å, Carlsson, J., & Linde, M. (2011, October 1). Exercise as migraine prophylaxis: A randomized study using relaxation and topiramate as controls. Retrieved May 13, 2015, from http://www.ncbi.nlm.nih.gov/pmc/articles/PMC3236524/

[669] Narin, S. (2003, September 1). The effects of exercise and exercise-related changes in blood nitric oxide level on migraine headache. Retrieved May 13, 2015, from http://www.ncbi.nlm.nih.gov/pubmed/12971707

[670] Khazaei, M. (2012). Chronic Low-grade Inflammation after Exercise: Controversies. Retrieved May 13, 2015, from http://www.ncbi.nlm.nih.gov/pmc/articles/PMC3586919/

[671] Barg, W., Medrala, W., & Wolanczyk-Medrala, A. (2010, October 5). Exercise-Induced Anaphylaxis: An Update on Diagnosis and Treatment. Retrieved September 14, 2015, from http://www.ncbi.nlm.nih.gov/pmc/articles/PMC3020292/

[672] Demystifying Meditation – Brain Imaging Illustrates How Meditation Reduces Pain. (2011, April 5). Retrieved May 13, 2015, from http://www.wakehealth.edu/News-Releases/2011/Demystifying_Meditation_Brain_Imaging_Illustrates_How_Meditation_Reduces_Pain.htm

[673] Schneider, R. (2012, November 13). Stress Reduction in the Secondary Prevention of Cardiovascular Disease. Retrieved May 13, 2015, from http://circoutcomes.ahajournals.org/content/5/6/750.long

[674] Goyal, M. (2014). Meditation Programs for Psychological Stress and Well-Being. Retrieved May 13, 2015, from http://www.ncbi.nlm.nih.gov/books/NBK180102/

[675] Sedlmeier, P. (2012, November 12). The psychological effects of meditation: A meta-analysis. Retrieved May 13, 2015, from http://www.ncbi.nlm.nih.gov/pubmed/22582738

[676] Hölzel, B., Carmody, J., Vangel, M., Congleton, C., Yerramsetti, S., Gard, T., & Lazar, S. (2012, January 30). Mindfulness practice leads to increases in regional brain gray matter density. Retrieved May 13, 2015, from http://www.ncbi.nlm.nih.gov/pmc/articles/PMC3004979/

[677] Nestoriuc, Y. (2007, March 1). Efficacy of biofeedback for migraine: A meta-analysis. Retrieved May 13, 2015, from http://www.ncbi.nlm.nih.gov/pubmed/17084028

[678] Navy SEALs Mental Training | The History Channel. (n.d.). Retrieved May 13, 2015, from https://www.youtube.com/watch?v=Ju4FojRkEKU

[679] Huang, T. (2008). A comprehensive review of the psychological effects of brainwave entrainment. Retrieved May 13, 2015, from http://www.ncbi.nlm.nih.gov/pubmed/18780583

[680] Plymouth State University. (n.d.). Retrieved May 13, 2015, from http://www.plymouth.edu

[681] Sun, T. (2013). The effects of binaural beat technology on physiological and psychological outcomes in adults: A systematic review protocol | Sun | The JBI Database of Systematic Reviews and Implementation Reports. Retrieved May 13, 2015, from http://joannabriggslibrary.org/jbilibrary/index.php/jbisrir/article/view/471/1276

[682] Noudeh, Y., Vatankhah, N., & Baradaran, H. (2012). Reduction of Current Migraine Headache Pain Following Neck Massage and Spinal Manipulation. Retrieved May 14, 2015, from http://www.ncbi.nlm.nih.gov/pmc/articles/PMC3312646/

[683] Hernandez-reif, M. (1998). Migraine Headaches are Reduced by Massage Therapy | International Journal of Neuroscience. Retrieved May 14, 2015, from http://informahealthcare.com/doi/abs/10.3109/00207459808986453?journalCode=nes

[684] Lawler, S. (2006). A randomized, controlled trial of massage therapy as a treatment for migraine. Retrieved May 14, 2015, from http://www.ncbi.nlm.nih.gov/pubmed/16827629

[685] FIELD, T. (2005). CORTISOL DECREASES AND SEROTONIN AND DOPAMINE INCREASE FOLLOWING MASSAGE THERAPY | International Journal of Neuroscience. Retrieved May 14, 2015, from http://informahealthcare.com/doi/abs/10.1080/00207450590956459

[686] Eraslan, D., Dikmen, P., Aydınlar, E., & İncesu, C. (2014, May 27). The relation of sexual function to migraine-related disability, depression and anxiety in patients with migraine. Retrieved May 15, 2015, from http://www.ncbi.nlm.nih.gov/pmc/articles/PMC4046390/

[687] Fukui, P. (2008). Trigger factors in migraine patients. Retrieved May 15, 2015, from http://www.ncbi.nlm.nih.gov/pubmed/18813707

[688] Frappier, J., Toupin, I., Levy, J., Aubertin-Leheudre, M., & Karelis, A. (2013, October 24). Energy Expenditure during Sexual Activity in Young Healthy Couples. Retrieved May 15, 2015, from http://www.ncbi.nlm.nih.gov/pmc/articles/PMC3812004/

[689] Hull, E. (2004, November 15). Dopamine and serotonin: Influences on male sexual behavior. Retrieved May 15, 2015, from http://www.ncbi.nlm.nih.gov/pubmed/15488546

[690] Migraine Headaches And Sexual Desire May Be Linked. (2006). Retrieved May 15, 2015, from http://www.sciencedaily.com/releases/2006/06/060609121759.htm

[691] Hambach, A. (2013). The impact of sexual activity on idiopathic headaches: An observational study. Retrieved May 15, 2015, from http://www.ncbi.nlm.nih.gov/pubmed/23430983

[692] Russo, E. (1998, May 1). Cannabis for migraine treatment: The once and future prescription? An historical and scientific review. Retrieved May 12, 2015, from http://www.ncbi.nlm.nih.gov/pubmed/9696453

[693] Stelt, V. (2001, September 1). Neuroprotection by Delta9-tetrahydrocannabinol, the main active compound in marijuana, against ouabain-induced in vivo excitotoxicity. Retrieved May 12, 2015, from http://www.ncbi.nlm.nih.gov/pubmed/11517236

[694] Mechoulam, R. (2002, February 1). Cannabinoids and brain injury: Therapeutic implications. Retrieved May 12, 2015, from http://www.ncbi.nlm.nih.gov/pubmed/11815270

[695] Russo, E. (2004). Clinical endocannabinoid deficiency (CECD): Can this concept explain therapeutic benefits of cannabis in migraine, fibromyalgia, irritable bowel syndrome and other treatment-resistant conditions? Retrieved May 12, 2015, from http://www.ncbi.nlm.nih.gov/pubmed/15159679

[696] Rheumatoid arthritis, cannabis based medicine eases pain and suppresses disease. (2005, November 11). Retrieved May 12, 2015, from http://www.medicalnewstoday.com/releases/33376.php

[697] Gable, R. (n.d.). The Toxicity of Recreational Drugs. Retrieved May 12, 2015, from http://www.americanscientist.org/issues/pub/the-toxicity-of-recreational-drugs/4

[698] Why Cannabis Stems Inflammation. (2008, July 22). Retrieved May 12, 2015, from http://www.sciencedaily.com/releases/2008/07/080720222549.htm

[699] Moreno, E. (2014, August 8). Targeting CB2-GPR55 receptor heteromers modulates cancer cell signaling. Retrieved May 12, 2015, from http://www.ncbi.nlm.nih.gov/pubmed/24942731

[700] Hashibe, M. (2006, October). Marijuana use and the risk of lung and upper aerodigestive tract cancers: Results of a population-based case-control study. Retrieved May 12, 2015, from http://www.ncbi.nlm.nih.gov/pubmed/17035389

[701] Welty, T., Luebke, A., & Gidal, B. (2014, October 1). Cannabidiol: Promise and Pitfalls. Retrieved September 15, 2015, from http://www.ncbi.nlm.nih.gov/pmc/articles/PMC4189631/

[702] Porter, B. (2013, December 1). Report of a parent survey of cannabidiol-enriched cannabis use in pediatric treatment-resistant epilepsy. Retrieved September 15, 2015, from http://www.ncbi.nlm.nih.gov/pubmed/24237632

[703] Magis, D. (2013). Safety and patients' satisfaction of transcutaneous Supraorbital NeuroStimulation (tSNS) with the Cefaly® device in headache treatment: A survey of 2,313 headache sufferers in the general population. Retrieved May 19, 2015, from http://www.thejournalofheadacheandpain.com/content/14/1/95

[704] Hua Tuo. (n.d.). Retrieved May 14, 2015, from http://en.wikipedia.org/wiki/Hua_Tuo

[705] Linde, K., Allais, G., Brinkhaus, B., Manheimer, E., Vickers, A., & White, A. (2011). Acupuncture for migraine prophylaxis. Retrieved May 14, 2015, from http://www.ncbi.nlm.nih.gov/pmc/articles/PMC3099267/

[706] Li, Y., Zheng, H., Witt, C., Roll, S., Yu, S., Yan, J., . . . Liang, F. (2012, March 6). Acupuncture for migraine prophylaxis: A randomized controlled trial. Retrieved May 14, 2015, from http://www.ncbi.nlm.nih.gov/pmc/articles/PMC3291669/

[707] Vickers, A. (2012, October 22). Acupuncture for Chronic Pain. Retrieved May 14, 2015, from http://archinte.jamanetwork.com/article.aspx?articleid=1357513

[708] My Radical Migraine-Banishing Acupuncture Success. (2012). Retrieved May 14, 2015, from http://www.xojane.com/healthy/curing-migraines-with-acupuncture

[709] Tuchin, P. (2008, May 27). A case of chronic migraine remission after chiropractic care. Retrieved May 14, 2015, from http://www.ncbi.nlm.nih.gov/pmc/articles/PMC2682939/

[710] Tuchin, P. (2000). A randomized controlled trial of chiropractic spinal manipulative therapy for migraine. Retrieved May 14, 2015, from http://www.ncbi.nlm.nih.gov/pubmed/10714533

Citations

[711] Holtzman, D., & Burke, J. (2007). Nutritional counseling in the chiropractic practice: A survey of New York practitioners. Retrieved May 14, 2015, from http://www.ncbi.nlm.nih.gov/pmc/articles/PMC2647073/

[712] Deaths after Chiropractic: A Review of Published Cases. (2010). Retrieved May 14, 2015, from http://www.medscape.com/viewarticle/726445_4

[713] A New, Evidence-based Estimate of Patient Harms Associated w... : Journal of Patient Safety. (2013). Retrieved May 14, 2015, from http://journals.lww.com/journalpatientsafety/Fulltext/2013/09000/A_New,_Evidence_based_Estimate_of_Patient_Harms.2.aspx

[714] Makary, M. (2012). How to Stop Hospitals From Killing Us, Medical errors kill enough people to fill four jumbo jets a week. Retrieved May 14, 2015, from http://online.wsj.com/news/articles/SB10000872396390444620104578008263334441352?mg=reno64-wsj&url=http://online.wsj.com/article/SB10000872396390444620104578008263334441352.html

[715] Migraine headache | University of Maryland Medical Center. (n.d.). Retrieved May 14, 2015, from http://umm.edu/health/medical/altmed/condition/migraine-headache

[716] Jürgens, T., Müller, P., Seedorf, H., Regelsberger, J., & May, A. (2012, March 3). Occipital nerve block is effective in craniofacial neuralgias but not in idiopathic persistent facial pain. Retrieved May 14, 2015, from http://www.ncbi.nlm.nih.gov/pmc/articles/PMC3311831/

[717] Saracco, M. (2011). Greater occipital nerve block in chronic migraine. Retrieved May 14, 2015, from http://www.ncbi.nlm.nih.gov/pubmed/20464617

[718] Caputi, C. (1997). Therapeutic blockade of greater occipital and supraorbital nerves in migraine patients. Retrieved May 14, 2015, from http://www.ncbi.nlm.nih.gov/pubmed/9100402

[719] Naja, Z. (2006). Repetitive occipital nerve blockade for cervicogenic headache: Expanded case report of 47 adults. Retrieved May 14, 2015, from http://www.ncbi.nlm.nih.gov/pubmed/17129309

[720] Mellick, L. (2006). Treatment of headaches in the ED with lower cervical intramuscular bupivacaine injections: A 1-year retrospective review of 417 patients. Retrieved May 14, 2015, from http://www.ncbi.nlm.nih.gov/pubmed/17040341

[721] Alp, I. (2013). Supraorbital and infraorbital nerve blockade in migraine patients: Results of 6-month clinical follow-up. Retrieved May 14, 2015, from http://www.ncbi.nlm.nih.gov/pubmed/23852904

[722] Occipital Nerve Block - Migraine.com. (n.d.). Retrieved May 14, 2015, from http://migraine.com/topic/occipital-nerve-block/

[723] McCormick, T. (2013). How to use Paraspinous Injections for Complex Headaches | Emergency Physicians Monthly. Retrieved May 14, 2015, from http://www.epmonthly.com/departments/clinical-skills/emrap/how-to-use-paraspinous-injections-for-complex-headaches/

[724] Cervicogenic headache. (n.d.). Retrieved May 14, 2014, from http://pain-medicine.med.nyu.edu/patient-care/conditions-we-treat/cervicogenic-headache

[725] Guyuron, B. (2014, June 10). A Discussion of "Critical Evaluation of Migraine Trigger Site Decompression Surgery". Retrieved May 14, 2015, from http://onlinelibrary.wiley.com/doi/10.1111/head.12370/full

[726] Occipital Nerve Block - Migraine.com. (n.d.). Retrieved May 14, 2015, from http://migraine.com/topic/occipital-nerve-block/

[727] Freeman, J., & Trentman, T. (2013, November 20). Clinical utility of implantable neurostimulation devices in the treatment of chronic migraine. Retrieved May 14, 2015, from http://www.ncbi.nlm.nih.gov/pmc/articles/PMC3838759/

[728] Guyuron, B. (2011). Five-year outcome of surgical treatment of migraine headaches. Retrieved May 14, 2015, from http://www.ncbi.nlm.nih.gov/pubmed/20966820

[729] Lisotto, C., Mainardi, F., Maggioni, F., & Zanchin, G. (2013, February 21). The comorbidity between migraine and hypothyroidism. Retrieved May 15, 2015, from http://www.ncbi.nlm.nih.gov/pmc/articles/PMC3620300/

[730] Amino, N. (1988). Autoimmunity and hypothyroidism. Retrieved May 15, 2015, from http://www.ncbi.nlm.nih.gov/pubmed/3066320

[731] Sategna-Guidetti, C. (1998). Autoimmune thyroid diseases and coeliac disease. Retrieved May 15, 2015, from http://www.ncbi.nlm.nih.gov/pubmed/9872614

[732] Redberg, R., & Smith-bindman, R. (2014, January 30). We Are Giving Ourselves Cancer. Retrieved May 15, 2015, from http://www.nytimes.com/2014/01/31/opinion/we-are-giving-ourselves-cancer.html?from=mostemailed&_r=1

[733] Ahmed, S., Jayawarna, C., & Jude, E. (2006). Post lumbar puncture headache: Diagnosis and management. Retrieved May 15, 2015, from http://www.ncbi.nlm.nih.gov/pmc/articles/PMC2660496/

[734] A Contaminated Lake Is Poisoning a Thai Village | VICE | United States. (2014). Retrieved May 15, 2015, from http://www.vice.com/read/a-contaminated-lake-is-poisoning-a-thai-village-855

[735] Teitelbaum, J. (2011). Iodine Deficiency - An Old Epidemic Is Back. Retrieved May 15, 2015, from http://www.psychologytoday.com/blog/complementary-medicine/201108/iodine-deficiency-old-epidemic-is-back

[736] Messina, M. (2006). Effects of soy protein and soybean isoflavones on thyroid function in healthy adults and hypothyroid patients: A review of the relevant literature. Retrieved May 15, 2015, from http://www.ncbi.nlm.nih.gov/pubmed/16571087

[737] Aamodt, A. (2008). Comorbidity of headache and gastrointestinal complaints. The Head-HUNT Study. Retrieved May 15, 2015, from http://www.ncbi.nlm.nih.gov/pubmed/18197884

[738] Mulak, A. (2005). Migraine and irritable bowel syndrome. Retrieved May 15, 2015, from http://www.ncbi.nlm.nih.gov/pubmed/16419571

[739] Cole, J., Rothman, K., Cabral, H., Zhang, Y., & Farraye, F. (2006). Migraine, fibromyalgia, and depression among people with IBS: A prevalence study. Retrieved May 15, 2015, from http://www.ncbi.nlm.nih.gov/pmc/articles/PMC1592499/

[740] Varga, E. (2005, May 17). Cardiology patient pages. Homocysteine and MTHFR mutations: Relation to thrombosis and coronary artery disease. Retrieved May 15, 2015, from http://www.ncbi.nlm.nih.gov/pubmed/15897349

[741] Gazerani, P. (2003). A correlation between migraine, histamine and immunoglobulin e. Retrieved May 15, 2015, from http://www.ncbi.nlm.nih.gov/pubmed/12641658

[742] Villa, G., Ceruti, S., Zanardelli, M., Magni, G., Jasmin, L., Ohara, P., & Abbracchio, M. (2010, December 10). Temporomandibular joint inflammation activates glial and immune cells in both the trigeminal ganglia and in the spinal trigeminal nucleus. Retrieved May 15, 2015, from http://www.ncbi.nlm.nih.gov/pmc/articles/PMC3017032/

[743] What are they? (Cluster Headaches). (n.d.). Retrieved May 15, 2015, from http://www.clusterheadaches.com.au/what-are-they.php

[744] Franco, A. (2010). Migraine is the most prevalent primary headache in individuals with temporomandibular disorders. Retrieved May 15, 2015, from http://www.ncbi.nlm.nih.gov/pubmed/20664830

[745] Minnesota Vikings WR Percy Harvin believes migraine problems are past. (n.d.). Retrieved May 15, 2015, from http://sports.espn.go.com/nfl/news/story?id=5568478

[746] Keller, D. (2013). CPAP Improves Migraine Burden in Patients With Sleep Apnea. Retrieved May 15, 2015, from http://www.medscape.com/viewarticle/806902

[747] David Anderson: Your brain is more than a bag of chemicals. (n.d.). Retrieved May 15, 2015, from https://www.youtube.com/watch?v=D9xJl4S6NsM

[748] Linde, M. (2013, June 24). Gabapentin or pregabalin for the prophylaxis of episodic migraine in adults. Retrieved May 15, 2015, from http://www.ncbi.nlm.nih.gov/pubmed/23797675

[749] Pfizer agrees record fraud fine. (2009, September 2). Retrieved May 15, 2015, from http://news.bbc.co.uk/2/hi/business/8234533.stm

[750] Last Week Tonight with John Oliver: Marketing to Doctors (HBO). (n.d.). Retrieved May 15, 2015, from https://www.youtube.com/watch?v=YQZ2UeOTO3I

[751] Dollars for Docs. (n.d.). Retrieved May 15, 2015, from https://projects.propublica.org/docdollars/

[752] Ergotamine. (n.d.). Retrieved May 18, 2015, from http://en.wikipedia.org/wiki/Ergotamine

[753] Walkembach, J., Brüss, M., Urban, B., & Barann, M. (2005, July 25). Interactions of metoclopramide and ergotamine with human 5-HT3A receptors and human 5-HT reuptake carriers. Retrieved May 18, 2015, from http://www.ncbi.nlm.nih.gov/pmc/articles/PMC1751187/

[754] Ergotamine medical facts from Drugs.com. (n.d.). Retrieved May 18, 2015, from http://www.drugs.com/mtm/ergotamine.html

[755] Gulbranson, S. (2002). Possible ergotamine-caffeine-associated delirium. Retrieved May 18, 2015, from http://www.ncbi.nlm.nih.gov/pubmed/11794425

[756] Bennett, J., & Klich, M. (2003). Mycotoxins. Retrieved May 18, 2015, from http://www.ncbi.nlm.nih.gov/pmc/articles/PMC164220/

[757] Ergotamine class for migraine headaches. (n.d.). Retrieved May 18, 2015, from http://migraine.com/migraine-treatment/ergotamine/

[758] Tfelt-Hansen, P. (2000). Ergotamine in the acute treatment of migraine: A review and European consensus. Retrieved May 18, 2015, from http://www.ncbi.nlm.nih.gov/pubmed/10611116

[759] Franconi, F. (2014). Gender and triptan efficacy: A pooled analysis of three double-blind, randomized, crossover, multicenter, Italian studies comparing frovatriptan vs. other triptans. Retrieved May 19, 2015, from http://www.ncbi.nlm.nih.gov/pubmed/24867845

[760] Thorlund, K. (2014). Comparative efficacy of triptans for the abortive treatment of migraine: A multiple treatment comparison meta-analysis. Retrieved May 19, 2015, from http://www.ncbi.nlm.nih.gov/pubmed/24108308

[761] Tfelt-Hansen, P. (2000). Triptans in migraine: A comparative review of pharmacology, pharmacokinetics and efficacy. Retrieved May 19, 2015, from http://www.ncbi.nlm.nih.gov/pubmed/11152011

[762] Common Drugs and Medications to Treat Migraine. (n.d.). Retrieved May 19, 2015, from http://www.webmd.com/drugs/condition-1116-Migraine.aspx?diseaseid=1116&diseasename=Migraine&source=0

[763] Laino, C. (n.d.). Too Many Heart Patients Getting Migraine Drugs. Retrieved May 19, 2015, from http://www.webmd.com/migraines-headaches/news/20110930/heart-concerns-with-migraine-drugs

[764] Non-steroidal anti-inflammatory drug. (n.d.). Retrieved May 18, 2015, from http://en.wikipedia.org/wiki/Non-steroidal_anti-inflammatory_drug

[765] Aleve (naproxen) for migraine headaches. (n.d.). Retrieved May 18, 2015, from http://migraine.com/migraine-treatment/aleve-naproxen/

[766] Ibuprofen User Reviews for Headache at Drugs.com. (n.d.). Retrieved May 18, 2015, from http://www.drugs.com/comments/ibuprofen/for-headache.html

[767] Advil migraine. (n.d.). Retrieved May 18, 2015, from http://migraine.com/migraine-treatment/advil-migraine/

[768] Guidelines for the management of paracetamol poisoning in Australia and New Zealand - explanation and elaboration. (n.d.). Retrieved May 18, 2015, from https://www.mja.com.au/journal/2008/188/5/guidelines-management-paracetamol-poisoning-australia-and-new-zealand-explanation

[769] Larson, A. (2005). Acetaminophen-induced acute liver failure: Results of a United States multicenter, prospective study. Retrieved May 18, 2015, from http://www.ncbi.nlm.nih.gov/pubmed/16317692

[770] Kirthi, V. (2013, April 30). Aspirin with or without an antiemetic for acute migraine headaches in adults. Retrieved May 6, 2015, from http://www.ncbi.nlm.nih.gov/pubmed/23633350

[771] Aspirin Side Effects in Detail - Drugs.com. (n.d.). Retrieved May 18, 2015, from http://www.drugs.com/sfx/aspirin-side-effects.html

[772] Star-Ledger, A. (2014). Cherry Hill woman sues Novartis over marketing of Excedrin pain medicines. Retrieved May 18, 2015, from http://www.nj.com/business/index.ssf/2014/01/cherry_hill_woman_sues_over_pricing_of_excedrin_pain_medicines_claiming_consumer_fraud.html

[773] Chlorpromazine (oral) medical facts from Drugs.com. (n.d.). Retrieved May 18, 2015, from http://www.drugs.com/mtm/chlorpromazine.html

[774] Behind the Thorazine Shuffle, the Criminalization of Mental Illness. (2012, March 16). Retrieved May 18, 2015, from http://jjie.org/behind-thorazine-shuffle-criminalization-of-mental-illness/

[775] Metoclopramide Injection - FDA prescribing information, side effects and uses. (n.d.). Retrieved May 18, 2015, from http://www.drugs.com/pro/metoclopramide-injection.html

[776] Prochlorperazine (oral) medical facts from Drugs.com. (n.d.). Retrieved May 18, 2015, from http://www.drugs.com/mtm/prochlorperazine.html

[777] Strenkoski-Nix, L. (2000, August 15). Pharmacokinetics of promethazine hydrochloride after administration of rectal suppositories and oral syrup to healthy subjects. Retrieved May 18, 2015, from http://www.ncbi.nlm.nih.gov/pubmed/10965395

[778] Phenergan Uses, Dosage & Side Effects - Drugs.com. (n.d.). Retrieved May 18, 2015, from http://www.drugs.com/comments/promethazine/for-nausea-vomiting.html

[779] Tigan Side Effects in Detail - Drugs.com. (n.d.). Retrieved May 18, 2015, from http://www.drugs.com/sfx/tigan-side-effects.html

[780] Raphael, G. (2006). Efficacy of diphenhydramine vs desloratadine and placebo in patients with moderate-to-severe seasonal allergic rhinitis. Retrieved May 18, 2015, from http://www.ncbi.nlm.nih.gov/pubmed/16680933

[781] Diphenhydramine Uses, Dosage & Side Effects - Drugs.com. (n.d.). Retrieved May 18, 2015, from http://www.drugs.com/diphenhydramine.html

[782] Gray, S. (2015). Strong Anticholinergics and Incident Dementia. Retrieved May 18, 2015, from http://archinte.jamanetwork.com/article.aspx?articleid=2091745

[783] Sudafed Nasal Decongestant Side Effects in Detail - Drugs.com. (n.d.). Retrieved May 18, 2015, from http://www.drugs.com/sfx/sudafed-nasal-decongestant-side-effects.html

[784] Dexamethasone Side Effects in Detail - Drugs.com. (n.d.). Retrieved May 18, 2015, from http://www.drugs.com/sfx/dexamethasone-side-effects.html

[785] Steroid-induced osteoporosis | University of Washington. (n.d.). Retrieved May 18, 2015, from http://courses.washington.edu/bonephys/opsteroid.html

[786] Solu-Medrol Side Effects in Detail - Drugs.com. (n.d.). Retrieved May 18, 2015, from http://www.drugs.com/sfx/solu-medrol-side-effects.html

[787] Opioid Prescriptions And Addictions Are On The Rise In The US (2013). Retrieved May 19, 2015, from

http://www.forbes.com/sites/alicegwalton/2013/09/16/opioid-prescriptions-skyrocket-while-pain-management-stalls/

[788] This Content Has Moved. (2015, April 1). Retrieved May 19, 2015, from http://www.cdc.gov/homeandrecreationalsafety/rxbrief/

[789] Popping Pills: Prescription Drug Abuse in America | NIH. (n.d.). Retrieved May 19, 2015, from http://www.drugabuse.gov/related-topics/trends-statistics/infographics/popping-pills-prescription-drug-abuse-in-america

[790] Injury Prevention & Control: Prescription Drug Overdose | CDC. (2015, April 3). Retrieved May 19, 2015, from http://www.cdc.gov/drugoverdose/index.html

[791] Evzio. (n.d.). Retrieved May 19, 2015, from http://www.goodrx.com/evzio

[792] Brennan, K. (2014). Symptom Codes And Opioids: Disconcerting Headache Practice Patterns In Academic Primary Care. (S41.003). Retrieved May 19, 2015, from http://www.neurology.org/content/82/10_Supplement/S41.003

[793] Benyamin, R. (2008). Opioid complications and side effects. Retrieved May 19, 2015, from http://www.ncbi.nlm.nih.gov/pubmed/18443635

[794] Migraine, narcotics, & rebound headaches. (2011, December 12). Retrieved May 19, 2015, from http://migraine.com/blog/migraine-narcotic-drugs-rebound-headaches/

[795] Levin, M. (2014). Opioids in headache. Retrieved May 19, 2015, from http://www.ncbi.nlm.nih.gov/pubmed/24127913

[796] Dodick, D. (2008). Reflections and speculations on refractory migraine: Why do some patients fail to improve with currently available therapies? Retrieved May 19, 2015, from http://www.ncbi.nlm.nih.gov/pubmed/18549360

[797] Krusz, J. (2000). Intravenous propofol: Unique effectiveness in treating intractable migraine. Retrieved May 19, 2015, from http://www.ncbi.nlm.nih.gov/pubmed/10759925

[798] Report: Joan Rivers died from too much Propofol. (2014). Retrieved May 19, 2015, from http://www.mercurynews.com/entertainment/ci_26910420/report-joan-rivers-died-from-too-much-propofol

[799] Krusz, J. (2006). Intravenous treatment of chronic daily headaches in the outpatient headache clinic. Retrieved May 19, 2015, from http://www.ncbi.nlm.nih.gov/pubmed/16499830

[800] Effectiveness of IV Therapy in the Headache Clinic for Refractory Migraines by Dr. John Claude Krusz and Teri Robert. Help for Headaches and Migraine Disease from Teri Robert, Writer and Patient Advocate. (n.d.). Retrieved May 19, 2015, from http://www.helpforheadaches.com/articles/iv-meds.htm

[801] Oxygen Therapy May Alleviate Cluster and Migraine Pain | National Headache Foundation. (2008, September 15). Retrieved May 15, 2015, from http://www.headaches.org/2008/09/15/oxygen-therapy-may-alleviate-cluster-and-migraine-pain/

[802] Cohen, A. (2009, December 9). High-flow oxygen for treatment of cluster headache: A randomized trial. Retrieved May 15, 2015, from http://www.ncbi.nlm.nih.gov/pubmed/19996400

[803] Ozkurt, B. (2012). Efficacy of high-flow oxygen therapy in all types of headache: A prospective, randomized, placebo-controlled trial. Retrieved May 15, 2015, from http://www.ncbi.nlm.nih.gov/pubmed/22560101

[804] Buchholz, D. (2002). *Heal your headache: The 1-2-3 program for taking charge of your pain.* New York: Workman Pub.

[805] Migraine Guide: Causes, Symptoms and Treatment Options. (n.d.). Retrieved May 19, 2015, from http://www.drugs.com/health-guide/migraine.html

[806] How anti-epileptic drugs work. (n.d.). Retrieved May 19, 2015, from http://www.epilepsysociety.org.uk/how-anti-epileptic-drugs-work#.VFuq_hb6a3U

[807] Topamax Side Effects in Detail - Drugs.com. (n.d.). Retrieved May 19, 2015, from http://www.drugs.com/sfx/topamax-side-effects.html

[808] Negro, A., & Martelletti, P. (2011, September 22). Chronic migraine plus medication overuse headache: Two entities or not? Retrieved September 15, 2015, from http://www.ncbi.nlm.nih.gov/pmc/articles/PMC3208042/

[809] Mathew, N. (2001). Antiepileptic drugs in migraine prevention. Retrieved May 19, 2015, from http://www.ncbi.nlm.nih.gov/pubmed/11903536

[810] Silberstein, S. (2004). Topiramate in Migraine Prevention: Results of a Large Controlled Trial. Retrieved July 4, 2015, from http://www.ncbi.nlm.nih.gov/pubmed/15096395

[811] Pancrazio, J. (1998). Inhibition of neuronal Na channels by antidepressant drugs. Retrieved May 19, 2015, from http://www.ncbi.nlm.nih.gov/pubmed/9435180

[812] Owens, M. (1997). Neurotransmitter receptor and transporter binding profile of antidepressants and their metabolites. Retrieved May 19, 2015, from http://www.ncbi.nlm.nih.gov/pubmed/9400006

[813] Owens, M. (1997). Amitriptyline Side Effects in Detail - Drugs.com. Retrieved May 19, 2015, from http://www.drugs.com/sfx/amitriptyline-side-effects.html

[814] Couch, J. (2011). Amitriptyline in the prophylactic treatment of migraine and chronic daily headache. Retrieved May 19, 2015, from http://www.ncbi.nlm.nih.gov/pubmed/21070231

Citations

[815] Dodick, D. (2009). Topiramate versus amitriptyline in migraine prevention: A 26-week, multicenter, randomized, double-blind, double-dummy, parallel-group noninferiority trial in adult migraineurs. Retrieved May 19, 2015, from http://www.ncbi.nlm.nih.gov/pubmed/19393844

[816] FDA Data Indicates Over 40,000 Homicides From Antidepressants. (2013). Retrieved May 19, 2015, from http://www.cchrnewengland.org/2013/08/30/fda-data-indicates-over-40000-homicides-from-antidepressants/

[817] Jackson, J. (2012). Botulinum Toxin A for Prophylactic Treatment of Migraine and Tension Headaches in Adults. Retrieved May 14, 2015, from http://jama.jamanetwork.com/article.aspx?articleid=1148201&quizId=3053&atab=7

[818] Saper, J. (2007). A double-blind, randomized, placebo-controlled comparison of botulinum toxin type a injection sites and doses in the prevention of episodic migraine. Retrieved May 14, 2015, from http://www.ncbi.nlm.nih.gov/pubmed/17716321

[819] Shuhendler, A. (2009). Efficacy of botulinum toxin type A for the prophylaxis of episodic migraine headaches: A meta-analysis of randomized, double-blind, placebo-controlled trials. Retrieved May 14, 2015, from http://www.ncbi.nlm.nih.gov/pubmed/19558252

[820] Watkins, T. (2010, October 15). FDA approves Botox as migraine preventive. Retrieved May 14, 2015, from http://www.cnn.com/2010/HEALTH/10/15/migraines.botox/

[821] Diener, H. (2010). OnabotulinumtoxinA for treatment of chronic migraine: Results from the double-blind, randomized, placebo-controlled phase of the PREEMPT 2 trial. Retrieved May 14, 2015, from http://www.ncbi.nlm.nih.gov/pubmed/20647171

[822] What To Expect From Treatment. (n.d.). Retrieved May 14, 2015, from http://www.botoxchronicmigraine.com/botox-treatment-expectations/

[823] Ramachandran, R. (2014). Therapeutic use of botulinum toxin in migraine: Mechanisms of action. Retrieved May 14, 2015, from http://www.ncbi.nlm.nih.gov/pubmed/24819339

[824] Naumann, M. (2004). Safety of botulinum toxin type A: A systematic review and meta-analysis. Retrieved May 14, 2015, from http://informahealthcare.com/doi/abs/10.1185/030079904125003962

[825] BOTOX Costs, Prices & Financing. (n.d.). Retrieved September 16, 2015, from http://www.docshop.com/education/dermatology/injectables/botox/cost

[826] $15 or $800: How Much Does Botox Cost? (n.d.). Retrieved May 14, 2015, from http://finance.yahoo.com/news/much-does-botox-cost-130059878.html

[827] Beta-Blockers for Migraine Headaches. (n.d.). Retrieved May 19, 2015, from http://www.webmd.com/migraines-headaches/beta-blockers-for-migraine-headaches

[828] Holroyd, K. (1991). Propranolol in the management of recurrent migraine: A meta-analytic review. Retrieved May 19, 2015, from http://www.ncbi.nlm.nih.gov/pubmed/1830566

[829] Propranolol Side Effects in Detail - Drugs.com. (n.d.). Retrieved May 19, 2015, from http://www.drugs.com/sfx/propranolol-side-effects.html

[830] D'Amico, D., & Tepper, S. (2008). Prophylaxis of migraine: General principles and patient acceptance. Retrieved May 19, 2015, from http://www.ncbi.nlm.nih.gov/pmc/articles/PMC2646645/

[831] Stovner, L. (2013, December 11). A comparative study of candesartan versus propranolol for migraine prophylaxis: A randomised, triple-blind, placebo-controlled, double cross-over study. Retrieved May 19, 2015, from http://www.ncbi.nlm.nih.gov/pubmed/24335848

[832] Tyrer, P. (1992). Anxiolytics not acting at the benzodiazepine receptor: Beta blockers. Retrieved May 19, 2015, from http://www.ncbi.nlm.nih.gov/pubmed/1348368

[833] Gerwig, M., Niehaus, L., Stude, P., Katsarava, Z., & Diener, H. (2012). Beta-blocker migraine prophylaxis affects the excitability of the visual cortex as revealed by transcranial magnetic stimulation. Retrieved May 19, 2015, from http://www.ncbi.nlm.nih.gov/pmc/articles/PMC3253148/?report=classic

[834] No more neuronal gibberish: How 100 billion nerve cells produce a clear thought or an action. (2015, January 15). Retrieved May 19, 2015, from http://www.sciencedaily.com/releases/2015/01/150115102746.htm

[835] New imaging method developed at Stanford reveals stunning details of brain connections | Stanford. (2010). Retrieved May 19, 2015, from http://med.stanford.edu/news/all-news/2010/11/new-imaging-method-developed-at-stanford-reveals-stunning-details-of-brain-connections.html

[836] Propranolol Side Effects in Detail - Drugs.com. (n.d.). Retrieved May 19, 2015, from http://www.drugs.com/sfx/propranolol-side-effects.html

[837] Straubhaar, B. (2006). The prevalence of potential drug-drug interactions in patients with heart failure at hospital discharge. Retrieved May 19, 2015, from http://www.ncbi.nlm.nih.gov/pubmed/16454536

[838] Thayer, A. (2014, August 18). Next-Gen Sequencing Is A Numbers Game | Chemical & Engineering News. Retrieved May 19, 2015, from http://cen.acs.org/articles/92/i33/Next-Gen-Sequencing-Numbers-Game.html

Citations

[839] Genetic Link To Migraine Found, In DNA Variant On Chromosome 8. (2010, August 30). Retrieved May 19, 2015, from http://www.medicalnewstoday.com/articles/199381.php

[840] Longoni, M. (2006). Inflammation and excitotoxicity: Role in migraine pathogenesis. Retrieved May 19, 2015, from http://www.ncbi.nlm.nih.gov/pubmed/16688611

[841] Yudkoff, M., Daikhin, Y., Horyn, O., Nissim, I., & Nissim, I. (2009, November 1). Ketosis and Brain Handling of Glutamate, Glutamine and GABA. Retrieved May 19, 2015, from http://www.ncbi.nlm.nih.gov/pmc/articles/PMC2722878/

[842] Anderson, P. (2014, July 3). Monoclonal Antibodies Promising for Migraine Prevention. Retrieved May 19, 2015, from http://www.medscape.com/viewarticle/827838

Made in the USA
Middletown, DE
10 April 2019